COMPLEMENTARY, ALTERNATIVE, AND INTEGRATIVE HEALTH

A MULTICULTURAL PERSPECTIVE

Edited by

Helda Pinzón-Pérez and Miguel A. Pérez

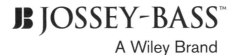

A Wiley Brand

Published by Jossey-BassA Wiley Brand
One Montgomery Street, Suite 1000, San Francisco, CA
94104-4594—www.josseybass.com

Jossey-Bass books and products are available through most bookstores. To contact Jossey-Bass directly call our Customer Care Department within the US at 800-956-7739, outside the US at 317-572-3986, or fax 317-572-4002.

Wiley publishes in a variety of print and electronic formats and by print-on-demand. Some material included with standard print versions of this book may not be included in e-books or in print-on-demand. If this book refers to media such as a CD or DVD that is not included in the version you purchased, you may download this material at **http://booksupport.wiley.com**. For more information about Wiley products, visit **www.wiley.com**.

Library of Congress Cataloging-in-Publication Data

Names: Pinzón-Pérez, Helda, 1966–, author. — Pérez, Miguel A., 1969–, author.
Title: Complementary, alternative, and integrative health : a multicultural perspective / Helda Pinzón-Pérez and Miguel A. Pérez.
Description: First edition. — San Francisco, CA : Jossey-Bass & Pfeiffer Imprints, Wiley, [2016] — Includes bibliographical references and index.
Identifiers: LCCN 2015051175 (print) — LCCN 2016001201 (ebook) — ISBN 9781118880333 (paperback) — ISBN 9781118880456 (epdf) — ISBN 9781118880425 (epub)
Subjects: — MESH: Complementary Therapies — Integrative Medicine — Cross-Cultural Comparison
Classification: LCC R733 (print) — LCC R733 (ebook) — NLM WB 890 — DDC 610—dc23
LC record available at http://lccn.loc.gov/2015051175

Cover design by Wiley
Cover image: © Subbotina Anna/Shutterstock

Printed in the United States of America

FIRST EDITION

PB Printing 10 9 8 7 6 5 4 3 2 1

The editors wish to dedicate this publication to their parents, Jesus Pinzón and Maria Vivas de Pinzón and Ricardo and Elena Pérez, as well as to our sister, Betty Calderon. Our work is a reflection of the values and work ethic we learned from each of them. To our children, Maria Elena, Kenneth, Daniel, and David, whom we hope will learn to value hard work in their search for excellence. We hope to teach them that the pursuit of excellence is a lifelong quest.

CONTENTS

PREFACE

In December 2014, in an omnibus budget measure signed by President Obama, Congress changed the name of the National Center for Complementary and Alternative Medicine (NCCAM) to the National Center for Complementary and Integrative Health (NCCIH) (NCCIH, 2015a). The editors and contributors of this volume welcome this change since it reflects the center's commitment to enhance public and scientific understanding of alternative, complementary, and integrative health practices, instead of only medical practices. Throughout this book, both names NCCAM and NCCIH will be utilized, depending on the terminology used by the bibliographical sources consulted.

This book emphasizes a new understanding of complementary and alternative medicine (CAM). It reflects an emphasis on complementary, alternative, and integrative health (CAIH) while recognizing the value that the term *CAM* has brought historically to our understanding of alternative models of care. In this book, the acronym CAM is replaced by CAIH to reflect the current understanding of complementary and integrative health. The acronym CAM will be utilized only when the bibliographical references consulted for this publication used that term.

Various names were considered for the title of this book, one of them being "Integrative, Complementary, and Traditional Health Practices," a term used by the American Public Health Association for one of its professional sections (2015). A second potential title was "Complementary, Alternative, and Integrative Health Care," which was used by the University of North Carolina at Chapel Hill (University of North Carolina at Chapel Hill School of Medicine, 2015). A third potential title was "Complementary and Integrative Medicine," which was used by the Mayo Clinic (2015) and the University of Texas MD Anderson Cancer Center (2015). Also considered was "Traditional and Complementary Medicine," used by the World Health Organization (WHO) in its 2013 document, "WHO Traditional Medicine Strategy 2014–2023." The editors chose to embrace the vision of the NCCIH and provide a more comprehensive perspective by using the term *complementary, alternative, and integrative health*, which places the emphasis on health and wellness rather than on the medical model. Although NCCIH refers to these practices as complementary and integrative health (CIH) approaches, the editors of this book added the word *alternative* in the acronym to acknowledge that consumers still use some of these practices as alternative forms of care.

In this book, the term *CAIH* is used to transition consumers and health professionals to the new terminology that may guide research and evidence-based practice in the future. Our hearts and scientific discovery remain committed to enhance the understanding of complementary, alternative, and integrative health approaches.

Why a Book on CAIH?

Multiple books have been published on CAM, but very few have captured the recent changes in the NCCIH and the new terms associated with traditional, complementary, alternative, and integrative health. This book responds to the need to train customers and health professionals on these recent changes. The editors and authors of this publication hope that this book begins to address this need.

This book also emphasizes the importance of the multicultural perspective of CAIH approaches. Multiple chapters of this book discuss the use of CAIH and CAM practices among various ethnic and cultural groups. Some sections emphasize the relevance of the concepts for health educators, since the editors are Master Certified Health Education Specialists and since all health professionals have a responsibility to educate the public on health-related issues.

Another reason for the publication of this book is the increasing use of complementary, alternative, and integrative health approaches worldwide and in the United States. Data from the WHO (2004) show that up to 80% of people in developing countries use traditional medicine as a primary source of healthcare. In the United States, results from the 2012 National Health Interview Survey indicated that 33.2% of US adults and 11.6% of US children age 4 to 17 used complementary health approaches (Clarke et al., 2015; NCCIH, 2015b). Despite their wide usage, however, CAIH and CAM practices continue to be misunderstood, are not always regulated, and are controversial among US healthcare practitioners.

A common concern expressed by detractors of CAIH is the lack of "scientific evidence" for many of the claims made by proponents, concerns that are heightened only by charlatans who sometimes employ deceptive marketing practices to lure unsuspecting consumers to try treatments that may in fact place their health status at risk. Proponents of CAIH point to the increasing body of evidence that supports the use of certain modalities such as acupuncture and tout fewer side effects as a reason for its use. Despite continuing controversies, there is agreement that more information is needed; that healthcare providers ought to be better versed in CAIH; and that consumers and healthcare providers must increase their communication related to CAIH. Currently, several efforts are under way to address these issues.

In the year 2000, WHO released the *General Guidelines for Methodologies on Research and Evaluation of Traditional Medicine* in an effort to maximize the proper utilization of traditional medicine, as well as to provide guidelines for research and evaluation initiatives on this topic. This official WHO publication set the framework for the scientific evaluation of CAIH and CAM and provided ethical guidelines for its evaluation and implementation.

In the United States, the need to improve communication between patients and providers has resulted in advocacy efforts to achieve that goal with very specific results. An important step in improving such communication is to train future generations of health professionals on CAIH. Howell (2012), a reporter from the Association of American Medical Colleges, discussed the value of incorporating CAM into the curriculum of medical schools to empower doctors to actively discuss with their patients the use of CAM. According to Howell, the emphasis on incorporating CAM training for health professionals began when the National Center for Complementary and Alternative Medicine launched the CAM Education Project in 1999.

This book aims to be a resource for students and health professionals to better understand CAIH approaches and translate that knowledge into more effective communication patterns with consumers. It is imperative that healthcare practitioners, including health educators, better understand the most common CAIH practices employed by individuals, since research results indicate that some populations employ CAM along with, and in some cases in lieu of, allopathic treatments. In addition, patients do not always reveal this information to their healthcare providers (NCCIH, 2015c).

Key Features of This Book

This book uses the acronym CAIH, which stands for complementary, alternative, and integrative health. This acronym collectively refers to common names used in the past and new emerging terms. The use of this acronym represents an attempt to reach consensus on the terminology to be used since there are multiple terms associated with the fields of traditional healing, alternative medicine, and integrative health, which can be confusing to both consumers and professionals alike. These terms show the transformation of the concepts and the evolution of our understanding of these fields. This book is based on the WHO's definition of complementary/alternative medicine, which is "the sum total of the knowledge, skills, and practices based on the theories, beliefs, and experiences indigenous to different cultures, whether explicable or not, used in the maintenance of health as well as in the prevention, diagnosis, improvement or treatment of physical and mental illness" (n.d., p. 1).

Since the classification of CAM therapies has varied throughout the years, this book groups CAM therapies into the divisions originally suggested by the NCCAM and integrates the new divisions currently proposed by the NCCIH. Initially, NCCAM (2014) divided CAM modalities into five categories: (1) alternative medical systems, (2) mind-body interventions, (3) biologically based treatments, (4) manipulative and body-based methods, and (5) energy therapies. Later, NCCAM grouped CAM practices into four categories: (1) natural products, (2) mind and body medicine, (3) manipulative and body-based practices, and (4) other CAM practices. This classification was revised again, and in 2015, NCCIH (2015b) divided complementary health approaches into three subgroups: (1) natural products, (2) mind and body practices, and (3) other complementary health approaches.

Most of the chapters in this book were written by a team of CAM practitioners and academicians working on CAIH. The combination of the real-life experience provided by CAM practitioners and the scientific approach given by university professors and other academicians in CAIH provides a unique approach to the reader's understanding of CAIH and CAM.

This edited volume is designed to provide a foundation to CAIH healing practices. It explores proven methods and provides a framework for questioning the efficacy of CAIH while exploring its use within a cross-cultural framework. Six chapters are dedicated to the exploration of CAIH in the racial and ethnic groups most commonly found in the United States. Since the current literature uses the term *CAM*, each chapter describes the CAM practices most often used by the selected racial and ethnic groups. A section titled *"Caveat Emptor"* is included in each chapter to remind readers that questions persist about CAIH and CAM. This book does not provide a detailed list of practices in each group, as doing so would take an entire encyclopedia. In addition to the racial/ethnic-specific chapters, the authors explore the most commonly used treatment methods and provide information on research literature to back up or deny their claims.

Each chapter in this book includes the following main sections: Learning Objectives, Introduction, Theoretical Concepts, Consumer Issues, Implications for Health Professionals, *Caveat Emptor*, Conclusion, Summary, Case Study, Key Terms, and References. A major emphasis of this book is the impact of the Affordable Care Act on CAIH practices. This topic is included primarily in the "Implications for Health Professionals" sections. The "*Caveat Emptor*" sections include regulatory and practical realities related to licensing and credentialing of healers in the corresponding chapter topics. The final chapter discusses the foundation for a new way of thinking about complementary and alternative medicine in the 21st century.

A basic premise of this publication is the inclusion of educational strategies designed to allow readers to critically analyze and evaluate CAIH practices, their impact in the healthcare system, and their association with the Affordable Care Act. In addition to a discussion on the different CAIH practices, each book chapter contains two sections designed to promote a better understanding of the practices included in the chapter. The "Summary" sections emphasize the main issues and concepts regarding traditional healing practices particularly relevant to each cultural and ethnic group. Similarly, the "Case Study" sections are designed to challenge the reader to be a critical consumer of CAIH services by analyzing a situation in light of the information contained in the chapter.

The editors hope that the information contained in this book helps improve the lives of consumers who read it. Consumers need to understand that much needs to be learned about the effective and safe use of non-mainstream healthcare practices including interactions with allopathic treatments. The purpose of this book is to provide a critical analysis of nonallopathic healing practices in the United States, their uses and limitations.

The editors also hope that the information contained herein be used to deliver more efficient and culturally appropriate healthcare services. It is hoped that US healthcare professionals, including health educators, will better understand the reasons, applications, and cultural context of CAIH practices.

An instructor's supplement is available at www.wiley.com/go/pinzonperez. Additional materials, such as videos, podcasts, and readings, can be found at www.josseybasspublichealth.com. Comments about this book are invited and can be sent to publichealth@wiley.com.

References

American Public Health Association. (2015). *Integrative, complementary, and traditional health practices*. Retrieved from https://www.apha.org/apha-com munities/member-sections/integrative-complementary-and-traditional-health-practices

Clarke, T. C., Black, L. I., Stussman, B. J., Barnes, P. M., & Nahin, R. L. (2015). *Trends in the use of complementary health approaches among adults: United States, 2002–2012*. National Health Statistics Report, No 79. Hyattsville, MD: National Center for Health Statistics.

Howell, W. L. (2012). *More medical schools offer instruction in complementary and alternative medicine*. Retrieved from https://www.aamc.org/newsroom/reporter/feb2012/273812/therapies.html

Mayo Clinic. (2015). *Complementary and integrative medicine*. Retrieved from http://www.mayoclinic.org/departments-centers/general-internal-medicine/minnesota/overview/specialty-groups/complementary-integrative-medicine

National Center for Complementary and Alternative Medicine. (2011). *What is complementary and alternative medicine?* Retrieved from http://nccam.nih.gov/health/whatiscam#informed

National Center for Complementary and Alternative Medicine. (2014). *NCCAM facts-at-a-glance and mission*. Retrieved from http://nccam.nih.gov/about/ataglance

National Center for Complementary and Integrative Health. (2015a). *Important events in NCCIH history*. Retrieved from http://www.nih.gov/about/almanac/organization/NCCIH.htm

National Center for Complementary and Integrative Health. (2015b). *What complementary and integrative approaches do Americans use?* Retrieved from https://nccih.nih.gov/research/statistics/NHIS/2012/key-findings

National Center for Complementary and Integrative Health. (2015c). *Time to talk about CAM: Healthcare providers and patients need to ask and tell*. Retrieved from https://nccih.nih.gov/news/2008/060608.htm

University of North Carolina at Chapel Hill School of Medicine. (2015). *Introduction to complementary, alternative, and integrative health care*. Retrieved from https://www.med.unc.edu/phyrehab/pim/education/principles-and-practices-of-alternative-and-complementary-medicine

University of Texas MD Anderson Cancer Center. (2015). *Complementary and integrative medicine*. Retrieved from http://www.mdanderson.org/patient-and-cancer-information/cancer-information/cancer-topics/cancer-treatment/complementary-medicine/index.html

World Health Organization. (2000). *General guidelines for methodologies on research and evaluation of traditional medicine*. Geneva, Switzerland. http://whqlibdoc.who.int/hq/2000/WHO_EDM_TRM_2000.1.pdf?ua=1

World Health Organization. (2004). *New WHO guidelines to promote proper use of alternative medicines*. Retrieved from http://www.who.int/mediacentre/news/releases/2004/pr44/en/

World Health Organization. (2013). *WHO traditional medicine strategy 2014–2023*. Retrieved from http://apps.who.int/iris/bitstream/10665/92455/1/9789241506090_eng.pdf?ua=1&ua=1

World Health Organization. (n.d). Traditional medicine: *Definitions*. http://www.who.int/medicines/areas/traditional/definitions/en/

ACKNOWLEDGMENTS

The editors wish to express their thanks first to God for the opportunity to work on this project, to the authors who have agreed to share their knowledge and experience through their contributions to this work, and to the staff at Jossey-Bass, especially our dearly departed friend Andy Pasternack, who encouraged us from the start to pursue this project. We would also like to thank the draft reviewers, Joyce Perkins and Michael Goldstein. They provided thoughtful and constructive comments on the complete draft manuscript. Most chapters in this book were written by a team of practitioners and academicians working on complementary, alternative, and integrative health. Our highest gratitude goes to the members of each team for their willingness to join efforts and learn from each other. The successful production of this work would not have been possible without each of them.

Dr. Helda Pinzón-Pérez is a professor in the Department of Public Health and School of Nursing at California State University, Fresno. She is a native of Colombia. Her research interests are international health as well as alternative medicine and integrative healing. Dr. Pinzón-Pérez has authored various articles on health and diversity. She has presented her research at multiple international conferences and has worked with colleagues from Colombia, Mexico, Ecuador, Costa Rica, the Dominican Republic, Uganda, India, and Thailand. She has received two Fulbright teaching and research awards—the first one in 2008 to work with a school of medicine in the Dominican Republic and the second one in 2016 to work with a school of public health in Peru. She has also been trained as a massage therapist.

Dr. Miguel A. Pérez is a health educator who specializes in international adolescent health issues, applied research, and cultural competence. Dr. Pérez has authored a textbook in health education, coedited a couple of books, and written several book chapters, in addition to over 40 peer-reviewed publications and numerous presentations at local, state, national, and international conferences, many based on his research on migrant and adolescent health risk behaviors in Colombia, El Salvador, the Dominican Republic, and Mexico. Dr. Pérez has received four Fulbright awards, two of them as a senior specialist in public/global health to work in Colombia and in South Africa dealing with drug prevention and HIV/AIDS education and prevention programs. In 2013 Dr. Pérez developed a health promotion and disease training program for nurses in Thailand.

Joel Arboleda Castillo is director of the Scientific Research Institute of the Universidad Central del Este in the Dominican Republic and professor of sociology at Universidad Autónoma de Santo Domingo. Mr. Arboleda is a PhD candidate in the sociology of globalization at the University of the Basque Country, Spain. He earned a master's degree in applied statistics in 2014 at Universidad Autónoma de Santo Domingo and a master's in the sociology of globalization at the University of the Basque Country in 2008. Mr. Arboleda's primary research interests include consequences of globalization on health and education issues in underdeveloped countries, impacts of migrations on public health, and social inequalities in health and education. Mr. Arboleda has several refereed publications.

Georgina Castle is a California licensed acupuncturist and herbalist. She earned a master's degree in traditional Oriental medicine from Emperor's College of Traditional Oriental Medicine, graduating with the highest honors. She is board certified by the National Commission for Acupuncture and Oriental Medicine as a diplomate in Oriental medicine. She is also a diplomate of acupuncture orthopedics certified by the National Board of Acupuncture Orthopedics. Prior to becoming an acupuncturist, she graduated from St. Mary's College of California with a bachelor of science degree in biology and earned a master's of public health degree in epidemiology at the University of California, Los Angeles. While at UCLA, she performed HIV and cancer research at the School of Public Health and facilitated data analysis at the Los Angeles County Department of Public Health. Ms. Castle provides a holistic approach to her patients' acupuncture experience through pulse analysis, herbal and nutritional therapies, cupping, and heat treatments. She specializes in neuromusculoskeletal pain management, fertility, and women's health issues. She has published articles on Chinese cupping and healthy habits of families.

Brandon M. Eggleston is an associate professor and lead faculty member of the online BS in Public Health program at National University, Costa Mesa, California. Dr. Eggleston earned his PhD from the University of Indiana,

Bloomington, and his master's in public health from Indiana University, Indianapolis. He has written five published peer-reviewed articles and a textbook on biostatistics as well as a workbook in the field of public health and health promotion. In addition to his published work, Dr. Eggleston has participated in 35 peer-reviewed professional conferences and made a number of invited presentations at the local, state, and national levels. Dr. Eggleston serves as a peer reviewer for the *International Journal of Yoga Therapy* and is an associate editor for the *International Journal of Health, Wellness, and Society.*

Peter Garcia is an assistant professor in the School of Nursing, California State University, Fresno. Dr. Garcia earned his Doctor in Nursing Practice (DNP) degree in health care systems leadership at the University of San Francisco and his master's degree in nursing with a nurse practitioner certification. He earned a bachelor's degree in nursing at Fresno State. Dr. Garcia's primary teaching and research interests focus on the role of the DNP in academia and nursing practices, evidence-based practices specific to surgical patients, and the role of holistic care for acute surgical clients. Aside from teaching, Dr. Garcia is a practicing nurse practitioner in Fresno, California, at a large private urologic center.

Cyndi Guerra is an assistant professor in the School of Nursing, California State University, Fresno. Dr. Guerra received her doctorate in nursing practice in health care systems leadership at the University of San Francisco, School of Nursing. She also served as an adjunct nursing faculty member at the university's master's in nursing program for the past four years and began teaching part time at Fresno State in 2012. She obtained her bachelor's degree, master's degree, and school nurse credential from Fresno State. Dr. Guerra was nominated as "Employee of the Year" at her previous place of employment. She currently serves as an executive board member for the Nancy Hinds Hospice Foundation. Dr. Guerra is an active member of the National Association of School Nurses, California School Nurses Organization, Sigma Theta Tau, and American Association of Nurse Practitioners.

Cheryl Hickey is an associate professor in the doctor of physical therapy program at California State University, Fresno. Dr. Hickey earned her EdD. in education at the University of California, Davis, and California State University, Fresno; and her MS in counseling, her MPT in physical therapy, and her BS in science at Fresno State. Dr. Hickey has taught at the college level for over 16 years. Her primary teaching and research interests include multicultural health with an emphasis on language barriers in physical therapy practice, cultural competency in health promotion, electrophysiology and muscle behavior, and patient–practitioner interaction with the role of the therapist as a teacher. Dr. Hickey has practiced clinical in physical therapy in the areas of acute care and oncology, outpatient orthopedics, and neuro-rehabilitation. She has publications in a section journal of the American Physical Therapy Association and in an international journal on the effect of language barriers in practice.

Amber Huhndorf is an Athabascan/Yupik from Nikiski, Alaska. She received her BS from Oregon State University. She has worked as a health educator and has planned, implemented, and evaluated health programs for her tribal wellness center. She is enrolled in the master's of public health program at California State University, Fresno, where she is investigating the Native community's readiness to address historical trauma for her master's thesis.

Monika Joshi is a registered nurse and a clinical ayurvedic specialist. She was a lieutenant, military nursing officer, and midwife in the Indian Army before moving to the United States in 1990. Ms. Joshi has worked in various hospital settings. She is a graduate of California College of Ayurveda and is also certified by the American Institute of Vedic Studies. She is a member of the National Ayurvedic Medical Association and the Association of Ayurvedic Professionals of North America. She is a sought-after speaker on various aspects of ayurveda. She has published a chapter about ayurveda in *Rose Lore: Essays in Semiotics and Cultural History*. Ms. Joshi was the first clinical ayurvedic specialist to have a practice in Central California. She has also worked as a field intern supervisor for the California College of Ayurveda, mentoring and supervising new graduates.

Vickie D. Krenz is a professor of public health at Fresno State and has been a faculty member for 25 years. She is recognized for her work in program planning and evaluation with a focus on tobacco prevention. She completed a bachelor's degree in Religions Studies, a master's degree in Philosophy and Religion, and a master's of Science in Public Health. She holds a PhD in health education from the University of Utah, Salt Lake City, Utah. Currently, she is the President of the Fresno State American Indian Faculty and Staff Association and is of Cherokee ancestry.

Raffy R. Luquis is an associate professor and program coordinator of the health education master's degree in the School of Behavioral Sciences and Education at Pennsylvania State University, Harrisburg. Dr. Luquis earned his PhD in health science at the University of Arkansas, and his MS in health education and BS in science at Pennsylvania State University. Dr. Luquis' primary teaching and research interests include multicultural health, cultural competency in health promotion, community health, program evaluation, and human sexuality. Dr. Luquis has had several refereed publications and more than 50 national, regional, and state presentations. He is a fellow of the former American Association for Health Education and the Research Consortium of the American Alliance for Health, Physical Education, Recreation, and Dance. Dr. Luquis earned the Master Certified Health Education Specialist credential from the National Commission for Health Education Credentialing in 2011.

Mariamma K. Mathai is currently a professor and associate director of Nursing at National University, Fresno campus. She is also professor emerita of nursing at California State University, Fresno, having spent 30 years teaching graduate and undergraduate students, including two terms as the chair of the department. Dr. Mathai earned her doctorate in nursing education and nursing administration and her master's in nursing education from Teachers College, Columbia University, in New York City. She received her BS in nursing from Kerala University, Trivandrum, India. Dr. Mathai has traveled extensively, visiting nursing schools and hospitals and making presentations about nursing and nursing education.

Steven B. Owens is a seasoned family medicine and public health–trained physician with expertise in minority health issues—health equity, disparities, and public health workforce recruitment and development. As the director of health equity for the Directors of Health Promotion and Education (DHPE), he provides technical assistance to state, local, and territorial departments of health to address health inequities by using public health systems and environmental change tools and geographic analysis of market research data to plan and inform effective health programs. Emphasizing health equity, he provides health department staff trainings on integrating social and behavioral determinants of health into projects and activities addressing chronic disease prevention and health promotion. Additionally, Dr. Owens oversees the placement of DHPE's health promotion and policy fellows at state departments of health. Prior to joining DHPE, Dr. Owens led the Diversity Initiative for United States Agency for International Development's Global Health Fellows program. Dr. Owens has provided capacity building and technical assistance in the area of HIV/AIDS and behavioral interventions for community-based organizations throughout the United States, US Virgin Islands, and Africa. Additionally, Dr. Owens has directed various health promotion programs in the areas of cancer prevention and research, aging, HIV/AIDS, hepatitis, nutrition, and minority health. He designs community programs to improve healthcare delivery and community-clinical linkages for vulnerable populations and serves as an external reviewer for the Centers for Disease Control and Prevention and other federal and state agencies. Dr. Owens is a certified Fascial Stretch Therapy group instructor, yoga practitioner, and distance runner. He earned his MD (medical doctorate) from the Brody School of Medicine at East Carolina University, his MPH (master's of public health) in international health policy and management from the Rollins School of Public Health at Emory University, and his master's degree in biology from Hampton University.

Gina Marie Piane has more than 30 years of experience in the public health field. Dr. Piane is a Certified Health Education Specialist and has experience working with diverse communities and patients of all ages and backgrounds. She taught students in the master's of public health program at Northern Illinois University and California State University, Long Beach, before moving to National University as the director of the master's of public health program. Dr. Piane conducts research in health behavior and international health. Her most current research studies investigate evidence-based interventions to reduce maternal mortality in sub-Saharan Africa. Dr. Piane is a faculty member of Delta Omega, the honor society for public health; the American Public Health Association; the Society for Public Health Education; and the Southern California Public Health Association. In addition to teaching and research, Dr. Piane has traveled extensively with students studying healthcare issues and systems in India, Thailand, Kenya, Tanzania, Zanzibar, Chile, Ecuador, and Brazil.

Kathleen Rindahl is an assistant professor of nursing at California State University, Fresno. Dr. Rindahl earned her DNP from Western University of Health Sciences, her MSN from Fresno State, and her BSM from California State University, Los Angeles. Dr. Rindahl also is a practicing nurse practitioner in an urgent care/family practice clinic. Her education and training includes public health nursing and school nursing and time as a Veteran Hospital Corpsman in the United States Navy. Dr. Rindahl's research focus includes rural and community health nursing and eating disorders, especially in early adolescents. She has been a guest speaker at local, national, and international conferences, presenting on topics in her areas of research.

Liliana Rojas-Guyler is an associate professor in the health promotion and education program at the University of Cincinnati. Dr. Rojas-Guyler earned her PhD in health and human behavior at Indiana University, and her MHSE in health education and her BS in health science at the University of Florida. Dr. Rojas-Guyler has taught at the college level for 18 years. Her primary teaching and research interests include Latino and vulnerable population health, multicultural health, and women's health. Dr. Rojas-Guyler has published over 20 articles in refereed journals and has made over 50 international, national, regional, and state presentations. She is a member of several professional organizations and is a board member of Eta Sigma Gamma, the national health education honorary society.

Dominick L. Sturz is an associate professor at California Baptist University, teaching various courses in public health and leading the development of their online master's of public health program. He is also a lecturer for the Department of Health Science at California State University, Fullerton, where he completed his undergraduate work and obtained his master's of public health degree in community health and disease prevention. Additionally, he has served as the director of educational program development for Choose Health Inc., a nonprofit that focuses on community health disparities, since 2008. Dr. Sturz obtained his doctor of public health in health education and promotion degree (DrPH) from Loma Linda University, where his research interests focused on spirituality, religion, and health. During his doctoral studies, he served the local community as a director of community health services and education for the Mexican Consulate in San Bernardino, California, and is currently a member of their Executive Planning Committee for their annual Bi-National Health Fair.

Prior to his work in academia, Dr. Sturz spent 10 years in the field of pharmaceuticals—working for Merck & Co., specializing in cardiovascular diseases, and then for Johnson & Johnson, specializing in mental health. During his time at Johnson & Johnson, he collaborated with the Department of Government Services, was a pharmacokinetic consultant in the development of specific pharmaceutical protocols for the California Department of Mental Health, led educational activities on state-wide county medical directors' conference calls, and developed a wellness program that subsequently was implemented in the California State Hospital system, gaining the attention of the Department of Health and Human Services and the Office of the Governor.

Pierre E. Wright has served as lecturer in the school psychology department at Howard University for over five years. Dr. Wright has over 15 years of experience in higher education, which includes outreach, research, evaluation, budget, and grants management. He has served in several executive leadership roles for national nonprofit organizations with missions to educate and advance the overall academic, social, and mental health of college students and their communities. He has published works in public health and education and maintains a special interest in HIV/AIDS education and risk reduction. Dr. Wright is also a Bikram Yoga studio owner. He is certified as a Fascial Stretch Therapist Level II, group stretch facilitator, and trained yoga therapist. As a result of strong practice and dedication to mind/body work, Dr. Wright has instructed yoga internationally and in cities around the United States. Currently Dr. Wright is working to establish a nonprofit organization to increase African American youth engagement in the practice of yoga and meditation to reduce and to promote optimal health. Dr. Wright continues to teach yoga at local school districts and churches and with civic groups attempting to mobilize health in their communities and regions.

Catherine L. Zeman has worked on sustainability and environmental health issues in a multitude of capacities through community organizing, as a consultant, and as a professor since 1990. Dr. Zeman received her PhD in preventive medicine with an emphasis on environmental and occupational health from the University of Iowa and a master's in environmental science from Southern Illinois University. Her undergraduate background includes degrees in nursing, biology, and anthropology. She also has a diploma in holistic health practice from the American College of Health Sciences. Dr. Zeman was a Fulbright Scholar to Romania on environmental health issues. She is the director of the Recycling and Reuse Technology Transfer Center at the University of Northern Iowa, where she oversees a staff of 10 student employees, researchers, and full- and part-time staff. She is a professor in the health division, School of Health, Physical Education and Leisure Services, at the University of Northern Iowa. She teaches classes in epidemiology, human diseases, environmental health, and environmental and occupational health regulations. Her research interests include nitrates in the environment and their impact on human health, immunity and exposure assessment, and international health disparities issues (primary), with secondary work in the areas of mind/body medicine, industrial ecology, and environmental sustainability.

Kara N. Zografos earned a bachelor of science in health science degree and a master's of public health degree from California State University, Fresno. She earned a doctorate in public health from Loma Linda University, receiving the Chancellor's Award for academic excellence upon graduation. She is currently an associate professor for the Department of Public Health at Fresno State, where she teaches courses at the undergraduate and graduate level. She is also the director of the master's of public health program. Her research interests include asthma, air pollution, and the relationship between religion and health. She is a member of the American Public Health Association and the Society for Public Health Education. Additionally, she is the Sunday School principal for the St. George Greek Orthodox Church in Fresno, California.

CHAPTER 1

EXPLORING COMPLEMENTARY, ALTERNATIVE, AND INTEGRATIVE HEALTH

Overview, Limits, and Controversies

Cyndi Guerra, Cheryl Hickey, and Helda Pinzón-Pérez

Today's health economics often drives the cost of modern medications, treatments, and therapies. Increasingly, these dynamics polarize the patient-consumer roles and alienate patients in the same system from which they seek care. Patients diagnosed with chronic disease, or illnesses, are particularly vulnerable to the economics of healthcare. For example, issues such as polypharmacy significantly escalate the cost of care for patients. As a result, patients are driven to seek other alternatives. Consequently, healthcare practitioners and health educators, whose patients have begun to explore more self-regulated and less expensive options afforded through complementary, alternative, and integrative health (CAIH) approaches, increasingly find themselves in need of knowledge related to these models of care. In today's society, these modalities can represent a more accessible treatment option and a lower financial burden for already economically challenged and chronically ill consumers.

Despite a young and limited body of formal research, as well as mixed conclusions regarding treatment efficacy, several motivations have fueled the patient/consumer's desire to use complementary and alternative treatments

LEARNING OBJECTIVES

At the completion of this chapter, students will be able to:

- Understand the importance of complementary, alternative, and integrative health (CAIH) and complementary and alternative medicine (CAM) in today's society.

- Differentiate current controversies between traditional medicine and complementary, alternative, and integrative therapies.

- Discuss strategies to bridge the gap between allopathic medicine and CAIH modalities.

- Provide an overview of CAM under the guidelines of the Affordable Care Act.

for addressing physical problems and for maintaining good health. This chapter explores the reasons patients/consumers are driven to engage in CAIH practices and the factors that have led to the continued historical prevalence of complementary and alternative medicine (CAM) use. It also provides a contemporary overview of CAIH, a discussion of modern controversies surrounding CAM, and the need for healthcare providers to increase their education related to CAIH modalities.

Throughout this chapter and the others in this book, the names National Center for Complementary and Alternative Medicine (NCCAM) and National Center for Complementary and Integrative Health (NCCIH) are both utilized due to the 2014 name change of the major federal organization related to CAIH and CAM in the United States. In addition, the term *Complementary, Alternative, and Integrative Health* will be used under the acronym CAIH to reflect an emphasis on health and wellness.

In this book, the acronym CAM is replaced by CAIH to adhere to the current emphasis on complementary and integrative health. Although NCCIH refers to these practices as complementary and integrative health (CIH) approaches, the editors of this book added the word *Alternative* in the acronym to acknowledge that consumers are still using some of these practices as alternative forms of care.

While we recognize the value that the denomination CAM (Complementary and Alternative Medicine) has brought historically to our understanding of traditional health and alternative models of care, the acronym CAM is currently being abandoned and will only be utilized in this book when used by the bibliographical references consulted for this publication. For additional clarification on the terms used in this book, please read the preface.

Theoretical Concepts

The National Center for Complementary and Alternative Medicine (NCCAM), known since December 2014 as the National Center for Complementary and Integrative Health (NCCIH), is the leading federal agency on CAIH approaches in the United States. It is one of the 27 institutes and centers of the National Institutes of Health within the US Department of Health and Human Services. Its mission is to "define, through rigorous scientific investigation, the usefulness and safety of complementary and integrative health interventions and their roles in improving health and health care" (NCCIH, 2015a). Throughout this book, both names (NCCAM and NCCIH) will appear according to the term used by the bibliographical references.

The NCCIH (2015a) defined *integrative health* as the incorporation of complementary approaches into mainstream healthcare, bringing conventional and complementary modalities together in a coordinated way. *CAM* is defined as the integration of biomedicine, complementary, and alternative modalities used together with safety and efficacy (NCCAM, 2009). According to NCCIH (2015a), "complementary" medicine is when a nonmainstream practice is used together with conventional medicine; "alternative" medicine is when a nonmainstream practice is used in place of conventional medicine.

Complementary, alternative, and integrative health is a term that includes complementary, alternative, and integrative approaches to prevent and manage disease as well as to maintain or restore health and wellness. This term is congruent with the 2014 name change of the National Center for Complementary and Alternative Medicine to the National Center for Complementary and Integrative Health. The NCCIH (2015a) defines complementary health approaches as practices and products of nonmainstream origin.

The classification of CAM therapies by the NCCAM and the NCCIH has varied throughout the years. Initially, NCCAM divided CAM modalities into five categories:

1. Alternative medical systems
2. Mind-body interventions
3. Biologically based treatments
4. Manipulative and body-based methods
5. Energy therapies

Later, NCCAM (2014) grouped CAM practices into four categories:

1. Natural products
2. Mind and body medicine
3. Manipulative and body-based practices
4. Other CAM practices

This classification was revised again. The NCCIH (2015a) divided complementary health approaches into three subgroups:

1. Natural products
2. Mind and body practices
3. Other complementary health approaches

Natural products include products such as herbs, botanicals, vitamins, minerals, probiotics, and dietary supplements. Mind and body practices include procedures and techniques such as yoga, chiropractic and osteopathic manipulation, meditation, massage therapy, acupuncture, tai chi, qi gong, healing touch, hypnotherapy, movement therapies (Feldenkrais method, Alexander technique, Pilates, Rolfing Structural Integration, and Trager psychophysical integration), and relaxation techniques (breathing exercises, guided imagery, and progressive muscle relaxation). Other complementary health approaches include traditional healers, ayurvedic medicine, traditional Chinese medicine, naturopathy, and homeopathy (NCCIH, 2015a).

Complementary, Alternative, and Integrative Approaches and CAM in Contemporary US Society and around the World

It is important for healthcare practitioners to have knowledge regarding the wide range of treatment modalities associated with CAIH. Understanding the role of CAIH in health management can be a powerful tool for practitioners and consumers. CAIH therapies can be instrumental in disease prevention and treatment. For this reason, many consumers are showing increasing preference for such practices that used to be called CAM (NCCAM, 2008).

Understanding or assisting patients in integrating CAIH modalities into their healthcare does not necessarily indicate acceptance on the part of the health educator or healthcare practitioner. Rather, it indicates a willingness to allow patients to have more autonomy and control over their care.

There has been an expansion of wellness programs in the United States over the last few decades, and many of these programs utilize CAIH modalities. Increasingly, such modalities have appealed to the US population because of some promising findings for improved health and wellness (Gebhardt & Crump, 1990). The concept of health awareness enabled people to be more proactive and responsible for their own health. Wellness programs, which surfaced decades ago, offered incentives to employees who chose to live healthier lifestyles and included initiatives such as weight loss and smoking cessation programs (Erfurt, Foote, & Heirich, 1992).

Other venues beyond the work setting also began in the 1990s to promote health and wellness programs for populations. Research reinforced the value of wellness programs by showing that they could improve health and, in some cases, reverse chronic conditions. Many occupational settings, such as community and state health departments, hospitals, universities, and schools, began to promote healthy lifestyle programs to gain long-term health benefits (Institute of Medicine of the National Academies [IOM], 2005; National Institute for Health Care Management Research and Educational Foundation, 2011).

As a result of strong public interest in natural treatment modalities, two governmental entities emerged: NCCAM in 1999, formerly known as the Office of Alternative Medicine [OAM], and the White House's Commission on Complementary and Alternative Medicine Policy in 2000. This commission was formed to aid in the creation of public policy regarding CAM and served as a beneficial force in assisting the public's safe and efficacious use of CAM (Health and Human Services, n.d.).

President Clinton appointed several physicians, nurses, PhDs, and CAM providers to serve on the White House's Commission on Complementary and Alternative Medicine Policy. Both the NCCAM and the White House's Commission were intended to make recommendations and advise on public policy regarding the safety and efficacious promotion of products labeled as CAM. The NCCAM proved, over time, to be the most important initiative that gave scientific credibility to CAM therapies. Currently, the NCCIH (2015a) promotes the development of scientific evidence that will "inform decision making by the public, by health care professionals, and by health policymakers regarding the use and integration of complementary and integrative health approaches."

Ultimately, the White House Commission introduced several guidelines in regard to CAM, including documented findings from research to support CAM use, product efficacy and safety for CAM-associated treatments, access to proper training for medical providers practicing CAM statewide, and increased dialogue among CAM providers and physicians practicing Western medicine (IOM, 2005).

This chapter examines US behaviors related to CAIH therapies; however, it is important to note that developments regarding CAM practices are not germane to the United States and that in fact, these efforts mirror what is happening on an international scale. For example, the use of CAM modalities has risen by 40% in patients with chronic illness and in primary care worldwide (Ben-Arye & Visser, 2012). The World Health Organization (WHO) reported that 70% to 80% of the population use CAM as their primary form of medicine (WHO, 2013).

To respond to the growing use of CAM practices around the world, WHO developed the *WHO Traditional Medicine Strategy 2014–2023*. In the document, the terms *traditional medicine* (TM) and *complementary medicine* (CM) were combined under the acronym T&CM. This strategy was developed as a result of the World Health Assembly resolution WHA.62.13 on traditional medicine to help nations around the world acknowledge "the potential contribution of TM to health, wellness and people-centered health care; (and promote) the safe and effective use of TM by regulating, researching, and integrating TM products, practitioners, and practice into health systems, where appropriate" (WHO, 2013, p. 11).

Use of CAM in the United States

Over the past few decades, the use of CAM has become increasingly appealing for US consumers, as documented by the National Health Interview Surveys (NHIS). The 2012 NHIS is currently the most comprehensive source of data on complementary and integrative health use in the United States. The NHIS Surveys are conducted by the National Center for Health Statistics from the Centers for Disease Control and Prevention. The surveys from 2002, 2007, and 2012 report data on CAM use among US populations (NCCIH, 2015b).

According to the NHIS, in 2012, 33.2% of US adults used complementary health approaches; the rates were 35.5% in 2007 and 32.3% in 2002. For children, the 2012 NHIS showed that 11.6% of US children aged 4 to 17 used complementary health approaches; in 2007, 12.0% used them. Aggregate results from a sample of 88,962 adults aged 18 and above in the 2002, 2007, and 2012 NHIS showed that the most common complementary health practice used among adults in the United States is natural products, such as nonvitamin, nonmineral dietary supplements (17.7% in 2012 and 2007; 18.9% in 2002), followed by deep-breathing exercises (10.9% in 2012; 12.7% in 2007; 11.6% in 2002). Yoga, tai chi, and qi gong were used by 10.1% of adults in 2012, 6.7% in 2007, and 5.8% in 2002 (NCCIH, 2015b).

The 2002 and 2007 surveys examined CAM use over a 12-month period. They showed an increase of 2.3% over a 2-year period for use of CAM therapies (from 36% to 38.3%) among adults ages 18 or older (NCCAM, 2008, 2013a).

The National Institutes of Health (NIH) reported in 2008 that approximately 12% of children in the United States were using a variety of complementary and alternative medicine treatments (Barnes, Bloom, & Nahin, 2008). Similarly, the National Health Survey reported that 38% of US adults used CAM therapies (Goldbas, 2012).

Data obtained by the NHIS indicated that there has been a substantial increase in out-of-pocket expenditures for self-care CAM therapies by US adults (Nahin, Barnes, Stussman, & Bloom, 2009); however, even more compelling was the fact that 629 million visits were made to CAM providers, which is an exceptionally high number compared to the 386 million who sought traditional medical services from primary care physicians annually (Gaylord & Mann, 2007). Another survey in 2007 found that 40% of Americans were using some form of CAM therapies (Nahin et al., 2009). Data compiled from 15 national centers for CAM show that consumers utilized such therapies largely based on their perceived positive effects and outcomes (Gaylord & Mann, 2007). Yet these are not the only motivators. According to research, consumers rate CAM therapies favorably as prevention tools and indicate that some therapies could be utilized safely to treat medical conditions (Gaylord & Mann, 2007).

It has been suggested that those who utilize CAM practices hold holistic values and beliefs because of their view of health from an integral perspective. Furthermore, those who use CAM are more likely to favor it, because it incorporates a health focus rather than an illness focus. CAM modalities increase the likelihood of improved outcomes, and CAM is effective for specific health problems, particularly chronic illnesses. Some of the chronic illnesses cited in the literature include cardiovascular disease, arthritis, and diabetes (Gaylord & Mann, 2007). The most frequently used CAM therapies are relaxation techniques, herbal medicine, massage therapy, and chiropractic services, which made up 42% of US patient consumption of CAM interventions (NCCAM, 2008).

Factors Leading to Increased Use of CAM

It is clear that CAM use is no longer contained to one small, well-defined segment of the US population. Studies have reported the use of CAM therapies among diverse socioeconomic, age, gender, and ethnic groups (NCCAM, 2008).

According to Clarke et al. (2015) in their discussion of trends in the use of complementary health approaches in the United States between 2002 and 2012, nonvitamin, nonmineral dietary supplements remained the most popular complementary health approach used. Yoga, tai chi, and qi gong use increased linearly in the three NHIS surveys in 2002, 2007, and 2012, with yoga accountable for an estimated 80% of the use prevalence.

Clarke et al. (2015) revealed that age and education are factors associated with an increased use of CAM. Older and more educated populations are more likely to use CAM. Between 2002 and 2012, an estimated 18.6% of adults with less than a high school diploma reported CAM use in 2002, and the figures were 18.9% in 2007 and 15.6% in 2012; 26.6% of adults with a high school diploma or equivalency diploma reported CAM use in 2002, 28.1%

in 2007, and 24.4% in 2012; 35.6% of adults with some college education reported CAM use in 2002, 41.3% in 2007, and 36.5% in 2012. In addition, 42.1% of those with a college degree or higher reported CAM use in 2002, 46.7% in 2007, and 42.6% in 2012 (Clarke et al, 2015). The remainder of this chapter focuses on data from the 2002 and 2007 NHIS. Later chapters in this book will present information reported by the 2012 NHIS.

According to the 2007 NHIS, women were more frequent CAM users, as were those with higher education levels and socioeconomic means. Data on the ethnic distribution of CAM use in the United States identified American Indian/Alaska Native CAM use to be as high as 50.3%, with Caucasians the next highest at 43.1%, followed by Asians at 39.9%, and Blacks and Hispanics at 25.5% and 23.7%, respectively (NCCAM, 2008).

Other groups in the United States that practice CAM do so because of their strong ancestral ties to these practices. These practices are often the only intervention individuals may know or are willing to consider. Some of these ancestral practices include traditional Chinese medicine, Indian ayurvedic medicine, herbal medicine, and shaman consultations. The association between ancestral practices and CAM exemplifies the strong CAM use among ethnic minority groups in the United States (NCCAM, 2008).

Early factors leading to the increased use of CAM were related to economic means, cultural predisposition, and specific health mind-sets; however, overall, contemporary CAM use seems to be moving away from patterned use toward a dispersed use that ranges from the elderly to the college age; from the highly educated to the less educated; from the higher socioeconomic groups to lower socioeconomic groups; and from migratory to American-born groups (Astin, 1998; IOM, 2005; NCCAM, 2007). The motivation for CAM use may vary from group to group. For example, immigrant individuals may use CAM simply because it is what they are familiar with and what they have access to. Asian Americans may favor traditional Chinese medicine practices that include acupuncture and acupressure because of previous positive cultural exposure to these practices (Astin, 1998; Synovitz & Larson, 2013).

As morbidity and mortality rates from chronic illnesses, such as diabetes, hypertension, and arthritis increase in the United States, many patients continue to look for therapies that improve health (Marks, Murray, Evans, & Estacio, 2011). Patients aspiring to improve their overall health may rely on CAM as a treatment option. For example, many of the current biomedical therapies do not manage chronic pain successfully. Several studies have shown yoga, acupuncture, massage, guided imagery, and chiropractic to be effective in pain relief (Goldbas, 2012).

Additionally, CAM therapies offer the autonomy element, which allows the patients to make informed decisions and choices in the management of their health. The integration of these methods promotes well-being and can lead to improved health (Marks et al., 2011). Early researchers on CAM, such as Kaptchuk and Eisenberg (1998), described four reasons that motivated use among the general public. The first reason is the association of CAM with natural and holistic methods of treatment. Many people today want to manage their health and disease patterns naturally, and they find in CAM an option to achieve this goal. Second is the concept of vitalism, or the belief that the body is capable of returning to optimal health naturally and through its own internal mechanisms. This perception supports the idea that energy from the body allows natural healing from within and that it is this natural ability that restores good health. Third is the concept of alternative medicine as a science. Alternative medicine is described as holistic and connects the physical, mental, spiritual, and emotional components of health. Biomedicine or traditional medicine focuses on the treatment of each subsystem; in contrast, CAM aims to treat the clients and their health as a whole unit. Fourth is the aspect of spirituality, which is defined in terms of a balance between the physical and the spiritual experience. This idea allows clients to connect the scientific side of medicine to the more personal, religious, or spiritual side and to make a connection with what is natural in the universe (Kaptchuk & Eisenberg, 1998).

Role of the Federal Government in CAIH

The leading governmental organization for CAIH and CAM in the United States is the NCCIH, which as mentioned before, was known until December 2014 as the NCCAM. This center traces its origins to 1991, when the US Congress passed Public Law 102-170, which provided $2 million in funding for fiscal year 1992 to establish an office in the NIH to investigate and determine the scientific value of promising unconventional medical practices. In 1992, Dr. Joseph J. Jacobs was named the first director of the Office of Alternative Medicine (OAM). In 1993, the NIH Revitalization Act of 1993 (PL 103-43) officially established the OAM within the NIH to facilitate the study of complementary and alternative medical practices as well as to educate the public on the results of related research (NCCIH, 2015c).

In October 1998, the NCCAM was established by Congress under Title VI, Section 601 of the Omnibus Appropriations Act of 1999 (PL 105-277). This bill amended Title IV of the Public Health Service Act and converted the OAM into an NIH center. In May 2007, the NCCAM created a Complementary and Integrative Medicine Council Service at the NIH

Clinical Center. In December 2014, Congress authorized the change in the name of this organization from National Center for Complementary and Alternative Medicine to the National Center for Complementary and Integrative Health (NCCAM, 2013b; NCCIH, 2015c).

Another governmental organization related to CAIH and CAM is the Food and Drug Administration (FDA), which is responsible for the regulation of all medications, finished dietary supplement products, and dietary ingredients sold in the United States. The Dietary Supplement Health and Education Act (DSHEA) of 1994 regulates dietary supplements. The regulations for dietary supplements are not the same as for drugs and over-the-counter (OTC) medications. Two key considerations should be noted in regard to dietary supplements. First, manufacturers do not have to prove that their supplements work. This is in contrast to prescription drug and OTC medications, for which manufacturers are obligated to prove that the medications are effective for their intended use. In addition, the FDA simply requires dietary supplement manufacturers to assure the safety of their products and not make untrue claims about their efficacy (FDA, 2015b).

According to the FDA, if a manufacturer does make a claim, it must also provide wording that suggests that the claim has not been evaluated by the FDA and that the product is not intended to diagnose, treat, or cure disease. A worrisome consideration is that dietary supplements do not give warnings as to possible side effects, when they could potentially be harmful, what can be the effects on surgical procedures, and what could be the results if taken in combination with over-the-counter medications or prescription drugs (NIH, 2013). The Federal Trade Commission (FTC) also has the responsibility to monitor some elements related to CAM use, specifically the truthfulness of ads published via internet, television, radio and print media (NIH, 2013).

The Affordable Care Act and CAM/CAIH

The future of CAM/CAIH under the Affordable Care Act (ACA) does not seem to be altogether clear. Some sources indicate that CAIH therapies may be covered by healthcare plans due to the lobbying efforts of groups such as the Integrative Healthcare Policy Consortium (IHCPC, 2013), among others. It appears that CAIH coverage may be directly determined by state regulations.

According to the Non-Discrimination in Health Care Provision of the Affordable Care Act, Section 2706(a), Title XXVII of the Public Health Service Act, patients ought to be protected in their rights to choose among a variety of healthcare providers, such as naturopathic physicians and acupuncturists. It also states that insurance plans cannot discriminate against providers who are acting within their scope of practice as determined by their licenses or certifications (American Association of Naturopathic Physicians, 2014; IHCPC, 2013).

Much of the future of CAIH inclusion and integration into the milieu of mainstream biomedicine in the United States may be based on two critical factors. First, CAIH interventions must establish their efficacy just as biomedicine has done and must do. Second, well-defined practice guidelines for research, for development, and for CAIH implementation must be established sustainably over time within society. For example, the addition of the OAM as an official branch of the NIH, within the Department of Health and Human Services in 1992, was an early step in the creation of a sustainable mechanism for the creation and dissemination of evidence about CAM. The establishment of the National Center for Complementary and Integrative Health will continue to provide guidance through the allocation of federal resources designed to conduct research that will guide decision making regarding coverage of CAIH and CAM practices under the ACA.

Consumer Issues

Ill people seeking any possible relief or cure are vulnerable to deception and are likely to use CAIH. The more serious the conditions, the more likely people are to use CAIH. If Western medicine has had very little benefit or no longer offers effective treatments, people tend to look for help elsewhere. These users of CAIH are more vulnerable to deception and misperception about the efficacy of these treatments. Consumers with chronic debilitating diagnoses, such as cancer, HIV, and diabetes, often use CAIH as a viable alternative.

These serious and chronic conditions have a high associated economic cost. This financial burden encourages patients to look toward CAM modalities as a hopeful and financially feasible possibility, which makes them more vulnerable to deception and misrepresentation (Gaylord & Mann, 2007).

Other groups that may be vulnerable to deception and misrepresentation are the poor and underprivileged groups within our society. These individuals may be vulnerable simply because they do not have access to the mainstream Western medical system, and their options are very limited. For example, new immigrants, minority groups, and lower socioeconomic groups have been found to be frequent users of CAM therapies. We do not know whether this comfort with CAM is due to preexposure or whether it is a simple manifestation of not having access to Western medical practices (Gaylord & Mann, 2007).

Quackery

Quackery, which is synonymous with health fraud, has been defined by the FDA (2015a) as:

> [T]he deceptive promotion, advertising, distribution or sale of articles, intended for human or animal use, that are represented as being effective to diagnose, prevent, cure, treat, or mitigate disease (or other conditions), or provide a beneficial effect on health, but which have not been scientifically proven safe and effective for such purposes. Such practices may be deliberate, or done without adequate knowledge or understanding of the article.

The major conditions in the United States in which quackery is most prominent are treatments for cancer, Alzheimer's, arthritis, and diabetes, as well as diagnostic tests, weight-loss products, and sexual performance products (FDA, 2009). Data from the FDA (2009) suggest that fraud and quackery attempts may in fact target many of the most vulnerable populations. In some cases, consumers are at risk of being taken advantage of monetarily and left without an intervention that offers any tangible benefit.

More worrisome, however, is that not only are people being taken advantage of financially, they also may be exposing themselves to unproven and damaging so-called "treatments" that may worsen their health status. Unproven treatments can cause physical harm and can leave patients physically impaired or even dead. For example, although shark cartilage was advertised as a natural cancer therapy, there is little to no evidence to support its effectiveness (FDA, 2009).

An example of these deceptive practices is illustrated in the case *United States* v. *Syntrax Innovations, Inc.* and described by the FDA (2008). In this case, a drug known as Triax Metabolic Accelerator was sold as a dietary supplement for weight loss. FDA scientists found that this drug represented a significant health risk because it contained triatricol, a potent thyroid hormone that is not classified as a dietary supplement according to the DSHEA and can carry a real risk for heart attack and stroke if not used properly. This case also brought class-action suits against three other dietary supplements that contained products not in compliance with DSHEA standards.

Box 1.1 presents some FDA recommendations to consumers in relation to CAM use. The FDA warns consumers that fraudulent products are not easy to identify and that it is important to consult with a doctor or healthcare professional before starting to use any new health product (FDA, 2013).

BOX 1.1   FDA TIPS TO HELP YOU IDENTIFY RIP-OFFS

- *One product does it all.* Be suspicious of products that claim to cure a wide range of diseases. A New York firm claimed its products marketed as dietary supplements could treat or cure senile dementia; brain atrophy; atherosclerosis; kidney dysfunction; gangrene; depression; osteoarthritis; dysuria (difficult urination); and lung, cervical, and prostate cancer. In October 2012, at the FDA's request, US marshals seized these products.

- *Personal testimonials.* Success stories, such as "It cured my diabetes" or "My tumors are gone," are easy to make up and are not a substitute for scientific evidence.

- *Quick fixes.* Few diseases or conditions can be treated quickly, even with legitimate products. Beware of language such as "Lose 30 pounds in 30 days" or "eliminates skin cancer in days."

- *"All natural."* Some plants found in nature (such as poisonous mushrooms) can kill when consumed. Moreover, numerous products promoted as "all natural" contain hidden and dangerously high doses of prescription drug ingredients or even untested active artificial ingredients.

- *"Miracle cure."* Alarms should go off when you see this claim or others like it, such as "new discovery," "scientific breakthrough," or "secret ingredient." If a real cure for a serious disease were discovered, it would be widely reported through the media and prescribed by health professionals—not buried in print ads, on TV infomercials, or on Internet sites.

- *Conspiracy theories.* Claims such as "The pharmaceutical industry and the government are working together to hide information about a miracle cure" are always untrue and unfounded. These statements are used to distract consumers from the obvious, common-sense questions about the so-called miracle cure.

Source: Food and Drug Administration (2013).

In order to better serve their constituents, health educators and medical providers now recognize the need for CAIH training and to incorporate holistic concepts in their professional practice (Ben-Arye & Frenkel, 2008; Ben-Arye, Frenkel, Klein, & Scharf, 2008). Medical providers must improve their knowledge of CAIH therapies because of the high number of patients in the United States who utilize CAIH therapies. One out of every five persons in the United States has a disability. Many patients who experience disabilities are likely to use CAM therapies to augment their current medical treatment, to decrease the progression of their illness or comorbidities, and/or to keep their current health at its optimal level (Okoro, Zhao, Li, & Balluz, 2011). Accordingly, as patient use increases, providers must be educated on CAIH therapies and how they can be integrated into a whole-treatment approach.

According to research reports, patients have a difficult time discussing their use of CAIH therapies with medical providers. While no literature exists, it is expected that the same holds true for discussions with health educators. Health educators are trained practitioners who promote individual and community health by planning, implementing, monitoring, and evaluating programs and interventions designed to improve health and encourage healthy lifestyles (National Commission for Health Education Credentialing, 2008). Health educators can serve as a source of information for individuals and communities on a variety of topics including CAIH. As more people are exploring the use and benefits of CAIH, health educators, like other healthcare professionals, must be knowledgeable about these healing modalities in order to educate the public they serve.

Research suggests that knowledge and usage of CAM by a group of clinical nurse specialists impacted their likelihood of recommending and integrating alternative treatments into their patient care. It was reported that those nurse specialists who used CAM personally were also likely to recommend it professionally. The therapies most recommended by clinical nurse specialists were humor and laughter, massage, prayer, acupuncture, and music therapy (Cutshall et al., 2010).

There are many reasons why patients may not be forthcoming with their provider regarding their CAIH use. Many patients feel it is not important for their provider to know or that the provider would not understand and/or would disapprove of their alternative therapy use. Some patients feel that the provider may discourage the use of CAM therapies (Ben-Arye et al, 2008). As a result, there is a need to further the patient-provider dialogue and enhance the partnership and trust that comes with shared care. Both of these factors—partnership in care and trust—would yield a more positive future outcome for patients (Gaylord & Mann, 2007).

Medical professionals have begun to incorporate the use of CAIH into their educational curriculum due to the increased interest and use of these therapies. Studies have shown that hospitals, medical programs, and insurance providers also have begun to increase their services in the area of CAM (IOM, 2005; National Institute for Health Care Management Foundation, 2011).

In May 2004, the Consortium of Academic Health Centers for Integrative Medicine began a foundation with the primary purpose of educating healthcare students in the area of CAM. As a result of the advocacy efforts of foundations such as the Consortium of Academic Health Centers, by 2010, 82 medical schools in the United States had incorporated CAM education into the curricula. The curricula in these programs includes theory, practice, and efficacy, and safety for patients (Bravewell Collaborative, 2010; Witt, Brinkhaus, & Willich, 2010). The proposed educational curriculum on CAM included different therapies and modalities and the integration of treatments in complementary and alternative medicine (Witt et al., 2010).

Other healthcare professions, such as psychology, social work, nursing, and pharmacy, have also begun to incorporate CAM education in their core curriculum (Tiralongo & Wallis, 2008). The objective of this education for healthcare providers is to increase their medical knowledge of CAM practices and to help them become comfortable with patient inquiries about CAM therapies. An ultimate goal is to enhance the scientific knowledge among traditional CAM providers to improve overall patient health via an open dialogue in which the client feels safe in disclosing CAM-related behaviors (Gaylord & Mann, 2007).

Limits and Controversies

Although CAIH use continues to grow among the general public, there is a lack of continuity and collaboration on the regulation, use, and efficacy of CAIH treatments among the medical community, patients, and policy-makers. Concerns have been expressed regarding the use of CAM and its effects on doctor-patient communication (Ben-Arye & Visser, 2012; Zhang, 2012). These challenges sometimes put patients and medical providers at odds with each other.

Patients may have compelling reasons for using CAM modalities. For example, one reason for CAM use is patients' dissatisfaction with Western medical approaches and their lack of a holistic emphasis on prevention and wellness (Gaylord & Mann, 2007). Most consumers want a treatment that does not focus solely on the illness but also on the psychological and social aspects that affect pathological processes. In addition, patients may be disappointed with the adverse side effects of mainstream treatments and their lack of efficacy. Yet the counterargument of using CAM approaches points to an ongoing controversy. Many CAM modalities lack strong empirical evidence to support their use. Health professionals, including health educators, need to find a balance in which cultural and scientific evidence are acknowledged and valued.

Another reason mentioned by patients who seek CAM treatments is the perception of autonomy that CAM gives them in managing their own symptoms. When using these modalities, patients feel they have more control over their health and their choices. In contrast to this perceived autonomy, patients may feel that the Western medicine approaches, which are based on the medical model, are the driving force in the delivery of today's healthcare in America (NCCIH, 2015d). Since most healthcare providers have been trained in the medical model, providers usually must struggle to find a middle ground between advocating for scientific approaches and acknowledging the value of CAM modalities.

Due to their dissatisfaction with Western approaches and a desire for holistic interventions, healthcare consumers often do not share their use of CAM with their providers, believing they could respond negatively to their use of alternative medicine therapy (Zhang, Peck, Spalding, Jones, & Cook, 2012). Patients also state that the physician's lack of CAM knowledge hinders patients' willingness to disclose CAM use. In addition, medical providers often do not ask if their patients are using CAM therapies, nor do patients believe that medical providers support the use of these therapies (Gaylord & Mann, 2007).

Patients today are more knowledgeable about their medical conditions and treatment options due to the Internet and social media. For this reason, there is a need for continued efforts toward educating the medical community, health educators, and consumers on appropriate sources of information. An increase in communication between allopathic medical providers, CAM providers, and patients is imperative to build partnerships based on a comprehensive understanding of the healthcare goals of both patient and primary-care providers (Ben-Arye & Vissar, 2012).

One of the major controversies surrounding the use of CAIH is the lack of evidence-based research to support its efficacy. The gold standard in biomedical research has been testing through the scientific method; however, this is not always possible with CAIH. Health educators and other healthcare practitioners ask whether research on CAIH therapies can be performed at the same level of safety and efficiency as research in biomedical therapies. The answer to this question is that in some cases it can, but in other cases it cannot because it will take major efforts to compile evidence. For example, according to Holt (2011), it can take around 10 years from the time regular research findings are published to the time they become a part of practice. In the case of CAM therapies, it can take even longer.

Not all research has supported the efficacy of CAM, particularly in the area of herbal medications. There is a very rapid growth in the use of herbals (Kraft, 2009). Thus, an increasing number of providers will encounter patients utilizing herbal medicines in all clinical settings (Zhang et. al, 2012). Similarly, herbal medications can interact with Western medications that patients are taking for their medical conditions (Kraft, 2009). Finally, many herbal medications have been shown to contain impurities, such as contaminants and long-term toxins (Kraft, 2009), and are advertised falsely. In addition, many herbal medications have been shown to contain contaminants not found in conventional Western medications, such as toxic metals, pesticides, and microbes (Zhang et. al, 2012). For example, the FDA (2014) has stated that US manufacturers of dietary supplements often do not meet standards in various ways. In addition, as mentioned, most CAM therapies are not regulated by the FDA.

The efficacy of many CAM therapies has been tested through randomized clinical trials (RCTs) and meta-analyses. Evidence points to some CAM therapies, such as the regular use of Omega-3, as being as safe and effective as medical therapies. CAM therapies usually cost less than conventional medications, ultimately decreasing the cost of healthcare in general (Holt, 2011).

In many cases, there is mixed or a lack of empirical evidence surrounding CAM therapies. Given the multitude of resources that show continued growth in CAM use, simply dismissing all of these therapies prematurely as being ineffective may do a disservice to patients (Holt, 2011).

Bridging the Gap

Bridging the gap between CAIH and Western medicine most likely requires work in three major fronts: (1) research on the efficacy of widely used CAIH interventions since currently there is not enough evidence; (2) education of both healthcare professionals and customers on the use of proven CAIH practices; and (3) a paradigm shift that allows for a collaborative plan of care including an integrated approach of CAIH and Western medical practices. Individuals often integrate CAIH therapies with Western medicine; however, on many occasions that integration happens without the knowledge and collaboration from the healthcare provider. A paradigm shift would allow for an integrated approach that actively involves patients and healthcare providers, hence reducing the likelihood of negative effects.

An important step is to create a collaborative dialogue between governmental and public agencies to develop initiatives that promote a reduction of the gap between the increasing use of CAM and the limited data supporting its efficacy (Segar, 2012; Synovitz & Larson, 2013). Gaylord and Mann (2007) suggested that there is a high growth rate in the area of CAM intervention research. For instance, a portion of the NIH budget is now allocated to the NCCAM (now known as the NCCIH), to perform further research on the efficacy of CAM interventions. Segar (2012) and Gaylord and Mann (2007) concluded that although there is a tremendous growth in CAM research, there are continued concerns as to whether evidence-based research through RCTs is an appropriate model to use with CAM modalities. Some believe that because RCTs are the gold standard in drug research, they also should be used in CAM research; however, other experts believe there are many reasons that CAM does not lend itself to RCTs. It is suggested that the placebo effect plays a strong role in CAM and that many of these therapies are perceived to be effective as a result of the placebo effect. The NCCIH plays a vital role in bridging the gap between CAIH and Western medicine. This center was created to define, with rigorous scientific investigation, the efficacy and safety of complementary and integrative health approaches (NCCAM, 2013a, 2013b). In addition, the center seeks to improve health and healthcare for the public who utilize CAIH practices and approaches. The center is working to fulfill its vision that scientific evidence informs decision making by the public, by healthcare professionals, and by health policymakers regarding the use and integration of these approaches (NCCAM, 2013a, 2013b). This institution represents the most organized government-supported effort to promote the safe and efficacious use of CAM modalities (Gaylord & Mann, 2007).

The NCCIH is closing the gap between CAIH and Western medicine, specifically in several key areas, including evidence-based research, public and provider education, and research agendas at home and abroad that incorporate scientific methodology. Finally, the center plays a critical role in disseminating current information regarding CAIH practices through research funding and publication of up-to-date information (NCCIH, 2015a).

With an organized infrastructure to promote research and disseminate it, the NCCIH will continue to create critical mechanisms to bridge the gap between traditional and Western medicine by stimulating research initiatives, training holistic care providers and Western medicine providers, and educating consumers. As the ACA is implemented, the NCCIH will most likely remain the major inspector and advocate for the successful promotion and protection of patients' options to use Complementary and Integrative practices and to be reimbursed for their use.

According to Gaylord and Mann (2007), critical education initiatives must be implemented. The first is to broaden core competencies attached to medical schools' curricula as they relate to CAIH practices. As discussed earlier in this chapter, some medical and nursing programs now include curricula related to CAM alongside allopathic training. In many cases, CAIH is linked to cultural competency, although this practice may be misleading since it stereotypes the use of CAM modalities and may not indicate that it is used by wide segments of the population. More curricula need to be developed on CAIH.

Another way to bridge the gap is increased communication between allopathic and CAIH practitioners. Improved communication should protect against the risk of drug interactions and negative effects that may result from the concomitant use of CAIH and Western medical practices. For example, better communication among patients, Western medical providers, and CAIH providers would avoid negative effects derived from the simultaneous use of prescribed and herbal medicines. Sometimes these two types of medicines may interact in a harmful manner.

In addition to the ongoing efforts to educate healthcare providers in medical schools about CAIH practices, there is also a drive to improve the communication between providers and patients. Both CAIH and conventional providers need to learn to be open and share information with respect to patient care, which will result in a significant improvement in customers' health status and the rapport built with the healthcare provider.

Caveat Emptor

Cognitive biases—emotional or psychological predispositions to utilize or support certain practices, in this case CAIH practices—can be quantified as a cultural exposure, a mainstream-media effect, and a health behavior preference (Gaylord & Mann, 2007). Cultural perspectives and personal experiences are major reasons cited as factors biasing individuals toward the use of CAM. Those healthcare consumers who are predisposed to use CAM interventions may have had a cultural experience that exposed them to such treatment. These individuals are more likely to support the use of CAM approaches in the future once they are integrated into mainstream healthcare (Cutshal et al., 2010). For example, American Indians on reservations who utilize Western medical facilities and recent Hispanic immigrants to the United States both use traditional cultural practices that are labeled as CAM modalities by mainstream practitioners (Gaylord & Mann, 2007). Therefore, cultures in which CAM usually is practiced tend to be more frequent users of CAM interventions. This may be true in part because of their predisposed cognitive bias to look favorably toward CAM based on past experience.

In addition, another practical reason CAM use has grown exponentially is due to media's role in developing a particular mind-set toward health practices in general. For example, the NIH and the Centers for Disease Control and Prevention have developed websites that contain a variety of resources to help consumers make informed decisions. The creation of these resources has been prompted by the increasing volume of information on the Internet regarding CAM therapies (NCCAM, 2013a).

Research about medical conditions and treatments once accessible only to physicians through medical journals is now accessible to the general public through media and the Internet. This exposure has catapulted the general public's understanding of healthcare options, such as CAM therapies. This relationship between growing media exposure and the ideas of quicker and promising natural treatments most likely has created a cognitive bias in the population. Many healthcare practitioners believe this cognitive bias is dangerous and consequently are developing educational programs to raise the general public's awareness of the risks of magical thinking and unreliable media-induced bias (NIH, 2013).

Several authors have suggested that another major cognitive bias has to do with health behavior preferences (Kraft, 2009). People attracted to CAM modalities tend to be populations who already practice healthy behaviors. These individuals are attracted to CAM practices because of their real or perceived holistic nature. Healthy, holistic, and natural approaches to care have been spurred by the discussion on the negative impact of Western approaches. As the general public has become more aware of the negative side effects associated with Western medical treatments, CAM has gained more attention.

Currently, there is growing advocacy for the inclusion of CAM in the educational curriculum of new generations of healthcare providers. There is also a growing movement for a comprehensive research agenda that provides evidence on the efficacy of CAM practices. The process of including CAM in medical school curricula and creating stronger regulatory standards must be formalized.

There is very little information on what will be covered under the ACA with regard to CAIH. Portions of the law, such as Section 2706, seem to indicate support for CAM coverage. In addition, while more research money is being allocated to study CAM practices, the traditional research designs, such as RCTs, are not always considered optimal for researching CAM therapies. A deeper discussion is needed as to how CAM would best be researched and what would be the best practice for integrating it into medical school and allied health curricula. Therefore, there is uncertainty as to the best practices for CAM research and didactic integration as well as a consistent and strong political support under the advent of the ACA (Integrative Healthcare Policy Consortium, 2013; Mader, 2013; Weeks, 2012).

Given these factors, the assurance that CAIH will continue to be integrated with mainstream medicine depends on the successful political support for an organized and comprehensive research agenda, the creation of formal educational standards, and the development of mechanisms for healthcare reimbursement for complementary, alternative, and integrative health practices.

Conclusion

Complementary, alternative, and integrative health (CAIH) is a term that can be used to denote the current complementary, alternative, and integrative approaches to prevent and manage disease and to maintain or restore health and wellness. The term *complementary and alternative medicine* (CAM) has had a historical significance but is now outdated since the name change of the National Center for Complementary and Alternative Medicine to National Center for Complementary and Integrative Health. Never before has there been a more organized initiative to integrate Complementary, Alternative, and Integrative Health (CAIH) into mainstream society and medicine. This initiative requires stronger regulatory standards for CAIH practices and more inclusive approaches. This chapter explored the reasons why patients and consumers engage in CAIH practices. It provided a contemporary overview of CAM and a cursory discussion of modern controversies surrounding its use. In addition, this chapter addressed the need for healthcare providers' education on the risks and benefits of CAIH, as they serve as primary resources for their patients.

Summary

- With the name change of the National Center for Complementary and Alternative Medicine (NCCAM) to National Center for Complementary and Integrative Health (NCCIH) in December 2014, a need for going beyond the term Complementary and Alternative Medicine (*CAM*) has arisen. The term *complementary, alternative, and integrative health* (CAIH) may be more appropriate, as it emphasizes health and wellness.

- Health educators and other healthcare practitioners are finding that many of their patients are exploring more self-regulated and less-expensive options afforded through CAIH.

- There is an increasing need to educate healthcare providers on CAIH modalities.

- The NCCIH, a subdivision of the National Institutes of Health, emphasizes the importance of incorporating complementary and integrative modalities with biomedicine in a safe and effective manner (NCCIH, 2015a).

- Understanding the role of CAIH in everyday treatments can be a powerful tool for practitioners. CAIH therapies can be instrumental in disease prevention and treatment. Many patients show an increased preference for CAIH practices (NCCAM, 2008).

- The integration of CAIH modalities by healthcare providers does not necessarily indicate acceptance, but rather indicates an overall willingness to allow patients to have more autonomy and control over their care.

- Research indicates that consumers rate CAM therapies favorably for use as prevention tools. People who utilize these approaches are likely to have holistic values and beliefs. Some CAM therapies can be utilized safely to treat specific medical conditions, while others can pose risks to health.

- Healthcare professionals have begun to incorporate CAM into the curriculum for training future practitioners due to patients' increased interest and use of CAM modalities. Studies have shown that hospitals, medical programs, and other interested parties have begun to increase their CAM services; however, more CAM curricula should be developed.

- It is important to instruct patients on FDA guidelines for protection when they use complementary and alternative products.

Case Study

Description

Chris is a 16-year-old high school junior. He currently is one of the highest-scoring athletes on his basketball team. Chris feels that wearing a balance wristband will give him increased strength, balance, and coordination. The wristband claims to work synergistically through the user's natural energy. Chris and his basketball friends ordered balance wristbands on the Internet.

Questions

1. What concepts or topics should be discussed with Chris about the CAIH modality he is using?

2. As a medical professional, would you share any personal bias you have about the product with Chris? Why or why not?

3. What valid resources or reputable websites would you give Chris for further education and information?

KEY TERMS

Affordable Care Act. Federal statute signed into law in March 2010 that contains two parts: the Patient Protection and Affordable Care Act (PL 111-148) and the Health Care and Education Reconciliation Act of 2010 (PL 111-152), intended to expand medical coverage to millions of economically challenged Americans and to make improvements to multiple programs, such as Medicaid and the Children's Health Insurance Program (CMS, n.d.).

Allopathic. Conventional medicine, also known as Western medicine (NCCIH, 2015a).

CAIH (complementary, alternative, and integrative health). Term used to denote complementary, alternative, and integrative approaches to prevent and manage disease as well as to maintain or restore health and wellness. This term is congruent with the 2014 name change of the National Center for Complementary and Alternative Medicine to National Center for Complementary and Integrative Health (NCCIH, 2015a).

CAM (complementary and alternative medicine). It refers to therapies not usually taught in US medical schools or generally available in US hospitals. They include a broad range of practices and beliefs, such as acupuncture, chiropractic care, relaxation techniques, massage therapy, and herbal remedies. They are defined by the National Center for Complementary and Integrative Health as a group of diverse medical and healthcare systems, practices, and products that are not generally considered to be part of conventional medicine (NCCIH, 2015a).

Cognitive biases. Tendencies to make decisions based on attachment to past experiences (Taylor, 2013). In this chapter, cognitive biases relate to experiences that would wrongfully change an individual's thought process toward using CAM.

Vulnerable groups. In regard to CAIH use, these groups include populations most likely to be taken advantage of because of serious chronic conditions. It also includes groups such as non-English speakers, children, or persons who are illiterate (NCCAM, 2012).

References

Astin, J. A. (1998). Why patients use alternative medicine: Results of a national study. *JAMA, 278*(19), 1548–1553.

Barnes, P. M., Bloom, B., & Nahin, R. L. (2008). Complementary and alternative medicine use among adults and children: United States, 2007. *National Health Statistics Reports*, No. 12. Hyattsville, MD: National Center for Health Statistics. Retrieved from http://nccam.nih.gov/news/camstats/costs

Ben-Arye, E., & Frenkel, M. (2008). Referring to complementary and alternative medicine—A possible tool for implementation. *Complementary Therapies in Medicine, 16*(6), 325–330. doi: 10.1016/j.ctim.2008.02.008

Ben-Arye, E., Frenkel, M., Klein, A., & Scharf, M. (2008). Attitudes toward integration of complementary and alternative medicine in primary care: Perspectives of patients, physicians and complementary health educator and healthcare practitioners. *Patient Education and Counseling*, *70*(3), 395–402.

Ben-Arye, E., & Visser, A. (2012). The role of health care communication in the development of complementary and integrative medicine. *Patient Education and Counseling*, *89*, 363–367.

Bravewell Collaborative. (2010). *The summit on integrative medicine and the health of the public*. Retrieved from http://www.bravewell.org/transforming_healthcare/national_summit

Centers for Disease Control and Prevention. (2006). *How to evaluate health information on the Internet*. Retrieved from ods.od.nih.gov/Health_Information/How_To_Evaluate_Health_Information_on_the_Internet_Questions_and_Answers.aspx.

Centers for Medicare and Medicaid Services. (n.d). Affordable Care Act. Retrieved from http://medicaid.gov/affordablecareact/affordable-care-act.html

Clarke, T. C., Black, L. I., Stussman, B. J., Barnes, M. A., & Nahin, R. L. (2015). Trends in the use of complementary health approaches among adults: United States, 2002–2012. *National Health Statistics Reports*, No. 79, 1–34. Hyattsville, MD: National Center for Health Statistics.

Cutshall, S., Derscheid, D., Miers, A. G., Ruegg, S., Schroeder, B. J., Tucker, S., & Wentworth, L. (2010). Knowledge, attitudes, and use of complementary and alternative therapies among clinical nurse specialists in an academic medical center. *Clinical Nurse Specialist*, *24*(3), 125–131.

Eisenberg, D. M., Davis, R. B., Ettner, S. L., Appel, S., Wilkey, S., Van Rompay, M., & Kessler, R. C. (1998). Trends in alternative medicine use in the United States, 1990–1997: Results of a follow-up national survey. *JAMA*, *280*(18), 1569–1575.

Erfurt, J., Foote, A., & Heirich, M. (1992). The cost-effectiveness of worksite wellness programs for hypertension control, weight loss, smoking cessation, and exercise. *Personnel Psychology*, *45*, 5–27.

Food and Drug Administration. (2008). *Inspection, compliance, enforcement, and criminal investigations*. Retrieved from http://www.fda.gov/iceci/enforcementactions/warningletters/2008/ucm1048298.htm

Food and Drug Administration. (2009)*. Draft report of quantitative risk and benefit assessment of consumption of commercial fish, focusing on fetal neurodevelopmental effects (measured by verbal development in children) and on coronary heart disease and stroke in the general population.* Retrieved from http://www.fda.gov/Food/FoodborneIllnessContaminants/Metals/ucm088794.htm

Food and Drug Administration. (2013). *6 tip-offs to rip-offs: Don't fall for health fraud scams.* Retrieved from http://www.fda.gov/ForConsumers/ConsumerUpdates/ucm341344.htm

Food and Drug Administration. (2014). *Development & approval process (drugs).* Retrieved from http://www.fda.gov/drugs/developmentapprovalprocess/default.htm

Food and Drug Administration. (2015a). *CPG sec. 120.500 health fraud—Factors in considering regulatory action.* Retrieved from http://www.fda.gov/iceci/compliancemanuals/compliancepolicyguidancemanual/ucm073838.htm

Food and Drug Administration. (2015b). *Dietary supplements.* Retrieved from http://www.fda.gov/Food/DietarySupplements/

Fontaine, K. L. (2011). *Complementary and alternative therapies for nursing practice* (3rd ed.). Boston, MA: Pearson.

Gaylord, S. A., & Mann, J. D. (2007). Rationales for CAM education in health professions training programs. *Academic Medicine, 82*(10), 927–933. doi: 10.1097/ACM.0b013e31814a5b43

Gebhardt, D., & Crump, C. (1990). Employee fitness and wellness programs in the workplace. *American Psychologist, 45*(2), 262–272.

Goldbas, A. (2012). An introduction to complementary and alternative medicine (CAM). *International Journal of Childbirth Education, 27*(3): 1–104. Retrieved from http://r.search.yahoo.com/_ylt=A0SO8ydr6pNW4dAAAgJXNyoA;_ylu=X3oDMTByb2lvbXVuBGNvbG8EZ3ExBHBvcwMxBHZ0aWQDBHNlYwNzcg--/RV=2/RE=1452563179/RO=10/RU=http%3a%2f%2fwww.icea.org%2fsites%2fdefault%2ffiles%2fJuly%25202012.pdf/RK=0/RS=J6XQ7nlbQDixM7eOAfzzsd9iYHc-

Health and Human Services. (n.d.). *White House Commission on Complementary and Alternative Medicine Policy.* Retrieved from http://www.whccamp.hhs.gov/fr1.html

Holt, S. (2011). Is evidence-based complementary and alternative medicine a contradiction in terms?—"No." *Focus on Alternative and Complementary Therapies, 16*(2), 117–119.

Institute of Medicine of the National Academies. (2005). Complementary and alternative medicine in the United States. Washington, DC: National Academies Press. Accessed at: https://www.ncbi.nlm.nih.gov/books/NBK83802/

Integrative Healthcare Policy Consortium. (2013). *Frequently asked questions about Section 2706.* Retrieved from http://www.ihpc.org/wp-content/uploads/section-2706-faq.pdf

Kantor, M. (2009). The role of rigorous scientific evaluation in the use and practice of complementary and alternative medicine. *Journal of the American College of Radiology, 6*(4), 254–262. doi: 10.1016/j.jacr.2008.09.012

Kaptchuk, T. J., & Eisenberg, D. M. (1998). The persuasive appeal of alternative medicine. *Annals of Internal Medicine, 129*(12), 1061–1065. doi: 10.7326/0003-4819-129-12-199812150-00011

Kraft, K. (2009). Complementary/alternative medicine in the context of prevention of disease and maintenance of health. *Preventive Medicine, 49*(2–3), 88–92.

Mader, L. S. (2013–2014). Will "Obamacare" affect natural healthcare in the United States? *Herbalgram-American Botanical Council, 100*, 86–89.

Marks, D. F., Murray, M., Evans, B., & Estacio, E. V. (2011). *Health psychology: Theory, research and practice* (3rd ed.). London, UK: Sage.

Nahin, R. L., Barnes, P. M., Stussman, B. J., & Bloom, B. (2009). Costs of complementary and alternative medicine (CAM) and frequency of visits to CAM practitioners: United States, 2007. *National Health Statistics Reports*, No. 18, 1–28. Hyattsville, MD: National Center for Health Statistics.

National Center for Complementary and Alternative Medicine. (2007). *Downloadable graphics on CAM use in the United States.* Retrieved from http://nccam.nih.gov/news/camstats/2007/graphics.htm

National Center for Complementary and Alternative Medicine. (2008). *The use of complementary and alternative medicine in the United States.* Retrieved from http://nccam.nih.gov/news/camstats/2007/camsurvey_fs1.htm#use

National Center for Complementary and Alternative Medicine. (2009). *Health information.* Retrieved from https://nccih.nih.gov/health

National Center for Complementary and Alternative Medicine. (2013a). *Complementary, alternative, or integrative health: What's in a name?* Retrieved from http://nccam.nih.gov/health/whatiscam

National Center for Complementary and Alternative Medicine. (2013b). *Finding & evaluating online resources on complementary health approaches.* Retrieved from http://nccam.nih.gov/health/webresources

National Center for Complementary and Alternative Medicine. (2011a). *What is complementary, alternative, or integrative health?* Retrieved from https://nccih.nih.gov/health/integrative-health#informed

National Center for Complementary and Alternative Medicine. (2011b). *Third strategic plan 2011–2014: Exploring the science of complementary and alternative medicine.* Retrieved from http://nccam.nih.gov/sites/nccam.nih.gov/files/about/plans/2011/NCCAM_SP_508.pdf

National Center for Complementary and Alternative Medicine. (2014). *NCCIH facts-at-a-glance and mission.* Retrieved from http://nccam.nih.gov/about/ataglance

National Center for Complementary and Integrative Health. (2015a). *Complementary, Alternative, or Integrative Health: What's in a Name?* Retrieved from https://nccih.nih.gov/health/integrative-health#informed

National Center for Complementary and Integrative Health. (2015b). *What complementary and integrative approaches do Americans use?* Retrieved from https://nccih.nih.gov/research/statistics/NHIS/2012/key-findings

National Center for Complementary and Integrative Health. (2015c). *Important events in NCCIH history.* Retrieved from http://www.nih.gov/about/almanac/organization/NCCIH.htm

National Center for Complementary and Integrative Health. (2015d). *Reasons people choose CAM and associated research.* Retrieved from https://nccih.nih.gov/training/videolectures/1/5

National Center for Complementary and Integrative Health. (n.d.). *Finding and evaluating online resources on complementary health approaches.* Retrieved from http://www.nccam.nih.gov/health/webresources

National Commission for Health Education Credentialing. (2008). *Health education profession*. Retrieved from http://www.nchec.org/credentialing/profession/

National Institute for Health Care Management Research and Educational Foundation. (2011, May). *Building a stronger evidence base for employee wellness programs*. Final document of meeting brief. Retrieved from http://r.search.yahoo.com/_ylt=AwrSbgwe8JNW9BEA4zJXNyoA;_ylu=X3oDMTByb2lvbXVuBGNvbG8DZ3E3ExBHBvcwMxBHZ0aWQDBHNlYwNzcg--/RV=2/RE=1452564639/RO=10/RU=http%3a%2f%2fwww.nihcm.org%2fpdf%2fWellness%2520FINAL%2520electonic%2520version.pdf/RK=0/RS=jBX9fIJdA5XlIE.rb3lxiBOAqYY-

National Institutes of Health. (2013, July 1). *Health information*. Retrieved from http://ods.od.nih.gov/Health_Information/ODS_Frequently_Asked_Questions.asp

National Institutes of Health, Office of Dietary Supplements. (n.d.). *Health information: Making decisions*. Retrieved from http://ods.od.nih.gov/Health Information/makingdecisions.sec.aspx

O'Brien, K. (2004). Complementary and alternative medicine: The move into mainstream healthcare. *Clinical and Experimental Optometry, 87*(2), 110–120.

Okoro, C. A., Zhao, G., Li, C., & Balluz, L. S. (2011). Use of complementary and alternative medicine among USA adults with functional limitations: For treatment or general use? *Complementary Therapies in Medicine, 19*(4), 208–215.

Segar, J. (2012). Complementary and alternative medicine: Exploring the gap between evidence and usage. *Health (London), 16*(4), 366-381. doi: 10.1177/1363459311425516

Synovitz, L. B., & Larson, K. L. (2013). *Complementary and alternative medicine for health professionals: A holistic approach to consumer health*. Burlington, MA: Jones & Bartlett Learning.

Taylor, J. (2013). *Cognitive biases are bad for businesses: Do you see irrationality in your business?*. Retrieved from https://www.psychologytoday.com/blog/the-power-prime/201305/cognitive-biases-are-bad-business

Tiralongo, E., & Wallis, M. (2008). Integrating complementary and alternative medicine education into the pharmacy curriculum. *American Journal of Pharmaceutical Education, 72*(4), 74.

Weeks, J. (2012). American Medical Association opposes nondiscrimination language supporting CAM practice in Affordable Care Act. . . plus more. *Integrative Medicine: A Clinician's Journal, 11*(5), 12.

Witt, C., Brinkhaus, B., & Willich, S. (2010). Future medical doctors need to be informed about CAM to ensure safe and competent patient care. *Tijdschrift voor Medisch Onderwijs, 29*(1), 87–89.

Wong, L., Toh, M. P., & Kong, K. H. (2010). Barriers to patient referral for complementary and alternative medicine and its implications on interventions. *Complementary Therapies in Medicine, 18*, 135–142.

World Health Organization. (2013). *WHO Traditional Medicine Strategy 2014–2023*. Geneva, Switzerland: WHO. Retrieved from http://apps.who.int/iris/bitstream/10665/92455/1/9789241506090_eng.pdf?ua=1&ua=1

Zhang, Y., Peck, K., Spalding, M., Jones, B., & Cook, R. (2012). Discrepancy between patient's use of and health providers' familiarity with CAM. *Patient Education and Counseling, 89(3)*, 399–404.

Zhang, J., Wider, B., Shang, H., Li, X., & Ernst, E. (2012). Quality of herbal medicines: Challenges and solutions. *Complementary Therapies in Medicine, 20(1–2)*, 100–106.

CHAPTER 2

MIND-BODY MEDICINE

Catherine L. Zeman

The Center for Mind-Body Medicine (CMBM, 2014) and the Institute of Medicine Committee on the Use of Complementary and Alternative Medicine (2005) identify over 100 different kinds of complementary and alternative medicine (CAM) modalities (Dupler, Odle, & Lerner, 2012). This chapter focuses on selected mind-body medicine (MBM) modalities that are addressed most frequently in the published literature and tracked by the National Center for Complementary and Integrative Health (NCCIH). The selected modalities include biofeedback, deep breathing, mindfulness meditation, transcendental (TM) meditation, tai chi, and yoga. Box 2.1 briefly describes some additional MBM modalities that the reader is encouraged to explore in more detail independently.

In order to develop an introductory understanding of MBM modalities for the health sciences, this chapter provides a broad overall introduction to and definition of MBM, an empirical description of the probable mechanisms of action of these modalities and the benefits using the allopathic/scientific paradigm, and delves into some of the more often researched therapies, including their patterns of use by specific racial/ethnic groups. Mind-body modalities are useful not only in managing disease; they also are crucial in restoring health and illness. This chapter concludes with a philosophical and empirical discussion that offers a rationale for healthcare professionals seeking to integrate these modalities into their professional

LEARNING OBJECTIVES

At the completion of this chapter, students will be able to:

- Identify the theoretical and scientific basis of autogenic therapy, color therapy, eye movement desensitization and reprocessing, humor therapy, Pilates, qi gong, shamanism, biofeedback, deep breathing, meditation, transcendental meditation, tai chi, yoga, and reiki.

- Discuss the stress response, new research areas focusing on stress and health, and the use of mind-body medicine (MBM) to ameliorate allostatic load (cumulative stress) and stereotype threat.

- Describe the placebo effect and the use of MBM as a trigger of this mind-body response.

- Identify benefits and risks associated with commonly used MBM modalities such as

(continued)

work with complementary, alternative, and integrative health (CAIH).

Theoretical Concepts

Overview

According to the NCCIH, mind-body medicine is a broad array of techniques and skills (modalities) that are taught by or delivered through an experienced practitioner and then perfected through repeated practice.

MBM is a distinct set of health approaches under the umbrella of CAIH and is broadly composed of modalities or specialized applications and epistemologies (philosophies) derived from a variety of Eastern and Western traditional healing practices from cultures around the world. Some of the most widely used mind-body techniques have deep roots in the cultural practices of the East and the West; for example, tai chi has origins in ancient China, sweat lodge purifications are common to a number of indigenous nations of the Americas, and transcendental meditation (TM) is a healing modality with origins in ayurvedic medicine.

Many of the MBM skills (i.e., meditation, biofeedback, tai chi) are designed to achieve greater control over heart rate, breathing, attitude and outlook, chronic pain, and the stress response. The reduction of cortisol levels and allevi-ation of chronic levels of stress that contribute to allostatic load (chronic, damaging stress) are both a major goal of and benefit of these approaches. Scientifically, the various MBM skills focus on attaining greater awareness of autonomic ner-vous system (ANS) functions as well as unconscious attitudes and beliefs that might contribute to self-defeating, unhealthy behavior. It is believed that by mastering the MBM modality and centering the mind and body, an individual can relieve chronic stress, change unhealthy behaviors, and ameliorate or lessen pain perception, all of which are related to a number of chronic diseases, such as depression, anxiety, high blood pres-sure, osteoarthritis pain, and obesity, among others (Bertisch, Wee, Phillips, & McCarthy, 2009).

BOX 2.1   VARIOUS MBM MODALITIES IN BRIEF

Autogenic therapy. Developed in 1932 by Dr. Johannes Schultz of Germany, this medita-tion practice drew its inspiration from both yoga and Eastern meditation traditions. Adherents spend 15 minutes daily invoking visualization techniques that focus on reducing stress and prompting the relaxation response (Shinozaki et al., 2010).

Color therapy. This modality can be traced back to the medieval era, when the Persian philosopher Avicenna (Latinized from, *Ibn-Sīnā*, 980–1037) wrote of the medical application of colored frequencies of light. This MBM was very popular in 19th-century American medicine and then fell out of favor. Recent research work is focusing on the blue wave spectrum of light for enhancing the effectiveness of chemotherapy and for treating infections (Ashby, 2007).

Eye movement desensitization and reprocessing (EMDR). This newer MBM modality has rapidly moved into the realm of accepted practice for the treatment of posttraumatic stress disorder. The American psychologist Francine Shapiro, developer of EMDR in the late 1980s, believes that the practice of guided recall along with specific eye movements allows traumatized individuals to release the traumatic event and integrate their experiences. This therapy has been so effective that it is now included in the best treatment practices of the Department of Defense and the American Psychiatric Association (Shapiro, 2009).

Humor therapy, laughter yoga, and laugh therapy. The use of humor and laughter to reduce stress and encourage healing, if combined with yoga poses and breathing, is termed laughter yoga. The connection between laughter and the ability to overcome emotional and physical challenges has been recognized since antiquity (Dolgoff-Kaspar, Baldwin, Johnson, Edling, & Sethi, 2012).

Pilates. An exercise and physical fitness system that involves concentration, control, centering of thought, precision in movement, and controlled breathing. It was developed in Germany by Joseph Pilates in the early 1900s (Pilates, Robbins, & Van Heuit-Robbins, 2012).

Qi gong. The practice of qi gong dates back over 4,000 years in China. It focuses on the cultivation of chi energy through the alignment of breath, movement, and awareness in a fashion similar to tai chi (Birdee, Wayne, Davis, Phillips, & Yeh, 2009).

Shamanism. A shamanistic practitioner enters altered states of consciousness, oftentimes with drumming, chanting, or ritual dances and sometimes with the use of psychotropic herbs or plants. The shaman's goal is to contact and interact with spiritual energies in order to influence divine events or to effect healing. The term has come to be very broadly applied to many indigenous spiritual practices (Winkelman, 2010).

MBM and Stress

To address the impact of MBM on the health status of individuals, a basic understanding of the stress response, allostatic load, and placebo effect are required. Humans regulate their responses to the environment through their central nervous system (CNS), peripheral nervous system and the voluntary and autonomic functions of those systems. The CNS and peripheral nervous system provide for conscious control of the body while the Autonomic Nervous System (ANS) with its sympathetic (encouraging the stress response) and parasympathetic (downregulating the stress response) branches coordinates responses with the endocrine system (Seeley, Stephens, & Tate, 2007). These branches of the nervous system coordinate systemic, instantaneous, and diffuse impacts to the brain, eyes, smooth and striated muscles, endocrine glands, excretory glands, heart, lungs, stomach, intestines, and bladder (Thibodeau & Patton, 2008). Hormone/neurotransmitters adrenaline, norepinephrine, and cortisol play the primary biochemical roles in these physiological responses (Lovallo, 2005; Seeley et al., 2007).

Stress, in the purely physiological sense, is the pushing of systems to and slightly beyond their physiological maximums. Without stress in this most basic sense, as well as physiological set points (minimums and maximums), physiological functioning would not be possible (Thibodeau & Patton, 2008). Research has shown that occasional stress is actually beneficial for physiological systems, improving performance and focus (Seeley et al., 2007). When the stress response is triggered, the sympathetic branch of the ANS floods the bloodstream with adrenaline, norepinephrine, and cortisol, providing high levels of glucose and shifting blood to the muscles and away from the organs. Physiological resources needed to fight or flee, which have become chronically activated, can work against health and well-being. Long-term, increased levels of stress hormones/neurotransmitters decrease cognitive function, increase blood pressure, move calcium out of the bone, free fats into the bloodstream, elevate blood sugar levels, and suppress the immune system (Thibodeau & Patton, 2008). Research also indicates that humans have the same response to an actual threat as to the *thought* of a threat, albeit not to the same degree (Thibodeau & Patton, 2008). Constant, unrelenting stress has been linked consistently to a wide range of acute diseases (e.g., a disease that develops quickly and is usually resolved relatively quickly, such as various infectious diseases) and chronic diseases (e.g., a disease that slowly develops over time and is marked by progressively worsening symptoms or periods of remission and exacerbation, such as high blood pressure, cardiovascular disease, autoimmune diseases, and diabetes). In some cases stress plays a causative role in diseases, and in other cases it triggers exacerbations or recurrences of the disease (Dupler et al., 2012).

Fast-paced society, time constraints, lack of social interaction, environmental stress, poverty, and outright discrimination add together for

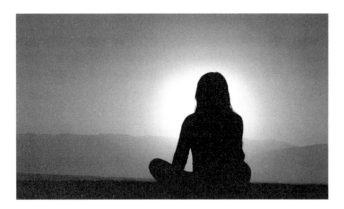

Figure 2.1   MBM modalities can aid in reducing the worst effects of a prolonged stress response.
Source: Centers for Disease Control and Prevention. Image 14023. Public Health Image Library, 2015.

minorities and socioeconomically disadvantaged groups. New research has illustrated how the stress response is relentlessly triggered (Carson et al., 2007); for example, research has focused on how stereotyped images of minorities and disenfranchised groups can trigger the stress response constantly in individuals (Levy & Sidel, 2006). Labeled *stereotype threat*, this disorder has been linked to cardiovascular disease in African American populations (Edwards, 2007; Pascoe & Richman, 2009). While these are areas of new and ongoing research, the potential ramifications are important to consider when working with minorities and other disadvantaged groups. Since MBM modalities aid in reducing the worst effects of the stress response, aiding clients in becoming aware of the sources of and comprehensive impacts of stressors in their lives and providing them with approaches to handling that stress are important parts of preventive health care, helping to create stress-resilient individuals (see Figure 2.1).

New Thinking about Mind-Body Medicine and the Placebo Effect

Outside of the obvious connection to providing clients with a means of managing stressors and the stress response more effectively, many MBM practitioners are interested in what the allopathic community calls the *placebo effect*. The placebo effect is the realization of benefit from a treatment intervention because the client expects the treatment to work, even in the absence of active biochemical compounds or with the use of "sham" surgery (Howick et al., 2013). The placebo effect is widely recognized in clinical trials (accounting for up to one-third of the positive benefits observed); individuals receive benefit from sham treatments (i.e., a "fake" surgery) or apparently inactive substances (i.e., a sugar pill) because they firmly believe in the treatment's effectiveness. Spontaneous remissions of chronic and sometimes serious medical conditions have been attributed to this effect. Therefore, the placebo effect can be triggered by the MBM modality and be an important healing force. While reversal of allostatic load is often pointed to as the major means of effectiveness for MBM modalities such as breathing, exercise, and meditation (i.e., yoga), other MBM modalities such as reiki seemingly have no current explanation for their benefits, outside of the placebo effect (Chopra, 1990; Howick et al., 2013; Lipton, 2005, 2008; Schmidt, 2012).

Modern science is beginning to understand what all indigenous healers must have seen as lesson 101 of their ethnoscientific practice—that the mind and body as separate entities is an illusion (Chopra, 1990; Dreher 2003; Suzuki & Knudtson, 1992; Winkelman, 2010). Consider the next quote by Chief Luther Standing Bear, a historical chief of the Teton Sioux Nation.

> From Wakan Tanka, the Great Spirit, there came a great unifying life force that flowed in and through all things—the flowers of the plains, blowing winds, rocks, trees, birds, animals—and was the same force that had been breathed into the first man. Thus all things were kindred, and were brought together by the same Great Mystery.
>
> —Quoted in Nerburn (1999, p. 15)

Most indigenous epistemologies and the MBM healing practices based on them (i.e., yoga, tai chi, shamanism) encompass distinct worldviews of practice that include consideration of the continuity of all life and the unity of mind-body through a concept of spirit, "energy," or life force. According to these traditions, this life force infuses every cell, molecule, and atom of the body. While the body in these traditions has its own unique energy field, that field is in resonance with the rest of life, with all of creation, and with the universe itself. It is a distinctly different view of the body from the allopathic perspective, which tends to envision the body as a collection of more mechanistic systems and as an individual biochemical and physical entity, not as an energetic field that is interrelated with all other fields. In ancient shamanic practices, for example, healers would attempt to repair energy damage through rhythmic chant, drumming, and herb use. In tai chi, the chi energy is thought to be freed and brought into balance by mindful movements and ordered breathing patterns (Wang, Collet, & Lau, 2004). Reiki healers claim to be able to sense "knots" or "tension" in this life-force energy, or qi, and to rebalance it (Gehrang, 2014).

Early pioneers in research and education concerning both the placebo effect and MBM, such as Larry Dossey and Deepak Chopra, both medical doctors, have repeatedly called for increased research into the area as well as education of medical and health professionals in MBM. Although many MBM benefits continue to be undervalued by mainstream, Western medical science, the voices of these pioneers have not been completely ignored. Ongoing research in the areas of neuroendocrinology, physiology, and biophysics has illustrated that the mind-body connection is more interdependent and important than previously acknowledged by Western science and allopathic medical theory (Bialek, 2012; Chang, Fisch, & Popp, 2010; Cohen & Popp, 1997). Dossey (2014) has called for modern medical and health practitioners to realize that they are entering a third era of medicine, one in which the role of the mind or consciousness must be recognized, welcomed, and integrated in patient treatment.

Modalities

The MBM modalities discussed in this section were selected for a detailed review, as they are the most commonly used and researched in the field. Proven uses are based on data derived from intervention studies (randomized controlled trials) supporting use of the modality in the application. The modalities have other uses; however, not all applications have been independently verified for effectiveness using empirically designed epidemiological studies. Case histories and testimonials often are cited as a reason that a particular MBM is used, but the gold standard is a scientifically controlled study. In addition to a brief overview of the modality and discussion of research support, the next sections provide the most current information on predominant patterns of use by racial/ethnic categories when it is available.

Biofeedback

Biofeedback refers to the use of technology to increase mindful awareness of bodily functions and to increase awareness of the effect of stress on those functions in order to relieve symptoms associated with chronic disease states that are related to stress triggers. Practitioners focus on functions that are below conscious awareness (unconscious), often entirely under control of the ANS. These functions include almost any physiological parameter that can be monitored in a way that allows the client to focus on the function and downregulate it, such as heart rate, blood pressure, skin temperature, and brainwave activity (Nezu, Nezu, & Xanthopoulos, 2011). The concept of becoming mindful of bodily functions—for example, breathing and heart rate—dates back thousands of years in the Eastern healing traditions of both yoga and tai chi. Western 19th-century researchers were aware of these practices, as knowledge of the functions and interactions between the CNS, the ANS, and the endocrine system were being formulated and refined. Also developing were an understanding of systems and systems theory (Bynum, 1994; Rifkin & Ackerman, 2011). Practitioners in medicine and psychology in the late 1960s first used the term *biofeedback* to describe the process of training a person to control ANS functions such as smooth muscle contraction and heart rate through the combined use of monitoring equipment and mindfulness (Moss, 1999).

Biofeedback has been proven effective for a variety of stress-triggered and related conditions as well as in certain rehabilitation applications, such as jaw pain related to chronic nerve impingement (temporomandibular disorder), migraine headaches, sphincter-control disorders, arthritis pain management, and rehabilitation following a cerebrovascular incident or stroke (Ernst & Posadzki, 2011; Kanjii, White, & Ernst, 2006). Few negative effects of biofeedback have been reported; one source noted only dizziness and disorientation as a possible side effect (Erns, Pittler, & Wider, 2006). However, practitioners are cautioned about biofeedback use with clients who might be delusional or suffering from psychosis or personality disorders, as such populations might find disturbing the notion that they could "control" previously unconscious bodily functions (Ernst et al., 2006).

A 2002 study, based on National Health Interview Survey (NHIS) data, examining CAM use in older adults found that biofeedback was not used with any degree of frequency outside of the White cultural group (Arcury, Suerken, Grzywacz, Bell, Lang, & Quandt, 2005). A 2011 study, however, indicated increased use of biofeedback by both Whites and African Americans (Su & Li, 2011) (see Figure 2.2). Little additional data exist on why a specific cultural group does or does not use a certain CAIH therapy, although conjectures about socioeconomic status, educational opportunities, and degree of acculturation have been proposed as reasons for the variation (Barner, Bohman, Brown, & Richards, 2010; Jones, 2001; Shah & Farrow, 2012).

Deep Breathing

In deep breathing, also called diaphragmatic breathing or belly breathing, clients are trained to use the abdominal muscles to perform effective breathing while relaxing. Maximum oxygenation of the body and clearing of the lungs through respiratory therapy is thought to be beneficial in

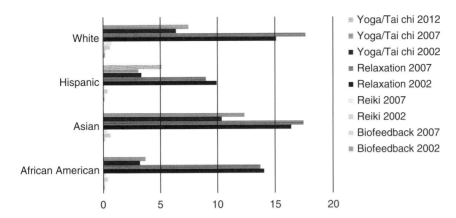

Figure 2.2   Percentage use of MBM modalities by race 2002, 2007, and 2012.
Sources: Arcury et al., 2005; Barnes, Bloom, & Nahin, 2008; Clark, Black, Stussman, Barnes, & Nahin, 2015; Su & Li, 2011.

reducing stress, promoting healing, and preventing pneumonia. Breathing exercises are well incorporated into medical practice as complements to surgical recovery following thoracic or abdominal surgery (Olsen & Anzen, 2012). Additionally, slow breathing exercises have been documented to reduce cardiovascular stress (Turankar et al., 2013); however, the benefits of deep breathing for specific, chronic health issues need additional research.

The category of deep breathing exercises was reported as the most utilized MBM modality across all cultural groups. When combined with meditation, it accounts for a majority of MBM use (excluding prayer) (Mind-Body Practices, 2010; Bishop & Lewith, 2010). In the 2002 NHIS survey, deep breathing was the MBM modality practiced by the largest percentage of all cultural groups (11.6% of all MBM), with 5.2% of African Americans, 11.1% of Asians, 4.2% of Hispanics, and 7% of Whites who used MBM (Arcury et al., 2005). In 2012 data from the NHIS, this remained true (deep breathing accounted for 10.9% of all MBM use) (Clark, Black, Stussman, Barnes, & Nahin, 2015).

Meditation and Transcendental Meditation

The Hindu Vedas contain the earliest written record of meditation as a spiritual technique for reflection and enlightenment. TM takes its unique style of meditation, involving a series of spoken chants or mantras and a focus on those sounds, from these Hindu spiritual traditions. TM is relatively new to the United States, having been introduced in the late 1950s to mid-1960s by Maharishi Mahesh Yogi, but the origins of this technique are found in Eastern spiritual practices (Goenka, 2003). The point of all the meditation techniques is to calm and focus the attention, to become aware of breathing patterns, to still the mind, and, if practiced within a faith tradition or set of spiritual teachings like TM, to gain enlightenment and transformation of consciousness.

In addition to being taught in general, meditation techniques are central to a number of different MBM modalities, including mindfulness meditation, progressive relaxation, and Qi gong. Research established the ability of long-term practitioners to influence various CNS and ANS functions, such as heart rate, brain wave pattern, and breathing (Benson, 1972; Kasala, Bodduluru, Maneti, & Thipparaboina, 2014; Telles et al., 2013).

Various researchers have examined the role that meditation can play in reducing anxiety and depression in college students, particularly nursing and medical students. Findings have shown net positive benefits (Shapiro, Astin, Bishop, & Cordova, 2005). What has been less well established is the link to direct medical benefit for specific health conditions outside of stress reduction; however, some positive results have been reported. Mixed results have been demonstrated for meditation for people with asthma and for the control of epilepsy, but reviewers have expressed concerns about the internal validity of study designs (Canter, 2003). A meta-analysis of over 800 studies illustrated a need for more standardized research and for improvement in study methodologies and sample sizes (Ospina et al., 2007). Ospina et al. (2007) reported that due to the small sample sizes and methodology of the reviewed studies, findings of effectiveness for health conditions outside of anxiety, depression, and blood pressure control were not consistently strong.

In regard to the use of meditation by specific cultural/ethnic groups, a study by Arcury et al. (2005) indicated that the racial/ethnic groups who were the heaviest users of this MBM modality were Asian cultural groups (5.5%), African Americans (4.1%), Whites (3.5%), and Hispanics (3.5%). When combined with the category of "deep breathing" in the Arcury et al. study, the meta-category of deep breathing/meditation became the MBM modality of choice across all racial/ethnic groups. In the 2012 data from the NHIS, a meta-category of deep-breathing/meditation would account for nearly 19% of all CAM use across all racial and ethnic categories, which is a larger percentage than supplements (17.7%) (Clark et al., 2015). Due to the increasing popularity of and potential applications for this modality, further research would be valuable to health practitioners.

Tai Chi

Tai chi is a martial arts form that some trace to Taoist monks from China in the 1100s. This source is somewhat disputed, as others see the origins of the practice as a fusion of Buddhist, Confucian, and Taoist thought originating in the royal Chen family of 1600s China (Kapes, 2013). The written record originated during the 1600s and described a martial arts form focused on slow fluid movement, a calm clear mind, and the notion that the yin (receptive) and yang (active) energies of the body are balanced (Henning, 1994). The client learns the basic moves of tai chi along, with breathing patterns associated with those moves, while clearing the mind to be in the moment. The movements are practiced two to three times a week for 15 to 30 minutes at a time. Research has documented the benefits of yoga for stress reduction and for increased flexibility and muscle tone (Kapes, 2013).

This MBM modality has been used by individuals dealing with depression, anxiety, effects of aging on mobility and muscle tone, osteoporosis, both rheumatoid and osteoarthritis, blood pressure problems, and a variety of stress-related gastrointestinal symptoms (Birdee et al., 2009; Ernst et al., 2006; Ernst & Posadzki, 2011). Research reviews have confirmed the value of the therapy for increased lower limb mobility and decreased pain in rheumatoid arthritis, as well as for increasing exercise endurance and fitness (Han et al., 2004). Although some studies have shown additional benefits, other studies have had no significant findings. A comprehensive review in 2004 noted the need for additional studies due to the conflicting findings and weak study designs predominating in the literature at that time (Wang et al., 2004). Su and Li (2011) reported on changing patterns of modality use across cultural/ethnic groups from 2002 to 2007 in the combined categories of yoga/tai chi and qi gong, noting that the use of these modalities was highest in Asian cultural groups (19%) and also increased in the African American (14.95%) and White (17.0%) cultural groups, while decreasing among Hispanics (−7.76%).

Yoga

Yoga is a stretching, meditation, and spiritual tradition of Eastern Indian origins dating back to the 400s to 500s BCE. The origins of yoga, like those of Tai chi, remain a topic of debate, but its association with Buddhism is clear (Singleton, 2010). The practice seeks to refine the body as a supple vessel for the life energy, or *prana*. This is done through a series of postures, structured stretches, and movements, as well as patterned breathing exercises in a calm meditative state. Clients practice about one hour, two to three times per week, with an experienced instructor.

As with Tai chi, benefits from yoga are seen with continued, consistent practice. The applications are many, and yoga has been used as a complementary therapy with many chronic conditions, stress, anxiety, depression, arthritis, and gastrointestinal problems, as well as to increase mobility and quality of life among elderly persons and to gain all the benefits usually associated with exercise (Ross & Thomas, 2010). Generally, studies have supported the use of yoga to improve outlook and function with certain mental (anxiety, depression) and chronic physical health concerns (e.g., arthritis) (Bartlett, Moonaz, Mill, Bernatsky, & Bingham, 2013; Srinivasan, 2013). Use among elderly persons has been found to be efficacious (with modifications taking into consideration mobility issues), but additional, larger studies are needed (Patel, Newstead, & Ferrer, 2012). Precautions and contraindications with the use of yoga are similar to Tai chi or any form of exercise.

Yoga and Tai chi are the most popular modalities used by Asian and White cultural groups (Barnes, Powell-Griner, McFann, & Nahin, 2004; Su & Li, 2011); however, findings from an analysis of the period 2002 to 2012, using recent NHIS data, indicated that there has been a positive linear increase in the percentage of Hispanics reporting the use of yoga. Data by all MBM modalities and all racial/ethnic groups was not released in this initial report, but the trend of increased Hispanic use of yoga as an MBM was evident (Clark et al., 2015) (see Figure 2.2).

Reiki

Mikao Usui is credited with the development of reiki ("mysterious atmosphere") in the early 1920s (Gehrang, 2014; Rousseau & Lardry, 2011). Usui was a Japanese Buddhist who believed that the *ki*, or universal energy, could be transferred from person to person through a skilled practitioner. Practitioners believe that the *ki* is weak or imbalanced in someone suffering from an illness and that reiki healers actually can draw infusions of *ki* energy through their bodies and transfer it via their hands into clients. Today there are two major branches of reiki practice, traditional Japanese and Western reiki, with healers attaining advancement through degrees of training in various reiki schools (Rousseau & Lardry, 2011).

Reiki has been used to treat fibromyalgia, pain, cancer pain, chemotherapy-associated illness, depression, and for general improvement of well-being (Thrane & Cohen, 2014). Research results have been mixed for its effectiveness, with some studies indicating benefits and others indicating no effect; for example, a study looking at burnout and anxiety control in nurses found reiki beneficial (Diaz-Rodriguez et al., 2011), while a study looking at postoperative pain control in pediatric patients found no benefit from reiki (Kundu, Lin, Oron, & Doorenbos, 2014). Another study conducted on chemotherapy outcomes found a beneficial impact for both trained reiki practitioners and sham (placebo) practitioners (Catlin & Taylor-Ford, 2011). Clearly, this MBM area would benefit from additional research of quality and rigorous design models, with larger numbers of participants in the studies.

In regard to the use of this modality by specific cultural/ethnic groups, Whites are the largest users of reiki, with about 28% growth in its use from 2002 to 2007 (Neiberg et al., 2011; Su & Li, 2011). In contrast to the growth in use by Whites, reiki use declined among African Americans, Hispanics, and Asians by 44% to 72% during the same time period (Neiberg et al., 2011; Su & Li, 2011).

Consumer Issues

Surveys of CAM use have been conducted since 1990. Surveys of CAIH use are still to be designed. In 1990, a sample of slightly more than 1,500 households was surveyed (Eisenberg et al., 1998; Lundgren & Ugalde, 2004). At that time, researchers discovered that 34% of those surveyed indicated that they were using CAM therapies of some form; that they were willing to largely spend out of pocket for the services (in 1990 dollars, it represented a financial impact of $13.7 billion, 75% out of pocket, which extrapolates to over $24 billion dollars in 2013 spending when accounting for inflation); and that 72% were not informing their medical doctors about the CAM use (Eisenberg et al., 1993; http://www.westegg.com/inflation/).

Additional surveys occurring in 1997, 1999, and 2002 (Eisenberg et al., 1998; Barnes et al., 2004; Mackenzie et al., 2003; Ni, Simile, & Hardy, 2002) represented a more accurate probability sample of the population. The 1999 data found that 28.9% of the sample used CAM of some form, with prayer accounting for the largest percentage of CAM use by modality at 13.7% (Ni et al., 2002). By 2004, again using a large sample through the NHIS, researchers found that CAM use, when prayer was included, had risen to 62% (36% excluding prayer). Again, prayer accounted for the largest modality being used (43%–24%, depending on prayer for self or others). Additional MBM modalities, such as meditation and yoga, also were tracked through NHIS (Barnes et al., 2004). CAM use and expenditures have only increased since those early surveys. The latest analysis of data from the NHIS in 2002 and 2007 indicated that 40% of Americans had utilized some form of CAM (excluding prayer) during the year surveyed (Barnes et al., 2008) and that over 34 million (16.6%) American adults had used some form of MBM (Barnes et al., 2008; Bertisch et al., 2009). According to 2012 data from the NHIS, 34% of American adults had used CAM during the reporting period (Clark et al., 2015).

Considering the financial impact of MBM, data from 2007 indicate that yoga, Tai chi, Qi gong, and relaxation therapies accounted for $4.3 billion of expenditures out of a total CAM expenditure of $13.9 billion (Nahin, Barnes, Stussman, & Bloom, 2009). Further, individual expenditures by those spending the most per year on CAM therapies were roughly $1,385 per capita in 2012—all of it out-of-pocket expenditures (Davis & Weeks, 2012; Nahin et al., 2009). These trends illustrate increasing use of CAM and MBM as a specific modality, even when the costs are not covered by insurance. It is clear that consumers continue to choose CAM and MBM modalities specifically to deal with chronic disease states involving physical and/or psychological discomfort. Consumers are also becoming aware of the importance of keeping their health and maximizing wellness as major health goals. In the future, consumers will actively look for MBM modalities that are CAIH oriented to lead them into this goal.

Implications for Health Professionals

Health practitioners must be knowledgeable about MBM modalities as they work with diverse groups. Furthermore, health educators and other healthcare providers working with culturally and ethnically diverse groups should strive for cultural competence when addressing health concerns and treatment choices (Pérez & Luquis, 2014). It is clear that many MBM modalities are being used; the use of many is increasing, depending on the cultural/ethnic group. Therefore, health practitioners must not only understand the use and applications of the modalities but also the proven benefits or risks associated with each. While most of the modalities covered in this chapter have few detrimental side effects, if used instead of proven treatments and for conditions for which no scientific evidence supports their use, they could be a detriment instead of a benefit to health. There is also no benefit for clients if health practitioners are unable to discuss the benefits and risks openly and freely in a culturally sensitive manner. It would be beneficial to develop a framework to guide practical applications of these MBM modalities.

Health practitioners in the nursing field may find it useful to consider these MBM modalities through the lens of the nurse's ways of knowing as proposed by Chinn and Kramer (2008). In their model, Chinn and Kramer identify the variety of ways that practitioners in the nursing field learn and integrate knowledge, personal knowing, and aesthetics. They suggest doing this through the lenses of ethics (obligation, the "right" thing to do) and empirics (scientific understanding), and last, through a synthesis of both areas that they term emancipatory knowing, where nurses are able to best support clients because they can integrate all of the ways of knowing and understanding first within themselves, and then pass that knowledge on to clients. For example, as a practitioner there is an obligation to "do no harm" that cannot be fulfilled if a comprehensive understanding of less invasive, safer modalities is not provided to a client, and conversely, if unsafe, untested approaches are not questioned. This model is comprehensive and shares an integrative approach with another model used by health practitioners in the community and public health area called the social ecological model. The social ecological model challenges public health practitioners to consider the entire social, interpersonal, and intrapersonal processes that affect individual health and well-being (see Figure 2.3). Like the MBM modalities themselves, these models challenge health practitioners to be integrative and holistic in their approach to understanding and supporting optimum health and well-being.

Perhaps these models could be used in conjunction with the suggestions of Zografos and Pérez (2014), when they state that in order for health workers to practice in a culturally competent fashion, they must "use their abilities in four areas—awareness, knowledge, experience, and skills—and be willing to make a commitment to a lifelong process of change" (p. 74). Using these four areas to guide professional practice combined with the integrative, analytical approaches developed by Chinn and Kramer and the social ecological model, health educators can ethically, safely, and effectively apply the concepts of cultural competency (listed in Box 2.2) when developing programs utilizing CAIH-MBM practices or working with different groups.

Health practitioners must become knowledgeable about MBM modalities and aware of their own biases in regard to MBM use. They should develop some practical experience with the MBM modalities and should rely on their training in needs assessment, advocacy, and evaluation to work on improving service delivery in this area. The National Commission for

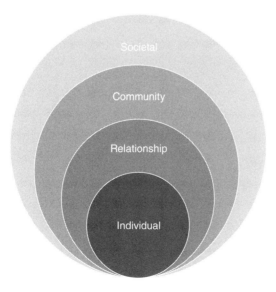

Figure 2.3   The social ecological model.
Source: Centers for Disease Control and Prevention (2015).

BOX 2.2   FRAMEWORK FOR WORKING WITH CLIENTS

1. Awareness
   a. Health professionals should become familiar with the cultural attributes and native languages of the groups they work with.
   b. Health professionals should also be familiar with typical stereotypes about the groups they work with, avoiding the pitfall of expecting every member of a specific cultural or minority group to fit that mold.
   c. Health professionals should be aware of their own biases, anxieties, and fears.

2. Knowledge
   a. Health professionals should be familiar with the various MBM modalities.
   b. Health professionals should be aware of cautions concerning the uses of MBM and the limitations of MBM as indicated in the research literature. They must also be aware that certifications for MBM practitioners and licensing requirements are neither consistent nor standardized from location to location in the United States (Lunstroth, 2006).
   c. Health professionals should be aware of demographic data on cultural group patterns of MBM use.
   d. Health professionals should understand and respect that some MBM is also based on spiritual concepts and respect those traditions (i.e., shamanism, yoga, prayer, Tai chi).

3. Experience
   a. Only by getting to know others of different cultural and identity groups will health educators begin to release their preconceived notions and rid themselves of anxieties and fears that might block genuine rapport.
   b. Experience working in multicultural settings and with various MBM modalities gives health professionals new insights for evaluating the effectiveness of programs and educational campaigns. Health professionals should use their experiences to improve their skills at evaluation.

4. Skills
   a. Health professionals should collect data and develop skills in the critical evaluation of MBM therapies.
   b. This can be guided by the National Commission for Health Education Credentialing competencies and should be grounded in practical experiences with ethnic/cultural groups and MBM.

Sources: Pérez & Luquis, 2014; Zeman et al., 2015.

BOX 2.3   IMPORTANT MBM RESOURCES

American Tai Chi and Qi gong Association. Provides training, certification, and general information about Tai chi and Qi gong.

http://www.americantaichi.org/

Association for Applied Psychophysiology and Biofeedback. A membership-based organization offering certification training and educational resources about biofeedback.

http://www.aapb.org/i4a/pages/index.cfm?pageid=1

International Center for Reiki Training. Offers information on all aspects of reiki, as well as the option of joining the Reiki Membership Association.

http://www.reiki.org/

National Center for Complementary and Integrative Health (NCCIH). The National Institutes of Health clearinghouse site for information on complementary and integrative approaches and the latest CAIH news and research findings.

https://nccih.nih.gov/

National Commission for Health Education Credentialing (NCHEC). Provides credentialing exams and works with other health professionals and educational organizations to ensure professional competency of the health educator workforce.

http://www.nchec.org/

National Health Interview Survey (NHIS). A nationally representative survey of health issues, conducted yearly since 1957 by the Centers for Disease Control and Prevention.

http://www.cdc.gov/nchs/nhis.htm

Transcendental Meditation (TM). The site founded and supported by the Maharishi Foundation, USA, that offers resources on and instruction in TM.

http://wwv.tm.org/

Yoga Alliance. This organization provides information on credentialing, training, and professional business practices in the United States.

https://www.yogaalliance.org/

Health Education Credentialing offers competency areas that can serve as guideposts to these activities. Box 2.3 includes a list of online resources on MBM.

Caveat Emptor

While many MBM modalities and practices have proven track records of effectiveness, particularly for stress-related chronic illness, the degree of success varies by the specific MBM modality studied and the condition for which it is used (Ernst et al., 2006). Health educators and other healthcare professionals need to understand which demographic groups favor specific modalities, what mind-body modalities entail, and the potential benefits of the modalities for the populations they work with. Furthermore, as health promoters and educators, practitioners need to evaluate potential risks and pitfalls to the use of mind-body modalities. Research conducted in 2008 indicates that the overall understanding of CAM on the part of health educators is relatively weak and that what is well understood are only the most commonly used modalities, such as massage therapy, chiropractic, and supplements (especially nutritional), which are not considered mind-body approaches (Johnson, Johnson, & Priestley, 2008).

It is important to keep in mind that the regulation of these mind-body modalities is fragmented in the United States. Certifications and training are organized mostly by professional organizations in some of the MBM areas, such as biofeedback, yoga and Tai chi, and reiki. In addition, there is no consistent professional regulation for MBM overall through state or federal professional licenses. In most instances, licensure is variable. Some states, such as Michigan, require that yoga training schools be licensed vocational schools, while other states allow for industry self-regulation through professional organizations (Lunstroth, 2006).

What this means for both consumers of CAIH-MBM and for health professionals is that there is no guarantee of the training or skill of the practitioners. As health professionals who may be asked about these therapies, we must convey this fact to clients. Most MBM practitioners are caring, committed professionals with certifications from their professional societies. Organizations and clients should be encouraged to inquire about a provider's certifications and training and to ask for references. Finally, clients should always be encouraged to share their use of MBM and discuss it with their healthcare providers. Healthcare providers should be aware of qualified and respected MBM practitioners in their areas to help clients make informed decisions. Similarly, consumers must realize that they should consult physicians or other appropriate healthcare practitioners before they start any MBM modality.

Conclusion

Ongoing research into the demographics and effectiveness of CAIH is needed to provide health educators and other health professionals with more detailed data concerning the use of MBM among various cultural/ethnic groups. Native Americans are particularly underrepresented in CAIH-MBM-specific research, yet they are some of the major users of CAM (Barnes et al., 2008). Further effectiveness research on the specific health conditions that are amenable to MBM modalities and proven benefits of the treatments are very much needed. Research to date indicates that the MBM modalities of CAIH offer generalized stress-reduction benefits for populations experiencing toxic stress loads. Research has also confirmed that MBM modalities are particularly effective in reducing stress. Thus, stress associated with stereotype threat experienced by many minority groups may be reduced through the use of MBM modalities. Further, in certain instances, the use of MBM modalities may serve to reconnect some cultural groups to their healing history and traditions.

Summary

- MBM is broadly composed of modalities (applied practices) and epistemologies (philosophies) derived from a variety of Eastern and Western traditional healing practices from cultures around the world, which are used to relieve chronic mental and physical diseases.
- Some of these approaches have been tested through epidemiological studies for efficacy and safety and have been found to be effective under specific circumstances and/or when used in combination with modern Western (allopathic) treatment methods.
- Possible modes of action include general stress reduction and reduction of allostatic load along with triggering of the placebo effect.
- Certain MBM modalities seem to be preferred by the majority of individuals in specific cultural groups, but broad overgeneralizations should be avoided when working with individual clients.
- Becoming culturally competent is an ongoing process of learning to be sensitive to other cultural and identity groups as well as becoming more aware of your own preconceptions.
- MBM modalities offer consumers the opportunity to keep their health and maximize wellness. MBM modalities are major approaches of CAIH.

Case Study

Description

Carmen is a health educator at a combined hospice and geriatric critical care facility. Recently, a relatively young (39-year-old male), Asian (Japanese American) client who suffered a sudden, critical, hemorrhagic stroke with major complications has been brought into the facility, as the medical team has determined that death is imminent. The extended family is quite distraught, as the sudden onset of the stroke did not provide anyone with closure. The constant presence of extended family and the highly emotional nature of the sudden loss have pushed the family and staff to an emotional edge. One family member has approached the staff about having a reiki practitioner come and work with the client during this time.

Questions

1. How would you explain reiki therapy to other health professionals?
2. Why might the family have been attracted to this MBM?
3. What benefits can you identify from the use of this therapy? What risks?
4. What role can a health professional have in regard to reiki use?
5. How could this instance be used as a teaching moment for increasing the CAIH-MBM competency of the staff?

KEY TERMS

Allostatic load. When chronic and unrelenting stressors create a situation of constant neural and neuroendocrine stimulation, overloading these bodily systems' ability to recover and negatively impacting other bodily systems (Lipton, 2008; Lovallo, 2005; Zeman et al., 2015).

Cultural competence. Ability to interact effectively with individuals from different races, ethnicities, cultures, and backgrounds (Pérez & Luquis, 2014; Zeman et al., 2015).

Cultural groups. Groups of individuals who share common cultural characteristics. This may or may not include individuals of different racial or ethnic groups (i.e., Americans share common cultural characteristics but may be of different ethnicities) (Pérez & Luquis, 2014; Zeman et al., 2015).

Mind-body medicine. A series of practices and an area of research that focuses on how the mind, emotional factors, mental factors, and spiritual practices can impact and influence health, well-being, and disease states (Cohen, 2006; Zeman et al., 2015).

Relaxation response. Triggering the parasympathetic branch of the autonomic nervous system through relaxation techniques, such as the mind-body medicine modalities of yoga and Tai chi, to downregulate the stress response. Doing so decreases the bloodstream levels of adrenaline, norepinephrine, and cortisol and leads to cardiovascular, respiratory, gastrointestinal, and psychological calming (Seeley et al., 2007; Zeman et al., 2015).

Stereotype threat. The stress caused when an individual of a minority or marginalized group encounters negative social stereotypes about his or her group, triggering the stress response (Edwards, 2007; Levy & Sidel, 2006; Zeman et al., 2015).

Stress response. When a physical or psychological threat is encountered, the sympathetic branch of the autonomic nervous system floods the bloodstream with adrenaline, norepinephrine, and cortisol, which provide high levels of glucose and shift blood to the muscles and away from the organs (Thibodeau & Patton, 2008; Zeman et al., 2015).

References

Arcury, T., Suerken, C., Grzywacz, J., Bell, R., Lang, W., & Quandt, S. (2005). Ethnic variation in complementary and alternative medicine use among older adults. *Gerontologist*, *45*, 264–265.

Ashby, N. (2007). *Simply color therapy*. New York, NY: Sterling/Zambezi.

Barner, J. C., Bohman, T. M., Brown, C. M., & Richards, K. M. (2010). Use of complementary and alternative medicine (CAM) for treatment among African-Americans: A multivariate analysis. *Research in Social and Administrative Pharmacy*, *6*(3), 196–208.

Barnes, P. M., Bloom, B., & Nahin, R. L. (2008). *Complementary and alternative medicine use among adults and children: United States, 2007* (12). Centers for Disease Control and Prevention. Retrieved from http://www.cdc.gov/search .do?q=Complementary+and+Alternative+Medicine&subset=nchs&sort=date% 3AD%3AL%3Ad1&oe=UTF-8&ie=UTF-8&ud=1&site=nchs&site=nchsamp;& btnG.x=0&btnG.y=0

Barnes, P. M., Powell-Griner, E., McFann, K., & Nahin, R. L. (2004). Complementary and alternative medicine use among adults: United States, 2002. *Vital Health and Statistics*, *343*, 1–19.

Bartlett, S. J., Moonaz, S. H., Mill, C., Bernatsky, S., & Bingham, C. O. (2013, October). Yoga in rheumatic diseases. *Current Rheumatology Reports*, *15*(387). Retrieved from doi: 10.1007/s11926-013-0387-2

Benson, W. R. (1972). The physiology of meditation. *Scientific American*, *226*, 84–90.

Bertisch, S. M., Wee, C. C., Phillips, R. S., & McCarthy, E. P. (2009, June). Alternative mind-body therapies used by adults with medical conditions. *Journal of Psychosomatic Research*, *66*(6), 511–519.

Bialek, W. (2012). *Biophysics: Searching for principles*. Princeton, NJ: Princeton University Press.

Birdee, G. S., Wayne, P. M., Davis, R. B., Phillips, R. S., & Yeh, G. Y. (2009). T'ai chi and Qigong for health: Patterns of use in the United States. *Journal of Alternative and Complementary Medicine*, *15*(9), 969–973.

Bishop, F. L., & Lewith, G. T. (2010, March 13, 2008). Who uses CAM? A narrative review of demographic characteristics and health factors associated with CAM use. *Evidence-Based Complementary and Alternative Medicine*, *7*(1), 11–28.

Bynum, W. F. (1994). *Science and the practice of medicine in the nineteenth century. Cambridge Studies in the History of Science*. New York, NY: Cambridge University Press.

Canter, P. H. (2003). The therapeutic effects of meditation. *Student British Medical Journal*, *11*, 176. Retrieved from http://dx.doi.org/

Carson, B., Dunbar, T., Chenhall, R. D., & Bailie, R. (2007). *Social determinants of indigenous health*. Crows Nest, NSW: Allen & Unwin.

Catlin, A., & Taylor-Ford, R. L. (2011, May). Investigation of standard of care versus sham Reiki placebo versus actual Reiki therapy to enhance comfort and well-being in a chemotherapy infusion center. *Oncology Nursing Forum, 38*(3), E212–E220. Retrieved from http://eds.a.ebscohost.com.proxy .lib.uni.edu/eds/detail?vid=5&sid=2fd50e4f-c7d2-4dac-ad35-7fa0a140c96d%40 sessionmgr4005&hid=4108&bdata=JnNpdGU9ZWRzLWxpdmU%3d#db=afh &AN=60297902

Centers for Disease Control and Prevention. (2015). The social-ecological model: A framework for prevention. Retrieved from http://www.cdc.gov/ ViolencePrevention/overview/social-ecologicalmodel.html

Center for Mind Medicine Practice. (2014). *What is mind-body medicine?* Retrieved from http://cmbm.org/about/what-is-mind-body-medicine/

Chang, J., Fisch, J., & Popp, F. (2010). *Biophotons* (2nd ed.). New York, NY: Springer Science & Business Media.

Chinn, P. L., & Kramer, M. K. (2008). *Integrated theory and knowledge development in nursing* (7th ed.). St. Louis, MO: Mosby Elsevier.

Chopra, D. (1990). *Quantum healing: Exploring the frontiers of mind/body medicine.* New York, NY: Bantam Books.

Clark, T. C., Black, L. I., Stussman, B. J., Barnes, P. M., & Nahin, R. L. (2015). *Trends in the use of complementary health approaches among adults: United States, 2002–2012.* Centers for Disease Control and Prevention, National Center for Health Statistics, No. 79. Washington, DC: National Center for Health Statistics, Centers for Disease Control and Prevention.

Cohen, H. M. (2006). *Healing at the borderland of medicine and religion.* A. M. Brandt & L. R. Churchill (Eds.). Chapel Hill, NC: University of North Carolina Press.

Cohen, S., & Popp, F. A. (1997). Biophoton emission of the human body. *Journal of Photocheistry and Photobiology, 40,* 187–189.

Committee on the Use of Complementary and Alternative Medicine by the American Public, Board on Health Promotion and Disease Prevention, Institute of Medicine of the National Academies. (2005). *Complementary and alternative medicine in the United States.* Washington, DC: National Academies Press.

Davis, M. A., & Weeks, W. B. (2012). The concentration of out-of-pocket expenditures on complementary and alternative medicine in the United States. *Alternative Therapies, Health and Medicine, 18*(5), 36–42.

Diaz-Rodriguez, L., Arroyo-Morales, M., Cantarero-Villanueva, I., Fernandez-Lao, C., Polley, M., & Fernandez-de-las-Penas, C. (2011). The application of reiki in nurses diagnosed with burnout syndrome has beneficial effects on concentration of salivary IgA and blood pressure. *Revista Latin-Americana de Enfermagem (RLAE), 19*(5), 1132–1138. Retrieved from http://eds.a.ebscohost.com.proxy .lib.uni.edu/eds/detail?vid=7&sid=2fd50e4f-c7d2-4dac-ad35-7fa0a140c96d%40 sessionmgr4005&hid=4108&bdata=JnNpdGU9ZWRzLWxpdmU%3d#db=afh& AN=69609870

Dolgoff-Kaspar, R., Baldwin, A., Johnson, S., Edling, N., & Sethi, G. K. (2012). Effect of laughter yoga on mood and heart rate variability in patients awaiting organ transplantation: A pilot study. *Alternative Therapies in Health and Medicine, 18*(5), 61–66.

Dossey, L. (2014). *One mind: How our individual mind is part of a greater consciousness and why it matters.* Carlsbad, CA: Hay House.

Dreher, H. (2003). *Mind-body unity: A new vision for mind-body science and medicine.* (eBook). Retrieved from http://ehis.ebscohost.com/eds/detail?vid=28&sid=44e729-d43b-4f51-a3d7-024c8bd5b5d2%40sessionmgr113&hid=1013d#db=cat01767a&AN=uni.b3563547

Dupler, D., Odle, T. G., & Lerner, B. W. (2012). Mind-body medicine. In K. Key (Ed.), *The Gale encyclopedia of mental health* (3rd ed., vol. 2, pp. 981–985). Detroit, MI: Gale, Cengage Learning.

Edwards, K. (2007). Health status, risk factors and unmet needs of diverse populations. *Journal of Cultural Diversity, 14*(1), 3.

Eisenberg, D. M., Davis, R. B., Ettner, S. L., Appel, S., Wilkey, S., Van Rompay, M., & Kessler, R. C. (1998). Trends in alternative medicine use in the United States, 1990–1997: Results of a follow-up national survey. *Journal of the American Medical Association, 280*(18), 1569–1575.

Eisenberg, D. M., Kessler, R. C., Foster, C., Norlock, F. E., Calkins, D. R., & Delbanco, T. L. (1993). Unconventional medicine in the United States: Prevalence, costs, and patterns of use. *New England Journal of Medicine, 328*(4), 246–252.

Ernst, E., Pittler, M. H., & Wider, B. (2006). *The desktop guide to complementary and alternative medicine: An evidence-based approach* (2nd ed.). Beijing, China: Mosby Elsevier.

Ernst, E., & Posadzki, P. (2011). Complementary and alternative medicine for rheumatoid arthritis and osteoarthritis: An overview of systematic reviews. *Current Pain and Headache Reports, 15*(6), 431–437.

Gehrang, T. (2014). *All about reiki: Your beginner's guide to discovering reiki, healing, self-treatments, attunements, your seven chakras, performing aura viewings, and the reiki symbols.* (Kindle edition). Retrieved from http://www.amazon.com/All-About-Reiki-Discovering-Self-Treatments-ebook/dp/B00632BHT2/ref=sr_1_17?ie=UTF8&qid=1397956125&sr=8-17&keywords=Reiki

Goenka, S. N. (2003). *Meditation now: Inner peace through inner wisdom.* Retrieved from http://site.ebrary.com/lib/rodlibrary/docDetail.action?docID=10647602

Han, A., Robinson, V., Judd, M., Taixiang, W., Wells, G., & Tugwell, P. (2004). Tai chi for treating rheumatoid arthritis. *Cochrane Database of Systemic Reviews, Article #CD004849.* Retrieved from www.uni.edu

Henning, S. (1994). Ignorance, legend and taijiquan. *Journal of the Chen Style Taijiquan Research Association of Hawaii, 2*(3). Retrieved from www.uni.edu

Howick, J., Friedemann, C., Tsakok, M., Watson, R., Tsakok, T., Thomas, J., Heneghan, C. (2013, May). Are treatments more effective than placebos? A systematic review and meta-analysis. *PLoS Clinical Trials, 10*(5), 1–8. Retrieved from 10.1371/journal.pone.0062599

Johnson, P., Johnson, R. D., & Priestley, J. L. (2008). A survey of complementary and alternative medicine knowledge among health educators in the United States. *American Journal of Health Education, 39*(2), 66–78.

Jones, J. (2001). Ethnicity may affect alternative, complementary therapy choices. *Journal of the National Cancer Institute, 93,* 1522–1523.

Kanjii, N., White, A. R., & Ernst, E. (2006). Autogenic training for tension type headaches: A systemic review of controlled trials. *Complementary Therapies in Medicine, 14*(2), 144–150.

Kapes, B. (2013). Tai chi. In *The Gale encyclopedia of nursing and allied health* (6th ed., pp. 3265–3268). Farmington Hills, MI: Gale.

Kasala, E. R., Bodduluru, L. N., Maneti, Y., & Thipparaboina, R. (2014). Effect of meditation on neurophysiological changes in stress mediated depression. *Complementary Therapies in Clinical Practice, 20*(1), 74–80. Retrieved from 10.1016/j.ctcp.2013.10.001

Kundu, A., Lin, Y., Oron, A. P., & Doorenbos, A. Z. (2014). Reiki therapy for postoperative oral pain in pediatric patients: Pilot data from a double blind, randomized clinical trial. *Complementary Therapies in Clinical Practice, 20*(1), 21–25.

Levy, B. S., & Sidel, V. W. (Eds.). (2006). *Social injustice and public health.* New York, NY: Oxford University Press.

Lipton, B. (2005). *The biology of belief: Unleashing the power of consciousness, matter, & miracles.* Santa Rosa, CA: Elite Books.

Lipton, B. (2008). From the microcosm of the cell to the macrocosm of the mind. *Lilipoh, 13*(54), 19–23. Retrieved from http://dx.doi.org/

Lovallo, W. R. (2005). *Stress & health: Biological and psychological interactions* (2nd ed.). London, UK: Sage.

Lundgren, J., & Ugalde, V. (2004). The demographics and economics of complementary alternative medicine. *Physical Medicine and Rehabilitation Clinics of North America, 15,* 955–961.

Lunstroth, J. (2006). Voluntary self-regulation of complementary and alternative medicine practitioners. *Albany Law Review, 70*(1).

Mackenzie, E. R., Taylor, L., Bloom, B. S., Hufford, D. J., & Johnson, J. C. (2003). Ethnic minority use of complementary and alternative medicine (CAM): A national probability survey of CAM utilizers. *Alternative Therapies in Health and Medicine, 9*(4), 50–56.

Mind-Body Medicine Practices in Complementary and Alternative Medicine. (2010). Retrieved from http://report.nih.gov/nihfactsheets/ViewFactSheet.aspx?csid=102&key=M#M

Moss, D. (1999). Biofeedback, mind-body medicine, and the higher limits of human nature. In D. Moss (Ed.), *Humanistic and transpersonal psychology: A historical and biographical sourcebook.* Westport, CT: Greenwood Press.

Nahin, R. L., Barnes, P. M., Stussman, B. J., & Bloom, B. (2009). Costs of complementary and alternative medicine (CAM) and frequency of visits to CAM practitioners: United States 2007. *National Health Statistics Report,* No. 18. Hyattsville, MD: National Center for Health Statistics.

National Center for Complementary and Integrative Health. (n.d.). https://nccih.nih.gov/health/mindbody

Neiberg, R. H., Aickin, M., Grzywacz, J. G., Lang, W., Quandt, S. A., Bell, R. A., & Arcury, T. A. (2011). Occurrence and co-occurrence of types of complementary and alternative medicine use by age, gender, ethnicity, and education among adults in the United States: The 2002 National Health Interview Survey (NHIS). *Journal of Alternative and Complementary Medicine, 17*(4), 363–370.

Nerburn, K. (1999). *The wisdom of the Native Americans*. Retrieved from www.amazon.com

Nezu, A. M., Nezu, C. M., & Xanthopoulos, M. S. (2011). Stress reduction in chronically ill patients. In R. J. Contrada & A. Baum (Eds.), *The handbook of stress science, biology, psychology, and health* (pp. 475–485). New York, NY: Springer.

Ni, H., Simile, C., & Hardy, A. M. (2002). Utilization of complementary and alternative medicine by United States adults: Results from the 1999 National Health Interview Survey. *Medical Care, 40*(4), 353–358.

Olsen, M. F., & Anzen, H. (2012, April). Effects of training interventions prior to thoracic or abdominal surgery: A systematic review. *Physical Therapy Reviews, 17*(2), 124–131.

Ospina, M. B., Bond, K., Karkhaneh, M., Tjosvold, L., Vandermeer, B., Liang, Y., . . . Klassen, T. P. (2007). *Meditation practices for health: State of the research*. AHRQ Publication No. 07-E010. Washington, DC: Government Printing Office.

Pascoe, E. A., & Richman, L. S. (2009). Perceived discrimination and health: A meta-analytic review. *Psychological Bulletin, 135*(4), 531–554.

Patel, N. K., Newstead, A. H., & Ferrer, R. L. (2012). The effects of yoga on physical functioning and health related quality of life in older adults: A systemic review and meta-analysis. *Journal of Alternative & Complementary Medicine, 18*(10), 902–917.

Pilates, J., Robbins, J., & Van Heuit-Robbins, L. V. (2012). *Pilate's evolution: The 21st century*. New York, NY: Presentation Dynamics.

Popp, F. A., Gu, Q., & Li, K. (1994). Biophoton emission: Experimental background and theoretical approaches. *Modern Physics Letters, 8*(21/22), 1269–1296.

Pérez, M. A., & Luquis, R. R. (2014). *Cultural competence in health education and health promotion* (2nd ed.). San Francisco, CA: Jossey-Bass.

Rifkin, B. A., & Ackerman, M. J. (2011). *Human anatomy: A visual history from the Renaissance to the Digital Age*. New York, NY: Abrams.

Ross, A., & Thomas, S. (2010). The health benefits of yoga and exercise: A review of comparison studies. *Journal of Alternative and Complementary Medicine, 16*(1), 3–12.

Rousseau, J., & Lardry, J. (2011). The history of reiki. *Kinesitherapie Revue, 112*, 28–31. Retrieved from http://eds.a.ebscohost.com.proxy.lib.uni.edu/eds/detail?vid=11&sid=2fd50e4f-c7d2-4dac-ad35-7fa0a140c96d%40sessionmgr4005&hid=4108&bdata=JnNpdGU9ZWRzLWxpdmU%3d#db=cin20&AN=2011070983

Schmidt, S. (2012). Can we help just by good intentions? A meta-analysis of experiments on distant intention effects. *Journal of Alternative and Complementary Medicine, 18*(6), 529–533.

Seeley, R. R., Stephens, T. D., & Tate, P. (2007). *Essentials of anatomy & physiology* (6th ed.). New York, NY: McGraw-Hill.

Shah, S. G., & Farrow, A. (2012). Trends in the availability and usage of electrophysical agents in physiotherapy practices from 1990 to 2010: A review. *Physical Therapy Reviews, 17*(4), 207–226.

Shapiro, R. (2009). *EMDR solutions II: For depression, eating disorders, performance and more.* New York, NY: Norton.

Shapiro, S. L., Astin, J. A., Bishop, S. R., & Cordova, M. (2005). Mindfulness-based stress reduction for health care professionals: Results from a randomized trial. *International Journal of Stress Management, 12,* 164–176.

Shinozaki, M., Kanazawa, M., Kano, M., Endo, Y., Nakaya, N., Hongo, M., & Fukudo, S. (2010). Effect of autogenic training on general improvement in patients with irritable bowel syndrome: A randomized controlled trial. *Applied Psychophysiology and Biofeedback, 35*(3), 189–198. Retrieved from 10.1007/s10484-009-9125-y

Singleton, M. (2010). *Yoga body: The origins of modern posture practice.* New York, NY: Oxford University Press.

Srinivasan, T. (2013). Bridging the mind-body divide. *International Journal of Yoga, 6(2),* 85.

Su, D., & Li, L. (2011). Trends in the use of complementary and alternative medicine in the United States: 2002–2007. *Journal of Health Care for the Poor and Underserved, 22*(1), 296–310.

Suzuki, D., & Knudtson, P. (1992). *Wisdom of the elders: Sacred native stories of nature.* New York, NY: Bantam Books.

Telles, S., Raghavendra, B., Naveen, K. R., Visweswaraiah, N. M., Krishnamurthy, S. K., & Subramanya, P. (2013). Changes in autonomic variables following two meditative states described in yoga texts. *Journal of Alternative and Complementary Medicine, 19*(1), 35–42. Retrieved from 10.1089/acm.2011.0282

Thibodeau, G. A., & Patton, K. T. (2008). *Structure & function of the body* (13th ed.). St. Louis, MO: Mosby Elsevier.

Thrane, S., & Cohen, S. M. (2014, Dec.). Review article: Effect of reiki therapy on pain and anxiety in adults: An in-depth literature review of randomized trials with effect size calculations. *Pain Management Nursing, 15*(4), 897–908. Retrieved from 10.1016/j.pmn.2013.07.008

Turankar, A. V., Jain, S., Patel, S. B., Sinha, S. R., Joshi, A. D., Vallish, B. N., & Turankar, S. A. (2013). Effects of slow breathing exercise on cardiovascular functions, pulmonary functions & galvanic skin resistance in healthy human volunteers—A pilot study. *Indian Journal of Medical Research, 137*(5), 916–921.

Wang, C., Collet, J. P., & Lau, J. (2004). The effect of t'ai chi on health outcomes in patients with chronic conditions: A systematic review. *Archives of Internal Medicine, 164,* 493–501.

Winkelman, M. (2010). *Shamanism: A biopsychosocial paradigm of consciousness and healing* (2nd ed.). Santa Barbara, CA: Praeger. Retrieved from http://ehis.ebscohost.com/eds/detail?sid=efa3d75b-3328-40ef-a171-e34124c64 bfb@sessionmgr15&vid=1#db=nlebk&AN=331909

Zeman, C. L., Hall, J., Depken, D. and Bocsan, I. (2015). Development, structure and impact of a ten year outreach and study abroad program in sustainability and environmental health disparities: University of Northern Iowa, the Iuliu Hatieganu University of Medicine and Pharmacy and the Romani of Pata Rat with a report on a cross-sectional, Romani environmental footprint study. In W. Leal (Ed.), *Transformative approaches to sustainable development at universities* (pp. 239–256). New York, NY: Springer. http://www.springer.com/ 978-3-319-08836-5

Zografos, K. N., & Pérez, M. A. (2014). Health disparities and social determinants of health: Implications for health education. In M. A. Pérez & R. R. Luquis (Eds.), *Cultural competence in health education and health promotion* (2nd ed., pp. 59–85). San Francisco, CA: Jossey-Bass.

CHAPTER 3

NATURAL COMPLEMENTARY AND ALTERNATIVE MEDICINE MODALITIES

Cheryl Hickey and Cyndi Guerra

The National Center for Complementary and Integrative Health (NCCIH), formerly known as the National Center for Complementary and Alternative Medicine (NCCAM), has created a list of terms that defines complementary, alternative, and integrative health (CAIH) modalities and related concepts. The depth of this list shows the expanding nature of complementary and alternative medicine practices and the rate at which the National Institutes of Health (NIH) continues to recognize the evolution of complementary, alternative, and integrative health. This chapter presents an overview of the most common approaches, discusses their value for health professionals, reviews practices related to consumer use, and discusses regulatory guidelines associated with natural CAIH modalities.

Theoretical Concepts

Overview

Natural CAIH modalities are intrinsically integrative since they tend not only to alleviate illness but also to promote health and wellness. The NCCIH has recognized the value of complementary and integrative health approaches including acupuncture; biofeedback; ayurveda; chiropractic care; deep breathing; energy healing; Feldenkrais; guided imagery; homeopathy; hypnosis; massage; meditation; naturopathy; nonvitamin; nonmineral natural products;

LEARNING OBJECTIVES
At the completion of this chapter, students will be able to:

- Identify the theoretical and scientific basis of homeopathy, naturopathy, fasting, herbal medicines, and dietary supplements.

- Define how natural complementary and alternative modalities are classified.

- Review the regulatory agencies for natural complementary and alternative medicine (CAM) modalities.

- Identify the efficacy of natural CAM practices based on research findings.

- Determine natural CAM modalities that are related to complementary, alternative, and integrative health.

Pilates; progressive relaxation; qi gong; reiki; tai chi; and yoga, among others (NCCIH, 2015a). Data from the 2012 National Health Interview Survey (NHIS) reveals that "17.7% of American adults had used a dietary supplement other than vitamins and minerals in the past year. These products were the most popular complementary health approach in the survey. The most commonly used natural product was fish oil" (NCCIH, 2015a).

Some of the key natural CAIH modalities, such as homeopathy, naturopathy, herbal medicine, and dietary supplements, have long histories that are culturally rooted. Naturopathic medicine, for example, can be traced back to the Hippocratic School of Medicine in 400 BC. Naturopathy had its origins in the United States and Europe in the early 1800s (College of Naturopathic Medicine, n.d.). Many patients report visiting naturopathic practitioners for a variety of medical reasons, such as basic primary care for their general health, as well as for chronic and acute illness (NCCAM, 2012c).

One of the most often used forms of CAIH is the category of herbal medicine and dietary supplements. According to the 2007 National NHIS report, an estimated $14.8 million was spent in the United States on CAIH modalities (NCCAM, 2009). This report also identified homeopathy and naturopathic medicine as the most commonly used CAM approaches nationwide.

Modalities

The NCCIH has established a classification of complementary and integrative health approaches to assist patients, practitioners, and the general public to make informed choices. In addition, this center has provided access to current research on CAIH practices and has directed its efforts toward educating consumers on wise practices and protecting themselves against unlawful and untruthful practices surrounding their utilization (NCCIH, 2015a,b,c; NCCAM, 2013d; NCCAM, 2012b).

Currently, the NCCIH classifies complementary practices into three major groups: (1) natural products, (2) mind and body practices, and (3) other complementary approaches (those that do not fit into either of the first two categories). Included in the third category are practices such as traditional Chinese medicine, homeopathy, naturopathy, ayurvedic medicine, and the practices of traditional healers (NCCIH, 2015d; NCCAM, 2013a, d; NCCAM, 2012b; College of Naturopathic Medicine, n.d.).

Natural CAM modalities include homeopathy, naturopathy, fasting, herbal medicine, and dietary supplements such as vitamins, minerals, and other natural products. This section reviews these five major categories, which have been cited by the NCCIH as being some of the most commonly used nationwide.

Homeopathy

The 2012 NHIS reported that an estimated five million adults and one million children used homeopathic treatments in the United States. This survey also revealed that 11.8% of children used homeopathy, but only 0.2% of these children received consultation with a homeopathic practitioner for their treatment (NCCIH, 2015b).

Homeopathy is a holistic approach to health that not only addresses illness but also prevents diseases (Loudon, 2006; NCCAM, 2015b). Homeopathy has a rich history in the ancient cultures of Chinese and Indian medicines. A more modern rebirth that eventually led the way to American use can be traced back to the German doctor Samuel Hahnemann during the 18th century. Homeopathy is based on three major concepts: the law of similars, individualized therapy, and the small or minimum dose remedy through dilution.

Law of Similars   Hahnemann felt that if a particular agent which caused a set of symptoms in a healthy person was given to an ill person, it could cure the disease. He fostered the idea that similar substances or agents can cure similar substances or agents, as was the case with quinine (Johnson & Boon, 2007; NCCIH, 2015a).

Individualized Therapy   Individualized therapy means that, because each person has a unique symptom pattern for an illness or the same disease is subtly different in each individual, the therapy must closely address variations from person to person. The law of similars along with the idea of minimum or small dose is based on the belief that major effectiveness of remedies can be obtained with the lowest dose possible by diluting and vigorously mixing the original substance with alcohol or water, in extremely small concentrations of the substance (Johnson & Boon, 2007; NCCIH, 2015a).

Small or Minimum Dose   Another principle associated with homeopathy is the law of minimum dose. According to this law, the lower the dose of the agent, the greater its effectiveness and the fewer its side effects. Many homeopathic remedies are prepared in such a way that no molecules of the original substance are noted in the compounds (NCCIH, 2015b). Homeopathic treatments are processed from plants, minerals, or animals. Some of the substances used in homeopathic treatments include belladonna, stinging nettle, and poison ivy, which are believed to activate a natural healing process. Homeopathic treatments are commercially available in different forms, such as tablets, ointments, gels, liquid drops, and creams (NCCIH, 2015b; Sutton, 2010).

Contemporary literature supports the principle of similar curatives and the use of ultra-high dilutions. Bellavite et al. (2015) documented an extensive list of cellular changes that have been established with increasing dilutions. These changes include increased apoptosis, which means the cell self-elimination damaged cells. Other changes are increased interferon-g production, decreased free radical production (a substance that can be harmful to tissues in the body), increased osteogenesis (or brittle bones), and increased or decreased expression of different groups of genes. Boldyreva (2011) also in part supports the importance of such physiological changes that occur in the body with ultra-high dilutions.

According to Bellavite et al. (2015), changes at the cellular level come in through one of three means: stimulation, inhibition, or differentiation. It is assumed that the higher the sensitivity to a regulatory factor, the lower the dose needed for effect. This is well documented for dilution of homeopathic remedies in a variety of cellular situations. Bellavite et al. offered the example of the regulatory capability that exists with nanoparticles, which is activated with diluted substances during dynamization or vigorous mixing of solutions. These particles may, in fact, lower the dose amount for regulating biologic events. If these lower doses can be specified, they can ward off subsequent negative effects that can come from excessive dosing.

Other examples are cited for prevention of breast cancer. Concepts such as detoxification, or clearing from the body accumulated toxins that are built up from environmental substances or viral or bacterial infections; antioxidant therapies to minimize oxidative stress in the body; and immune enhancement through the use of mushroom extracts, thymus extracts, and colostrum are also cited in the literature (Longevity Health Center, 2015). For example, Bellavite et al. (2015) indicated that even infinitesimal changes in molecules that bind to receptors can make a substantial difference in the efficiency of their role or even result in opposing outcomes. One such relationship exists with the use of tamoxifen, a substance that shows an estrogen-opposing activity in breast tissue, but can exhibit an estrogen-like behavior in other body tissues.

Under supervision of a trained medical professional, many homeo-pathic remedies are found to be safe, effective, and causing no serious adverse effects. In addition, no major drug interactions have been reported by the United States Food and Drug Administration (FDA) when the homeopathic treatment has been provided by a trained healthcare worker

(NCCAM, 2013a); however, it is important to recognize that adverse effects can arise in any CAIH therapy, including homeopathy.

In the United States, the FDA regulates homeopathic drugs but does not evaluate their efficacy and safety (NCCIH, 2015a). The FDA can and does allow the distribution of certain homeopathic drugs without prior approval. A current list developed in the Homeopathic Pharmacopeia of the United States (HPUS) contains a description of active ingredients that are legally accepted and can be sold as homeopathic products in the country. The FDA also requires that homeopathic remedies have the following information within the product packaging:

An appropriate label on the outside of the medication

Proper indications and/or diagnosis for the illness being treated

A list of all the ingredients

The dilution of the active ingredients

Correct dispensing dose of the homeopathic medication
    (NCCAM, 2009)

A few homeopathic products have been promoted as "homeopathic immunizations" and have been marketed as a substitute for traditionally recommended childhood immunizations. The NCCIH (2015b), however, continues to support the Centers for Disease Control and Prevention's (CDC) current recommendations for childhood vaccinations and immunizations. The FDA (2015) also advises that patients consult a healthcare professional regarding the use of any complementary and alternative treatments. Doing this ensures proper and efficient coordination of the individual's healthcare by his or her healthcare provider.

Consumers should always discuss the use of any homeopathic treatment with medical providers. Consumers should also be encouraged to follow the CDC's recommended immunization schedule. If consumers are pregnant or nursing, they should be encouraged to consult with a medical provider before starting the use of any homeopathic treatment or any product marked as natural.

Naturopathy

Naturopathy is an alternative medical system which proposes that there is a healing power in the body that establishes, maintains, and restores health (NCCIH, 2015b). The approach of naturopathy emphasizes the patient's role as a respondent and activist in his or her healthcare and well-being. Practitioners work with patients with the goal of supporting their personal power through treatments such as nutrition and lifestyle counseling, dietary supplements, medicinal plants, exercise, homeopathy, and treatments from traditional Chinese medicine (NCCAM, 2012c).

Naturopathic medicine focuses much of the patient's health on the responsibility for his or her own well-being. Through education by a naturopathic provider, the patient adheres to a healthy lifestyle, a healthier diet, and an overall health prevention plan for life. In fact, the word *naturopathy* comes from the Greek word that means "nature disease" and encompasses the belief that nature (e.g., one's own body processes) has an innate ability to heal itself or heal disease (NCCAM, 2012c).

Naturopathic medicine aims to strengthen the body's immune system. According to the 2007 NHIS, an estimated 729,000 adults and 237,000 children used a naturopathic treatment in 2006 (NCCAM, 2012c). According to the NCCAM (2012c), naturopathic remedies are found to be relatively safe and have a low risk of side effects compared to some conventional medical treatments. In addition, these remedies have limited interference with conventional medications (NCCAM, 2012c).

A study supported by the NCCAM (2008) reported on a group of 70 warehouse workers experiencing low back pain that occurred during daily job duties. Naturopathic therapies, such as acupuncture, exercise, and diet modification, were initiated and were found to have positive results. The naturopathic therapy was beneficial to employers since it reduced medical expenses for both employer and employee, and resulted in fewer injuries and less employee absenteeism, and benefited employees by increasing quality of life.

A study by Herman, Szczurko, and Cooley (2008) also supported several benefits to using naturopathic medicine, including being a less costly and less invasive treatment than Western medicine. In this study, the naturopathic modalities of exercise, relaxation techniques, and acupuncture were studied in low back pain, among patients who were warehouse workers. The study showed that the naturopathic remedies were more successful and cost effective compared to pain medication and other Western medical treatments.

Naturopathy practitioners believe first in doing no harm. In addition, they believe strongly in patient education aimed at helping consumers take responsibility for their own health. Naturopaths believe that disease is a normal occurrence. They believe in treating the whole person and all factors that can contribute to illness. These factors may be spiritual, emotional, physical, mental, and environmental (NCCAM, 2012c).

Another principle of naturopathy is that health promotion and prevention of disease are critical. It is the practitioner's role to assist patients in understanding their risk factors and preventing subsequent illness. Factors such as lack of exercise or poor diet can disrupt the body's homeostatic function. Naturopathic practitioners believe that living healthier lifestyles will promote optimal health in patients and prevent potential diseases (NCCIH, 2015d).

A third principle promoted by naturopathic practitioners is the healing power of nature and the body's natural processes. It is a naturopathic belief that the body has its own innate capability to heal itself and restore health. This is done by the body's own defenses, such as the immune system. The advent of natural approaches, such as rest and diet, can help the body's systems heal themselves (NCCAM, 2012c).

In addition, naturopathic practitioners believe that germs are not the causative agent of diseases. Based on these ideas, they do not seek to treat the symptoms but the underlying disease. For example, if the disease is seen as an accumulation of toxins in the body as caused by stress, the stress would need to be addressed, not the symptoms that manifest stress (Synovitz & Larson, 2013; Dunne, Benda, Kim, Mittman, Barrett, Snider & Pizzommo, 2005). Toxins can come in the form of accumulated substances in the body, such as alcohol or cholesterol from a poor diet. Therefore, practitioners need to treat the underlying causes of diseases, not the symptoms. Symptoms are viewed as positive indicators that the body is self-healing and undergoing recovery or accommodating to the pathological condition.

Naturopathic providers believe that their role is to support the patient's own body in its ability to keep or restore health, and they are trained to see illness as a disruption of the body's normal functions. To naturopathic providers, health is the body's ability to return to normal homeostatic function; therefore, they view the patient as a whole and try to achieve an understanding of the totality of factors that create illness.

Some treatments of naturopathic medicine are herbal medicines, dietary changes, counseling, hydrotherapy, physical medicine, exercise therapy, and lifestyle counseling (NCCAM, 2012c). Naturopathic treatments focus on the innate ability to restore and maintain health by balancing the functions of various body systems, such as the immune system and the endocrine system. In order to attain equilibrium in these systems, naturopaths encourage patients to use natural elements, such as sunlight, air, water, rest, and exercise (Synovitz & Larson, 2013).

Naturopathic providers seldom treat their patients with medications and perform more therapeutic measures with their patients. Therapeutic measures include promoting normal sleep patterns, balancing dietary needs, and using dietary supplements or herbal medicines. Naturopaths use education and guidance to encourage patients to take responsibility for healthier lifestyles, leading to an increased function of the body, which could mean, for example, less joint pain or a decrease in symptoms that were once present (Fontaine, 2013).

Fasting

In the strictest definition, fasting, also known as dry fasting, means a brief period of abstinence from food and the continued drinking of water. Fasting therapy has been associated with religious and spiritual practices for centuries, and it continues to be practiced among many religions. It is believed that fasting therapy strengthens the mind and increases one's spiritual focus (Hartman, 2012). In some religions, individuals refrain from food and drink during specific hours of the day and during certain times of the year; in others, individuals may fast for a period of up to 24 hours in order to pray and meditate to increase spirituality.

From a naturopathic standpoint, fasting often is seen as a type of detoxification. Some have endorsed it as a therapy for cancer or other conditions. Although fasting therapy is not clearly defined by the NCCIH, it has been identified as a natural modality to restore health and treat medical illnesses. Fasting therapy is believed to be a therapeutic modality to treat acute and chronic illnesses. The development of fasting in the United States began as early as the 20th century. Fasting methods consist of water and teas, followed up by enemas and exercise (Hartman, 2012).

Fasting has been used to treat cancer in place of traditional Western medicine. A qualified physician, such as an oncologist, may use fasting and juice therapy along with the usual cancer treatments. A bulletin by the National Cancer Institute (2012) indicated that a University of Southern California doctor found that a few days of fasting can protect normal cells in lab animals from the effects of chemotherapy drugs; however, it did not protect cancer cells, inferring that fasting prior to chemotherapy may have a protective effect on normal cells while allowing chemotherapy to kill the cancerous cells. Patients who voluntarily abstain from food and consume particular fruits and vegetable juices believe that this modality will cleanse and detoxify the internal body (Hartman, 2012). Those who ascribe to this type of fast believe that juices assist the immune system to function and detoxify the body by resting the physiological systems and increasing physical healing.

The American Cancer Society (ACS) did not agree with the fasting and juicing modalities and felt that there are no scientific bases for detoxification as a cure for cancer. Some risks and adverse effects of fasting therapies are anemia, dizziness, tiredness, low blood pressure, and irregular heartbeat. Fasting may also interfere with medical conditions, such as diabetes, due to increased glucose levels and issues related to increased acidity and irritation in the lining of the stomach (Hartman, 2012; Ziberter & Ziberter, 2014; Kanazawa & Fukudo, 2006).

Given some of the risks just listed, adverse effects from fasting are a concern. For instance, even though animal studies such as the one done by Lee et al. (2012) indicated positive effects in animals, such studies have not been replicated in humans. Lee et al. subjected mice with cancer to short-term starvation or fasting for up to 48 to 60 hours and found that the mice had less normal cell destruction after receiving chemotherapy than mice that ate normally before receiving chemotherapy.

Beyond fasting as a cancer intervention, studies have been performed on the effect of dietary restriction (commonly known as caloric restriction [CR] and intermittent fasting [IF]) on brain plasticity, and fasting to restrict calorie intake and its effect on obesity and disease risks that accompany obesity (such as hypertension and diabetes).

Studies have examined the effect of fasting via skipping breakfast, extreme fasting with a period of starvation, or fasting with caloric restrictions and have found positive results (Ziberter & Ziberter, 2014; Kanazawa & Fukudo, 2006; Michalsen, Hoffmann, Moebus, Backer, Langhorst, & Dobos, 2005). Furthermore, it is suggested that lack of breakfast can be a metabolic advantage. In fact, studies have suggested that skipping breakfast (or dinner) leads to a decreased caloric intake and therefore a decrease in obesity, and therefore, a lower rate of overall disease processes ultimately associated with obesity (Ziberter & Ziberter, 2014). The Ziberter and Ziberter study also suggested that as long as there are significant occasional breaks between meals to allow for ketosis (or normal metabolic process) and lipolysis (breakdown of fat) with the corresponding lower calorie intake, there will be less risk of obesity and other diseases.

Research supports the idea that dietary factors can promote positive effects on brain plasticity. For example, dietary interventions including CR seem to promote synaptic metabolic reactions to oxidative damage. They also appear to affect the number, structure and function of synapses. Likewise, CR has been shown to reduce abdominal fat mass, increase insulin sensitivity, and reduce levels of proinflammatory cytokines, reactive oxygen species, and blood lipids (Murphy, Dias, & Thuret, 2014).

Herbal Medicine

Herbal medicines are defined as remedies coming from plants. Plant components that can be included are roots, stems, flowers, seeds, and other elements. Plant substrates that also can be utilized are chemicals pulled from the plant's structure. Examples of these applications include an agent to add scent (aromatherapy), a therapeutic medical treatment, and seasoning for foods.

Herbs and spices are subsets of a larger group, known as botanicals, which are valued for their medicinal or therapeutic properties including flavor and scent. Spices are used to flavor and for their aromatic properties in seasoning, whereas herbs are plants used to maintain or improve health via their phytomedical properties. Herbs can be used in conjunction with each other or alone. Herbs can be sold dried or fresh, or as chemical extracts from the plant. Many herbs are also incorporated in cosmetic products to enhance fragrances and appearance. For example, cinnamon may make a cosmetic have an appealing odor. Also, prescription products may contain herbs to enhance their chemical properties (Synovitz & Larson, 2013). Among some of the most popular herbs are gingko biloba, St. John's wort, garlic, soy, and kava kava. A fair amount of scientific evidence supports their efficacy and notes their risks.

It is important to note that there are safety concerns surrounding herbal therapies. Two commonly cited safety issues include various forms of herbal toxicity and the presence of contaminants in herbs. For example, development of nephropathy, end-stage renal failure, and prophylactic kidney removal have been linked to the herb *Aristolochia fangchi* in some patients. Urothelial carcinoma also has been associated with some herbs. This cancer is related to DNA structural changes via the aristolochic acid found in herbs. Other common toxic components of herbal medicines are pyrrolizidine alkaloids, which are found in certain plants and are used as additives in herbal medicines. In addition, foreign-prepared herbs, which may not be regulated in the same way as US-produced herbs, can contain processing contaminants, such as heavy metals and other substances (Bent, 2008).

Dietary Supplements

Dietary supplements—vitamins, minerals, and nonvitamin, nonmineral natural products—can be classified as a botanicals if they meet the guidelines set forth in the Dietary Supplement Health and Education Act (DSHEA) of 1994. Under the DSHEA, products deemed to be dietary supplements are those that include one or more of these ingredients: vitamins, minerals, herbs or other botanicals, amino acids, or substances intended to supplement the diet by increasing dietary intake. The DSHEA also stipulates that the product must not be represented for use as a conventional food or as a sole meal, and it must be labeled as a dietary supplement (US FDA, 2009a; National Institutes of Health, 1994). According to the FDA, items classified as dietary supplements must be taken by mouth in the form of pill, capsule, gelcaps, tablet, or liquid. Botanicals in general can be in many forms, including fresh or dried, liquid or solid extracts, tablets, capsules, powder, tea bags, and others (NCCAM, 2013c; University of Maryland Medical Center, 2013; US FDA, 2009b; US FDA 2009c).

Nonvitamin, nonmineral natural products are taken by mouth and contain dietary ingredients (other than vitamins and minerals) intended to supplement the diet. Other botanical products include soy or flax products and dietary substances such as enzymes and glandulars. Among the most popular forms of botanical products reported in the 2012 NHIS are echinacea, ginseng, flaxseed, and fish oil (NCCAM, 2013d). Garlic, for example, has been used to treat fevers, sore throats, digestive ailments, hardening of the arteries, and other health problems and conditions (US FDA, 2009b; NCCAM, 2013c; University of Maryland Medical Center, 2013).

Nonvitamin, nonmineral dietary supplements were the most commonly used CAM modality reported by the 2007 and 2012 NHIS (17.7%) and the 2002 NHIS (18.9%). The most commonly taken of these supplements reported in the 2007 and 2012 NHIS were fish oil, glucosamine, chondroitin, or a combination supplement (Clarke et al., 2015).

There are too many herbal medicines and dietary supplements to describe individually in this chapter. Table 3.1 presents a summary of the most commonly used dietary supplements and herbal medicines available. This table is not comprehensive. For detailed and up-to-date information on the scientific properties, uses, and risks of supplements, consult the US National Library of Medicine (MedlinePlus) at http://www.nlm.nih.gov/medlineplus/ and the NCCIH at https://nccih.nih.gov. These federal agencies provide information for consumers and scientists. A comprehensive description of herbs or botanicals with common names, evidence-based information, potential side effects, cautions, and additional resources can be found at https://nccih.nih.gov/health/herbsataglance.htm. It is important to check these resources and consult with a trained health provider prior to the use of any herbal medicine or dietary supplement.

Consumer Issues

In recent years, global and US regulatory guidelines have increased for medications and CAM therapies. The growing use of herbal medications combined with their increased advertisement and accessibility online has led to more regulatory action in the form of more product labeling and more consumer education efforts.

Safety concerns with herbal medications can arise from areas that are not necessarily a concern with well-regulated, traditional, pharmaceutical medications prescribed by medical doctors. In addition, although many herbal medications do not show a pattern of harm, there is still a risk mostly associated with the self-prescription behavior of clients. Often patients lack adequate knowledge about the potential side effects of herbal

Table 3.1 Applications of Some of the Most Commonly Used Dietary Supplements, Herbal Medicines, and Nonvitamin, Nonmineral Natural Products

Commonly Used Dietary Supplements and Herbal Medicines	Uses	Scientific Evidence to Support Use	Possible Side Effects or Interactions with Use
Fish oil/Omega 3/DHA	Fish oil is considered good for the neurological system. It is found in mackerel, tuna, salmon, anchovy, and trout. Supplements can be coupled with calcium, iron, and vitamins A, B1, B2, B3, C, or D. Applied to a wide range of varying levels of pathologies. Some effectiveness is noted for cardiac and circulatory systems.	The Natural Center for Complementary and Integrative Health provides information on fish oil as effective for high triglycerides; likely effective for heart disease; and possibly effective for high blood pressure, rheumatoid arthritis, menstrual pain, attention-deficit/hyperactivity disorder, Raynaud's syndrome, stroke (moderate amounts only), osteoporosis, atherosclerosis, kidney problems, bipolar disorder, psychosis, weight loss, endometrial cancer, age-related eye disease, and asthma in children (not adults).	Low doses seem safe. High doses may create complications, such as decreased immune system responses and risk of bleeding.
Glucosamine	Two types exist: glucosamine hydrochloride and glucosamine sulfate. The primary use is for osteoarthritis, knee pain, rheumatoid arthritis, back pain, and glaucoma.	The Natural Medicines Comprehensive Database indicates insufficient evidence on glucosamine hydrochloride.	Side effects include gastrointestinal symptoms, such as gas and cramps. Glucosamine may interfere with some cancer medications, and it is not recommended for use with warfarin, if undergoing surgery, or with medications for diabetes or asthma.
Echinacea	Utilized as an antiviral to combat the cold or the flu.	A 2007 meta-analysis reviewing 14 studies indicated favorable results with echinacea for decreasing both duration and severity of colds.	Side effects are not common; however, gastrointestinal effects and rashes have been noted. Allergic reactions to items in the daisy family of plants are more likely to occur with use. Anaphylaxis is possible.

Flaxseed	Used to treat arthritis, to prevent cancer, as a laxative, and for breast pain, hot flashes, and high cholesterol.	There is mixed evidence about its effects. Some studies indicate flaxseed may reduce the risk of some cancers and that it may be beneficial for some heart diseases, particularly lowering cholesterol in individuals with high starting cholesterol, as well as for postmenopausal women.	Few side effects. May possibly lower the body's ability to absorb medications. Not recommended for use when taking with other conventional oral medications.
Ginseng	Lowers blood glucose levels and benefits immune function. Research is under way for insulin resistance, cancer, and Alzheimer's disease.	Compiled research does not completely support the positive benefits associated with ginseng; however, much of this research is based on small studies and laboratory research, not human studies.	Side effects may include headaches, sleep problems, and gastrointestinal problems. Allergic reactions are possible.
Gingko biloba	Used for memory enhancement. Also used in the treatment of dementia, intermittent claudication, and tinnitus.	Large, recent studies (some lasting for six years) have not indicated increases in memory or decrease in dementia.	Side effects may include: possibility of nausea, gastrointestinal upset, diarrhea, dizziness, or allergic skin reactions. It is not recommended for people with bleeding disorders or with pending surgery because it can increase bleeding. Raw seeds contain gingkotoxin, which can lead to seizures and death. An animal study has shown that long-term use can lead to tumor formation.

(continued)

Table 3.1 Applications of Some of the Most Commonly Used Dietary Supplements, Herbal Medicines, and Nonvitamin, Nonmineral Natural Products (*continued*)

Commonly Used Dietary Supplements and Herbal Medicines	Uses	Scientific Evidence to Support Use	Possible Side Effects or Interactions with Use
Garlic supplements	Used to treat high cholesterol, heart disease, and high blood pressure. Used in the prevention of stomach and colon cancers.	Studies indicate that garlic may lower blood pressure slightly, particularly for those who have hypertension. Although some studies indicate regularly consumed garlic may lower the risk of some cancers, a long-term study on stomach cancer did not find an effect.	Use of garlic supplements appears safe. Garlic odor of breath and body can occur with use. Other side effects may include heartburn, upset stomach, possible allergic reactions, or thinning blood (similar to aspirin). Garlic supplements interfere with the HIV drug saquinavir.
Coenzyme Q-10	Occurs naturally in the body. It functions to transform food into energy and is a powerful antioxidant. (Antioxidants fight damage caused by free radicals.)	Some (mostly animal) studies have indicated a positive effect on the immune system in helping resist some infections. Some (mostly animal) studies have indicated that it may prevent some types of cancers. Use may decrease the effect of heart damage from cancer drugs.	May not work well or mix safely with other treatments. The effect on patients undergoing chemotherapy needs to be evaluated more.

Sources: Adapted from Barrett et al. (2002); Bent (2008); National Center for Complementary and Alternative Medicine (2012b, 2013b, c, 2015e); National Library of Medicine (2011, 2013a,b); Shah, Sander, White, Rinaldi, & Coleman (2007); University of Maryland Cancer Center (2015); and Van Kampen, Baranowski, Shaw, & Kay (2014).

medications, the risk of overdose, and the possibility of interaction with over-the-counter and prescribed medications. In rare cases, there is a potential for harm due to the herbal medication itself (WHO, 2002). Moreover, patients who self-prescribe herbal medications often do not share this knowledge with their physicians. Consequently, interactions can arise with prescribed medications.

The regulation of homeopathy in the United States is not uniform from state to state. Variations in regulatory laws result in homeopathic practices that differ from region to region. Often, if an individual is a licensed medical practitioner (e.g., a medical doctor or registered nurse), he or she can legally practice homeopathy. It is also true that in some states, nonlicensed professionals practice homeopathy (NCCIH, 2015b).

Naturopathy as a practice in the United States has various types of practitioners: naturopathic physicians, traditional naturopaths, and other healthcare providers who practice and offer naturopathic care. The titles by which they are known vary from naturopathic physicians to naturopathic doctors (NCCAM, 2012c).

Research surrounding homeopathic practices is difficult because of the lack of uniformity in its practice and the lack of drug standardization in homeopathic remedies. Remedies may also be more tailored to the individual and not suited for study in large, controlled types of research designs.

Homeopathic preparations are regulated under the Federal Food, Drug and Cosmetic Act, although even today the FDA does not evaluate the effectiveness and safety of homeopathic remedies (US FDA, 2015). Currently, the FDA is evaluating the regulation effectiveness of homeopathic products, but no decisions were in place as of the time of this writing.

The FDA (NCCAM, 2012b) also requires that homeopathic remedies have all of the following information within the product packaging:

An appropriate label on the outside of the medication

Proper indications and/or diagnosis for the illness being treated

A list of all the ingredients

The dilution of the active ingredients

Correct dispensing dose of the homeopathic medication

Enforcement policies for homeopathic treatments are addressed in the FDA's policy guide titled "Conditions under Which Homeopathic Drugs May Be Marketed" (CPG 7132.15) (NCCIH, 2015a).

The Center for Food Safety and Applied Nutrition (CFSAN) has determined that certain key products are popular with those who attempt to defraud the public. These products include those that affect weight loss, sexual performance, memory loss, and serious diseases such as cancer, diabetes, heart disease, arthritis, and Alzheimer's (US FDA, 2014a,c,e). The FDA provided following guidelines for consumers when using natural CAM products:

1. Awareness of a product that claims to treat multiple conditions.

2. Products that use personal testimonies about unrealistic success.

3. Products that indicate quick cures.

4. Products that indicate they are all natural as a primary selling point. *All natural* does not always mean safe or effective because naturally occurring elements can be dangerous and poisonous.

5. Things that are referred to as new or breakthrough or as having secret undiscovered ingredients.

6. Products that claim the government and/or pharmaceutical companies have hidden information about their curative nature (US FDA, 2014d).

A key piece of historical legislation that protects consumers is DSHEA, which allows consumers access to the products they desire while giving the public some protection against dietary supplements that may have potential harmful effects. A by-product of the DSHEA law was mandatory labeling of CAM products with lists of ingredients. Supplements have a postmarket evaluation if they contain well-known ingredients and a 75-day premarket notification for items that contain new ingredients. For new ingredients, the manufacturer is required to submit citations that establish reasonable arguments as to why the supplement is expected to work and evidence of reasonable safety (US Department of Health and Human Services [DHHS], 2011; US FDA, 2014a,e; WHO, 2014).

In conclusion, it is important to be aware of certain considerations when contemplating the use of homeopathic, naturopathic, and dietary supplement treatments. As advised by all professional health organizations and the NCCIH, it is important to always discuss the use of any new medication, whether they are dietary supplements or other conventional medication prescriptions by healthcare providers, with your primary medical provider. It is also advised that individuals continue to follow the immunization schedule recommended for children and adults by the CDC. Natural practices such as fasting are closely related to CAIH since they are used to promote health and wellness. Although fasting is usually seen as safe, it is important to remember that no CAIH modality is completely free of risk. Consultation with a healthcare provider is always advised, especially if the consumer is pregnant or nursing.

Implications for Health Professionals

Health professionals play a major role in educating the public about natural CAIH products. The advocacy role of health practitioners in the development of research that provides evidence on the safety, benefits, and risks of natural products should be evident. They should also be active participants in the enactment of legislation that protects consumers from quackery. Health professionals should become familiar with the regulatory and legislative processes related to natural CAIH modalities.

The FDA sets guidelines for the quality standards of dietary supplements. The guidelines are meant to promote purity, accuracy of strength, and composition. It is also the intent of the standards to prevent wrongful ingredients, such as contaminants, and to prevent mislabeling of dietary supplements. In addition, the FDA conducts inspections of facilities that manufacture dietary supplements. Within the United States, major independent entities (e.g., US Pharmacopeia, ConsumerLab, and National Science Foundation International) evaluate the integrity of dietary supplement products. A product bearing the seal of approval of these entities is said to be guaranteed as properly manufactured, free of harmful levels of contaminants, and with accurate amounts of active ingredients as posted on the label. However, these independent assessments do not guarantee the safety or effectiveness of any dietary supplement (US DHHS, 2011; US FDA, 2014c,e).

Federal oversight and regulation of dietary supplements is different from those for prescription or over-the-counter drugs. One major difference is that drugs must be approved by the FDA before they can be placed on the market. This is not the case for dietary supplements. Although supplement manufacturers are required to have evidence that the product is safe and that the label claims are accurate, they do not have to provide this information prior to marketing the product. Once a product is placed on the market, the FDA does monitor it and will take legal steps against manufacturers and websites that market supplements if they are perpetuating false claims, such as attesting to be a curative agent for any type of disease or if the product is deemed to be unsafe for humans consumption as determined in part by currently regulated substance codes and laws (US DHHS, 2011; US FDA, 2014a,c,e).

Even though dietary supplement use has increased, few instances of harmful results have been reported, yet the FDA takes action when appropriate. In 2014, the FDA instituted a mandatory recall of a weight-loss pill intervention to ensure consumer safety. The presence in the pills of two substances, sibutramine and phenolphthalein, compelled the recall. Sibutramine and phenolphthalein were once FDA approved; however, there have been recent concerns that phenolphthalein could be carcinogenic, and sibutramine was associated with an increased risk of seizures, heart attacks, arrhythmia, and strokes. Sibutramine is considered a controlled substance that had been approved for the treatment of obesity; since it is a controlled substance, however, it cannot be included in dietary supplements (US FDA, 2014a,b,c,d,e).

Several groups ensure the safety of natural products. CFSAN regulates dietary supplements. The Federal Trade Commission (FTC) regulates false and misleading health claims. The NCCIH also plays a major role in the development of evidence on CAIH efficacy and in determining how CAIH protocols could be integrated into Western medicine approaches. A major challenge for health professionals is to work cooperatively with these agencies. Patients who choose CAM remedies may require their health professionals to incorporate natural CAM remedies alongside the traditional medical model to achieve what the patient feels would be best for his or her well-being. Once natural CAM remedies are utilized for health maintenance, they can be considered CAIH approaches.

Caveat Emptor

Although natural products have a reputation of being safe, they still carry risks that must be minimized through guidelines and policies. The need for regulatory mandates to increase the safety of natural CAIH products is of particular interest for health professionals, including health educators. Given the growth in the use of natural products, it is important to ask what role the government plays in interacting with the consumer, the products, and those who manufacture the supplements. This section describes the role of some agencies that have oversight authority and regulatory power on natural CAIH products.

The FDA is an agency within the Department of Health and Human Services that oversees the relationships between consumers and manufacturers. It is seen as protecting the public by ensuring the safety and efficacy of drugs, biological products, and medical devices, as well as the food supply. This agency regulates and monitors the development of medicines that are effective and safe and assists the public by providing the most accurate science-based information on medicines and foods. Its scope of practice includes natural CAIH products such as herbal medicines and dietary supplements (US DHHS, 2011; US FDA, 2009b; US Pharmacopeia, n.d.).

CFSAN within the FDA plays a primary role in advocating for the education of the public on dietary supplements and alternative products. The Federal Food, Drug, and Cosmetic Act of 1938 provided specifications prohibiting false therapeutic claims for medications and controlled product advertising (US FDA, 2012). In addition, the act was the original act from which all modern legal amendments that govern the use of herbal medication and dietary supplements are derived (World Intellectual Property Organization, 2014).

The Dietary Supplement Health and Education Act (DSHEA) recognized that the use of dietary supplements would continue to grow as a result of several factors, including lack of health insurance, lack of faith in Western medicine, and the diversification of the US population. It acknowledged that one motivation for Americans to use dietary supplements was most likely because of their view that supplements can be a less costly and a potentially healthier means to mitigate the side effects and costs of Western medical treatment. Since the passage of the DSHEA, the government began developing a formal mechanism to educate and empower consumers. Its efforts may have broadened consumers' choices and health outcomes, based on the premise that the government's role should be to promote sound scientific evidence regarding the use of dietary supplements (US FDA, 2009b).

Recognizing that the dietary supplement industry was now a strong part of the US economy, the government wanted to choose a course that would not impose unreasonable restrictions. Its position was meant to enable, not disable, US consumers and to allow them access to safe products (US FDA, 2009b).

The 1994 law defined a dietary supplement as a product (not including tobacco) that was meant to supplement the diet and that contained one or more of the following elements: vitamins, minerals, herbs or other botanicals, or amino acids, and that were used to increase total dietary intake. The act further cited various acceptable forms of ingestion for dietary supplements.

According to the 1994 act, statements for dietary supplements may be made if "the statement claims a benefit related to a classical nutrient deficiency disease and discloses the prevalence of such disease in the United States; describes the role of a nutrient or dietary ingredient intended to affect a structure or function in humans; characterizes the documented mechanism by which a nutrient or dietary ingredient acts to maintain such structure or functional characteristic, or describes in general the well-being gained from consumption of a nutrient or dietary ingredient." (US FDA, 2009b).

In addition, the law required that statements put forth by manufacturers must be substantiated as truthful and not misleading. If manufacturers make a claim, that claim must contain the mandatory disclosure statement. Labeling that make claims about affecting the structure or function of the body or well-being or makes claims about addressing nutrient deficiency diseases must have a disclaimer, such as "The FDA has not evaluated the claim and the product is not intended to diagnose, treat, cure, or prevent any disease" (US FDA, 2009b, para. 3).

The FDA promotes a user-friendly approach to educating the consumer when it comes to fraudulent health products. As defined by the FDA (2014a,c,e), a fraudulent product is one that is deceptively touted as being effective against a disease or health condition, but has no scientific proof to support its effectiveness and safety. The FDA indicates that fraudulent advertisements may be found in many venues, including television infomercials, the Internet, and retail stores. Fraudulent products entail more risk than just lost money; they can be damaging and even life-threatening (WHO, 2014).

The FDA partners with a myriad of other agencies of academic and regulatory nature and monitors both research and reports of adverse effects from dietary supplements. The FDA has an adverse event reporting system, which began to compile data in 2003 (US DHHS, 2011; US FDA, 2014b,e; WHO, 2014).

Conclusion

CAIH modalities include homeopathy, naturopathy, fasting, herbal medicines, dietary supplements, and other natural products. Because many areas of CAIH are much less regulated than Western medicine approaches, and because much of the population who use CAIH may do so voluntarily and in a self-monitored way, there is ample opportunity for quackery and for consumers to be exploited. The need for consumer education, legislation, and regulatory guidelines for natural CAIH products is essential. The role of the NCCIH, the FDA, the FTC, and CFSAN in educating and advocating for consumers' protection is evident. Global challenges arise in the use of natural CAIH modalities. Societal concerns regarding the use of these practices include the development of regulatory approaches, the assessment of product efficacy, and the guarantee of quality control or consistency with the delivery of a given intervention.

Summary

- Modalities such as homeopathy, naturopathy, fasting, herbal medicines, dietary supplements, and other natural products have been labeled in the past as natural CAM therapies.

- "Natural" does not mean free of risks. CAIH modalities can cause side effects and drug interactions.

- Homeopathic remedies are regulated by the US Food and Drug Administration, but they are not assessed consistently for safety or effectiveness.

- Naturopathic medicine aims to strengthen the body's immune system.

- Herbal remedies, dietary supplements, and restrictive diets can be harmful if not used under the supervision of a well-trained practitioner.

- Fasting means a brief period of abstinence from food and water, although there are variations in fasting. It is believed that fasting therapy strengthens the mind and increases the individual's spiritual focus. Some risks of fasting have also been noted.

- A major challenge for health professionals is to utilize CAIH remedies to go beyond illness management to the achievement of well-being.

- Consumers should tell their healthcare providers about any natural CAIH modality they are using to ensure coordination of care, to reduce risks, and to maximize safety.

Case Study

Description

Sally has struggled with her desire to lose weight most of her life. She has tried various diets with very little success and no permanent results. Sally feels desperate to find a solution to her unwanted weight. She currently has hypertension and is borderline diabetic. Sally feels guilty when she discusses her weight with her physician. Although her physician is always supportive, she feels ashamed that every time she goes to see her healthcare provider, she has not made any progress toward losing weight. While browsing the Internet, Sally saw an advertisement for a weight-loss supplement. The advertisement stated that the product is guaranteed to cause weight loss until the client has reached an optimal weight. It lists several personal testimonials from satisfied customers. The advertisement indicates that the product is all natural and that it is embedded with a breakthrough miracle fat-burning substance. Sally purchases the items and begins taking the pills. At her next visit with her doctor, Sally does not tell her physician that she is taking the supplement because she is afraid that her doctor will not agree with it.

Questions

1. Based on this case, what advertisement elements are of concern based on the FDA's guidelines for consumers purchasing dietary supplements? Please list and explain.

2. What actions has Sally taken that could be harmful to her health?

3. What policies can be enacted to make dietary supplements into CAIH products that can be used to enhance health and well-being?

KEY TERMS

Dietary supplement. Defined by the Dietary Supplement Health and Education Act as a product that is intended to supplement the diet; it contains dietary ingredients, such as vitamins, minerals, herbs, other botanicals, and amino acids; is intended to be taken by mouth; and has been labeled as a dietary supplement (NCCIH, 2015e).

Fasting. Abstinence from food and liquids with the purpose of improving health. Fasting therapy has been associated with religious and spiritual practices. It is believed that fasting therapy strengthens the mind and increases one's spiritual focus (Hartman, 2012; Ziberter & Ziberter, 2014; Kanazawa & Fukudo, 2006).

Herbal medicine. Also called botanicals or phytotherapy. It is one type of dietary supplement that uses plant or plant derivatives for therapeutic purposes (MedlinePlus, 2015).

Homeopathy. An alternative medical system that originated in Germany at the end of the 18th century which is based on two major theories: "Like cures like," which states that an illness can be cured by a substance that produces similar signs and symptoms in healthy individuals, and the "law of minimum dose," which is based on the belief that major effectiveness of remedies can be obtained with the lowest dose possible (NCCIH, 2015b).

Naturopathy. Medical system that evolved in Europe during the 19th century. It is based on the recognition of the healing power of nature and the ability of the body to maintain and restore health. Naturopathic treatments are natural and believed to often be less invasive than some conventional medical therapies (NCCIH, 2015d).

References

Altunc, U., Pittler, M. H., & Ernst, E. (2007). *Homeopathy for childhood and adolescent ailments: Systematic review of randomized clinical trials. Mayo Clinic Proceedings, 82*(1), 69–75. Retrieved from http://www.ncbi.nlm.nih.gov/pubmed/17285788.

Barrett, B. P., Brown, R. L., Locken, K., Maberry, R., Bobula, J. A., & D'Alessio, D. (2002). Treatment of the common cold with unrefined echinacea: A randomized, double-blind, placebo-controlled trial. *Annals of Internal Medicine, 137*(12), 939–946. Retrieved from http://www.ncbi.nlm.nih.gov/pubmed/12484708

Bellavite, P., Signorini, A., Marzotto, M., Moratti, E., Bonafini, C., & Olioso, D. (2015). Cell sensitivity, non-linearity and inverse effects. *Homeopathy, 104*, 139–160.

Bent, S. (2008). Herbal medicine in the United States: Review of efficacy, safety and regulations. *Journal of General Internal Medicine, 23*(6), 854–859.

Boldyreva, L. (2011). An analogy between effects of ultra-low doses of biologically active substances on biological objects and properties of spin supercurrents in superfluid ^{3}He-B. *Homeopathy, 100*(3), 187–193.

Clarke, T. C., Black L. I., Stussman B. J., Barnes, P. M., & Nahin, R. (2015). Trends in the use of complementary health approaches among adults: United States, 2002–2012. *National Health Statistics Reports No. 79*. Hyattsville, MD: National Center for Health Statistics.

College of Naturopathic Medicine. (n.d.). *What is naturopathy?* Retrieved from www.naturopathy-uk.com/home/home-what-is-naturopathy/

Dunne, N., Benda, W., Kim, L., Mittman, P., Barrett, R., Snider, P., & Pizzorno, J. (2005). Naturopathic medicine: What can patients expect? *Journal of Family Practice, 54*(12), 1067–1072.

Fontaine, K. L. (2013). *Complementary & alternative therapies for nursing practice* (3rd ed.). Englewood Cliffs, NJ: Prentice Hall.

Hartman, K. (2012, February 8). *Fasting might boost chemo's cancer-busting properties.* Retrieved from http://www.scientificamerican.com/article/fasting-might-boost-chemo/

Herman, P. M., Szczurko O., & Cooley K. (2008). Cost-effectiveness of naturopathic care for chronic low back pain. *Alternative Therapies in Health and Medicine, 14*(2), 32–39.

Homeopathic Pharmacopœia of the United States. (2013). *2013 HPUS web site updates.* Retrieved from http://www.hpus.com/updates2013.php

Johnson, T., & Boon, H. (2007). Where does homeopathy fit in pharmacy practice? *American Journal of Pharmacology Education, 71*(1), 1–8.

Kanazawa, M., & Fukudo, S. (2006). Effects of fasting therapy on irritable bowel syndrome. *International Journal of Behavioral Medicine, 13*(2), 214–220.

Lee, C., Raffaghello, L., Brandhorst, S., Safdie, F., Bianchi, G., Marin-Montalvo, A., . . . Longo, V. (2012). Fasting cycles retard growth of tumors and sensitize a range of cancer cell types to chemotherapy. *Science Translational Medicine, 4*(124).

Longevity Health Center. (2015). *A naturopathic perspective on breast cancer.* Retrieved from http://www.longevityhealthcenter.com/naturopathic-breast-cancer-healing.php

Loudon, I. (2006). A brief history of homeopathy. *Journal of the Royal Society of Medicine, 99*(12), 607–610. Retrieved from www.ncbi.nlm.nih.gov/pmc/articles/PMC1676328

MedlinePlus. (2015). *Herbal medicine.* Retrieved from http://www.nlm.nih.gov/medlineplus/herbalmedicine.html

Michalsen, A., Hoffmann, B., Moebus, S., Dacker, M., Langhorst, J., & Dobos, G. (2005). Incorporation of fasting therapy in an integrative medicine ward: Evaluation of outcome, safety, and effects of lifestyle adherence in a large prospective cohort study. *Journal of Alterntive and Complementary Medicine, 11*(4), 601–607.

Murphy, T., Dias, G. P., & Thuret, S. (2014). Effects of diet on brain plasticity in animal and human studies: Mind the gap. *Neural Plasticity, 2014.* Article ID 563160.

National Cancer Institute. (2012). *NCI Cancer Bulletin.*

National Center for Complementary and Alternative Medicine. (2008). *Study points to cost-effectiveness of naturopathic care for low-back pain.* Retrieved from http://nccam.nih.gov/research/results/spotlight/070708.htm

National Center for Complementary and Alternative Medicine. (2009). *Americans spent $33.9 billion out-of-pocket on complementary and alternative medicine.* Retrieved from http://nccam.nih.gov/news/2009/073009.htm

National Center for Complementary and Alternative Medicine. (2012a). Downloadable graphics on CAM use in the United States. Retrieved from http://nccam.nih.gov/news/camstats/2007/graphics.htm

National Center for Complementary and Alternative Medicine. (2012b). Herbs at a glance: Flaxseed and flaxseed oil. Retrieved from https://nccih.nih.gov/health/flaxseed/ataglance.htm

National Center for Complementary and Alternative Medicine. (2012c). *Naturopathy: An introduction.* Retrieved from https://nccih.nih.gov/node/2413#hed1

National Center for Complementary and Alternative Medicine. (2013a). *Complementary, alternative, or integrative health: What's in a name?* Retrieved from http://nccam.nih.gov/health/whatiscam

National Center for Complementary and Alternative Medicine. (2013b). *Herbs at a glance: Garlic.* Retrieved from http://nccam.nih.gov/sites/nccam.nih.gov/files/Herbs_At_A_Glance_Garlic_06-15-2012_0_0.pdf

National Center for Complementary and Alternative Medicine. (2013c). *Herbs at a glance: Gingko.* Retrieved from http://nccam.nih.gov/sites/nccam.nih.gov/files/Herbs_At_A_Glance_Gingko_06-10-2013.pdf

National Center for Complementary and Alternative Medicine. (2013d). *Using dietary supplements wisely.* Retrieved from http://nccam.nih.gov/health/supplements/wiseuse.htm

National Center for Complementary and Integrative Health. (2015a). *Complementary, alternative, or integrative health: What's in a name?* Retrieved from https://nccih.nih.gov/health/integrative-health

National Center for Complementary and Integrative Health. (2015b). *Dietary and herbal supplements.* Retrieved from https://nccih.nih.gov/health/supplements

National Center for Complementary and Integrative Health. (2015c). *Homeopathy: An introduction.* Retrieved from https://nccih.nih.gov/health/homeopathy

National Center for Complementary and Integrative Health. (2015d). *Naturopathy.* Retrieved from https://nccih.nih.gov/health/naturopathy

National Center for Complementary and Integrative Health. (2015e). *Omega-3 supplements: In depth.* Retrieved from https://nccih.nih.gov/health/omega3/introduction.htm

National Institutes of Health. (1994). Dietary Supplement Health and Education Act of 1994. Public Law 103-417. Retrieved from https://ods.od.nih.gov/About/DSHEA_Wording.aspx

National Library of Medicine. (2011). *Glucosamine sulfate.* MedlinePlus. Retrieved from http://www.nlm.nih.gov/medlineplus/druginfo/natural/807.html

National Library of Medicine. (2013a). *Ginseng.* MedlinePlus. Retrieved from http://www.nlm.nih.gov/medlineplus/druginfo/natural/967.html

National Library of Medicine. (2013b). *Glucosamine hydrochloride.* MedlinePlus. Retrieved from https://www.nlm.nih.gov/medlineplus/druginfo/natural/747.html

Shah, S. A., Sander, S., White, C. M., Rinaldi, M., & Coleman, C. I. (2007). Evaluation of echinacea for the prevention and treatment of the common cold: A meta-analysis. *Lancet Infectious Diseases, 7*(7), 473–480. Retrieved from http://www.ncbi.nlm.nih.gov/pubmed/17597571

Sutton, A. (2010). *Complementary and alternative medicine* (4th ed.). Detroit, MI: Omnigraphics.

Synovitz, L. B., & Larson, K. L. (2013). *Complementary and alternative medicine for health professionals: A holistic approach to consumer health.* Burlington, MA: Jones & Bartlett.

University of Maryland Medical Center. (2013). *Complementary and alternative medicine guide.* Retrieved from http://umm.edu/health/medical/altmed/

University of Maryland Medical Center. (2015). *Coenzyme Q10.* http://umm.edu/health/medical/altmed/supplement/coenzyme-q10

US Department of Health and Human Services. (2011). *National Institute of Health: Office of Dietary Supplements.* Retrieved from http://ods.od.nih.gov/HealthInformation/DS_WhatYouNeedToKnow.aspx

US Food and Drug Administration. (2009a). *Dietary Supplement Health and Education Act of 1994.* Retrieved from https://ods.od.nih.gov/About/DSHEA_Wording.aspx

US Food and Drug Administration. (2009b). *Dietary supplement safety act: How is FDA doing 10 years later.* Retrieved from http://www.fda.gov/newsevents/testimony/ucm113767.htm

US Food and Drug Administration. (2009c). *Selected amendments to the FD&C Act.* Retrieved from http://www.fda.gov/RegulatoryInformation/Legislation/SignificantAmendmentstotheFDCAct/default.htm

US Food and Drug Administration. (2012). *FDA history—Part II.* Retrieved from http://www.fda.gov/AboutFDA/WhatWeDo/History/Origin/ucm054826.htm

US Food and Drug Administration. (2014a). *New Life Nutritional Center dietary supplements: Recall—undeclared drug ingredients.* Retrieved from http://www.fda.gov/safety/medwatch/safetyinformation/safetyalertsforhumanmedicalproducts/ucm390685.htm

US Food and Drug Administration. (2014b). *Recall—firm press release.* Retrieved from http://www.fda.gov/Safety/Recalls/ucm390693.htm

US Food and Drug Administration. (2014c). *6 tip-offs to rip-offs: Don't fall for health fraud scams*. Retrieved from http://www.fda.gov/ForConsumers/ConsumerUpdates/ucm341344.htm

US Food and Drug Administration. (2014d). *Tips for dietary supplement users*. Retrieved from http://www.fda.gov/Food/DietarySupplements/UsingDietarySupplements/ucm110493.htm#risks

US Food and Drug Administration. (2014e). *Tips for older dietary supplement users*. Retrieved from http://www.fda.gov/Food/DietarySupplements/UsingDietarySupplements/ucm110493.htm

US Food and Drug Administration. (2015). *Dietary supplements*. Retrieved from http://www.fda.gov/Food/DietarySupplements/

US Pharmacopeia. (n.d.). *The regulation of homeopathic medicine*. Retrieved from http://www.hpus.com/regulations.php

Van Kampen, J. M., Baranowski, D. B., Shaw, C. A., & Kay, D. G. (2014). Panax ginseng is neuroprotective in a novel progressive model of Parkinson's disease. *Experimental Gerontology, 50*, 95–105.

World Health Organization. (2002). *Program on traditional medicine. WHO traditional medicine strategies, 2002–2005*. Geneva. Retrieved from http://herbalnet.healthrepository.org/handle/123456789/2028

World Intellectual Property Organization. (n.d.). *Federal Food, Drug, and Cosmetic Act (FD&C Act)*. Retrieved from http://www.fda.gov/RegulatoryInformation/Legislation/FederalFoodDrugandCosmeticActFDCAct/default.htm

Ziberter, T., & Ziberter, E. Y. (2014). Breakfast: To skip or not to skip? *Frontiers in Public Health, 2*. doi: 10.3389/fpubh.2014.00059

CHAPTER 4

MANIPULATIVE AND BODY-BASED PRACTICES

Kathleen Rindahl, Helda Pinzón-Pérez, and Georgina Castle

According to the 2012 National Health Interview Survey (NHIS), 33.2% of US adults use complementary health approaches. For children, the 2012 NHIS showed that 11.6% of US children ages 4 to 17 received complementary health approaches (National Center for Complementary and Integrative Health [NCCIH], 2015a,i). In 2007, about 12% of the children and 38% of adults participating in the US NHIS survey used some modality of CAM (Barnes, Bloom, & Nahin, 2008). One CAM modality that has experienced important growth is the area of manipulative and body-based practices, specifically therapies that use manual movement of one or more body parts to improve imbalances of joints, soft tissues, and the circulatory and lymphatic system (National Institute of Medicine, 2013; Raby Institute, 2011). This chapter addresses some of the most commonly used manipulative and body-based practices and their applications as complementary, alternative, and integrative health (CAIH) modalities.

Theoretical Concepts

Overview

In 2011, the National Center for Complementary and Alternative Medicine (NCCAM) officially defined *manipulative and body-based practices* as CAM modalities that involved movement of one or more parts of the human body. This classification was based on the 2007 NHIS and included CAM modalities such as chiropractic,

LEARNING OBJECTIVES

At the completion of this chapter, students will be able to:

- Identify the theoretical and scientific basis of massage therapy, acupuncture, acupressure, and chiropractic therapy.

- Describe selected modalities of manipulative and body-based practices.

- Identify the history of selected therapeutic methods for massage therapy, acupuncture, acupressure, and chiropractic.

- Discuss the benefits and risks associated with massage therapy, acupuncture, acupressure, and chiropractic.

- Analyze the research studies conducted on massage therapy, acupuncture, acupressure, and chiropractic.

(continued)

osteopathic manipulation (to move muscles and/or bones by hand), massage, and movement therapies (Barnes et al., 2008; NCCAM, 2013f).

In 2013, the NCCAM modified this classification and called it *mind and body practices.* It included a group of procedures and techniques such as acupuncture, massage therapy, meditation, movement therapies, relaxation techniques, spinal manipulation, tai chi, qi gong, yoga, healing touch, and hypnotherapy. The *movement therapies* included the Feldenkrais method, Alexander technique, Pilates, Rolfing Structural Integration, and Trager psychophysical integration. The *relaxation techniques* category included breathing exercises, guided imagery, and progressive muscle relaxation (NCCAM, 2013e).

In 2015, the National Center for Complementary and Integrative Health (NCCIH), formerly known as NCCAM, defined mind and body practices as approaches that "may be used to improve health and well-being or to help manage symptoms of health problems" (2015f). This definition confirms that mind and body practices could be classified as CAIH approaches. Manipulative and body-based practices are currently included in the classification of mind and body approaches. According to the NCCIH (2015f), "Mind and body approaches most commonly used by adults include yoga, chiropractic or osteopathic manipulation, meditation, and massage therapy."

According to the NCCIH (2015i), the popularity of some mind and body practices, such as massage, decreased substantially between 2007 and 2012. Among adults, the use of massage therapy was 8.3% in 2007 and only 6.9% in 2012. According to the 2012 NHIS, 0.7% of children used massaged therapy. For chiropractic approaches, the 2012 NHIS showed that 8.4% of adults and 3.3% of children use chiropractic care (NCCIH, 2015i). For acupuncture, the 2012 NHIS indicated that 1.5% of adults used this form of CAIH; in the 2007 NHIS an estimated 1.4% and in the 2002 NHIS an estimated 1.1% used acupuncture (NCCIH, 2015g). Other mind-body practices included in the 2012 NHIS were yoga (9.5% of adults and 3.1% of children) and meditation (8.0% adults and 1.6% children).

The 2007 NHIS found that an estimated 18 million adults and 700,000 children had used massage therapy in 2006 (NCCAM, 2013a). In addition, approximately 150,000 children had used acupuncture in 2006, an increase of approximately 1 million more users between 2002 and 2007 (NCCAM, 2013a,b). The survey also revealed that 8.6% of adult participants (more than 18 million) and 3% of children (more than 2 million) had used chiropractic or osteopathic manipulation during the year preceding the survey (NCCAM, 2013a,c,d). Given their prevalent use among US populations, this chapter focuses on massage therapy, acupuncture, acupressure, and chiropractic care as major manipulative and body-based modalities that were included in the 2007 and 2012 NHIS.

Modalities

Massage Therapy

History and Overview of Massage

The NCCIH (2015e) defined massage therapy as the systematic manipulation of muscles and other soft tissues of the body by pressing and rubbing through the hands, fingers, forearms, elbows, or feet of a trained therapist. The goal of massage therapy is to promote the health and well-being of the individual (Fontaine, 2011; NCCIH, 2015e). This definition clearly describes the nature of this type of therapy as a CAIH practice since it emphasizes the value of massage as an integrative modality to maximize health and wellness.

The therapeutic process of massage can include stroking, kneading, compressing, rocking, applying friction, vibration, percussion, pressure, and/or movement of the body or body parts within the normal anatomical range of movement. Massage techniques are applied by the therapist's hands, fingertips, forearm, elbow, and in some cases feet. Some therapies include the use of massage devices that imitate or potentiate the human touch. Typically massage therapy is delivered with the use of lubricants, such as oil or cream, to decrease the friction between the client's skin and the therapist's touch. Some massage therapies incorporate the use of hot and cold stones for muscle relaxation as well as salt rubs or herbal preparations to provide stimulating friction to exfoliate the skin. Some therapists may add aromatherapy in the healing sessions (Coughlin, 2002; Nelson, 2010). It is important to note that massage therapy does not include spinal manipulation or physical therapy.

The use of therapeutic touch to help promote healing has its roots in almost every culture throughout history. References to the use of massage as a healing art have been identified in the Tibetan and Chinese cultures as early as 3000 BCE (Fontaine, 2011; Rost, 2009). The earliest illustration of the use of massage therapy was found in Egyptian tomb paintings dating back to approximately 2500 BCE (R. Calvert, 2002). The practice of massage was a part of everyday life in Roman and Greek history (Synovitz & Larson, 2013). Citizens were known to frequent public bathhouses where they received rubbings with aromatic oils (R. Calvert, 2002; Fontaine, 2011). Roman soldiers were attended to by specifically assigned and specially trained professional masseuses who would rub them before and after battle (R. Calvert, 2002; Synovitz & Larson, 2013); even condemned criminals, the gladiators, were rubbed down prior to entering the arena for a fight to the death (Nutting & Dock, 1907). Evidence of massage as a prescribed treatment to promote healing is found in historical texts and seems to have been prescribed by physicians such as Hippocrates and Galen (J. Calvert, 2011; Fontaine, 2011).

Despite its strong benefits as a healing therapy in many cultures, massages were viewed as an act of sexual promiscuity in some societies, especially in regard to their use in Roman public bathhouses (Braun & Simonson, 2008). The rise of Christianity afforded religious leaders the leverage to stop the use of the public baths and subsequently the practice of massage. Those who continued to offer massages, particularly women, were deemed to be practicing witchcraft and were brutally punished (Braun & Simonson, 2008).

Ironically, the survival of massage as a therapeutic touch modality can be attributed to the Catholic Church, which allowed nuns who cared for the sick to be trained in massage therapy (J. Calvert, 2011; Nutting & Dock, 1907). The teaching of therapeutic massage remains rooted in nursing practice, as evidenced by Florence Nightingale's description of massaging the patient at the time of sleep in her *Notes on Nursing* (1859). In the 1920s, massage techniques were integrated in the nursing curriculum in the United States in Pennsville and New York. Nurses taking state licensure exams were required to be knowledgeable about massage techniques in order to pass (R. Calvert, 2002). The nursing practice of nighttime back rubs for hospital patients was widely practiced until the early 1980s. The introduction of technological advances and increased demands on nurses' time made comfort techniques, such as back rubs, no longer a part of routine care (Fontaine, 2011).

In the United States, the 1970s brought on a movement for therapeutic massage to be used outside of hospital settings as a way to reduce stress (R. Calvert, 2002; Synovitz & Larson, 2013). Despite the establishment of a professional organization for massage practitioners in 1943, massage therapy was not widely recognized as a true profession. In 1958 the organization American Association of Masseurs and Masseuses (AAMM) was renamed as the American Massage & Therapy Association (AM&TA),

which legitimatized the profession as the science of health and healing through human touch. In 1983 AM&TA revised their name by omitting the "&," becoming the American Massage Therapy Association (AMTA, 2010).

There are approximately 100 different types and techniques of massages; some are specific to a particular culture or geographical region (Huebscher & Shuler, 2004). For example, massages can be categorized as Eastern or Oriental and as Western. Eastern massages focus energy and use pressure points, and Western massages focus on soothing and relaxation techniques (Synovitz & Larson, 2013). This chapter focuses primarily on the common types of massages offered in the United States, such as executive massage, myofascial release, pregnancy massage, reflexology, Rolfing, sports massage, Swedish massage, Thai massage, and trigger point massage (AMTA, 2014; Herring & Roberts, 2002).

Types of Massage

Chair Massage or Executive Massage

The chair massage or executive massage technique uses a specially designed massage chair in which the fully clothed client sits comfortably, with a doughnut-shaped pillow supporting the client's head and face. This seated massage focuses on the head, neck, back, arms, and hands, using integrated massage techniques such as shiatsu, trigger point therapy, and Swedish massage. Sessions typically last between 10 and 20 minutes and focus on reducing people's anxiety levels (Field, 2002; Fontaine, 2011; Shulman & Jones, 1996). In this type of massage, mobile massage therapists offer massage services for employees in the workplace, which prompted the name *executive massage* (Palmer, 1998). Typically, this type of massage is offered in airports and shopping malls, as a convenient and affordable massage (R. Calvert, 2002; Fontaine, 2011; Palmer, 1998).

Myofascial Release

Myo- is a Greek root word for muscle, and *fascia* is the elastic connective tissue wrapped around muscles and other parts of the body (Fontaine, 2011; Stedman, 2011). Myofascial release is a type of whole-body therapy that is first preceded by a comprehensive evaluation and diagnostic workup by a certified myofascial therapist. The therapist performs a visual and tactile examination of the patient's soft tissues and fascial layers. These therapists must have advanced training from a licensed massage therapist, physical therapist, and/or occupational therapist. Treatment includes release of myofascial restrictions identified by the therapist by palpation of tissue that may feel hot, hard, and sensitive. Gentle sliding pressure is applied in the direction of the restriction to stretch the tissues. The stretching of tissues and the heat imparted by the practitioner's hands are thought to help produce a softer consistency of fascial tissues, releasing stored tensions and increasing mobility (Manheim, 2007; Riggs, 2007; Tozzi, Bongiorno, & Vitturini, 2011).

Myofascial release therapy is considered effective for some individuals for the treatment of muscle strain and sprains, headache, and chronic pain (Riggs, 2007; Castro-Sanchez et al., 2011; Tozzi et al., 2011). Despite documented positive effects of myofascial therapy, evidence-based research specifically on the diagnostic process and the treatment of myofascial therapy could not be identified (Remvig, Ellis, & Patijn, 2008). Myofascial therapy is contraindicated in malignancy, cellulitis, hematomas, infections, circulatory impairment, and rheumatoid arthritis, as it may cause additional risk for these patients (Fontaine, 2011).

Pregnancy Massage

Pregnancy massage therapy is focused on pregnant women (prenatal) and women after giving birth (postpartum). It addresses the special needs of pregnant women, such as discomfort in the low back, feet, and legs. This type of massage is usually done with the woman in a side-lying position and focuses on the neck, arms, hands, back, pelvis, legs, and feet. There is no evidence-based research that directly identifies massage as a risk during pregnancy; however, some physicians will not recommend massage therapy during the first trimester, due to the risk of miscarriage (Fontaine, 2011; Stager, 2009). In addition, there is very limited evidence-based research on the benefits of massage during pregnancy. However, one study, which specifically identified women who received massage therapy for 16 weeks during their pregnancy, reported decreased anxiety, depression, and reported leg and back pain. In addition, compared to those who did not receive massages, those who did had evidence of higher dopamine and serotonin levels in their blood. Serotonin and dopamine are hormones that help individuals sleep better and have a general overall feeling of wellness (Field, Diego, Hernandez-Reif, Schanberg, & Kuhn, 2004).

Reflexology

Reflexology has its roots in Asian, Native American, Indian, European, Egyptian, Middle Eastern, and South American cultures (Field, 2009). This type of massage focuses on the pressure points of the feet, hands, and ears corresponding to the reflex zones of the body (Fontaine, 2011). Figures 4.1 to 4.3 illustrate the pressure points located on the hands, feet, and ears and their correlation to the connected body system or organs.

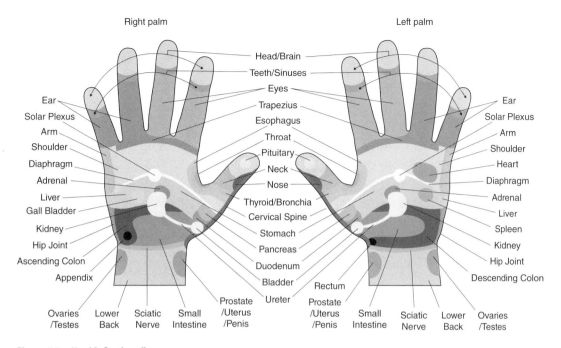

Right palm   Left palm

Head/Brain
Teeth/Sinuses
Eyes
Ear   Ear
Trapezius
Solar Plexus   Solar Plexus
Esophagus
Arm   Arm
Throat
Shoulder   Shoulder
Pituitary
Diaphragm   Heart
Neck
Adrenal   Diaphragm
Nose
Liver   Adrenal
Thyroid/Bronchia
Gall Bladder   Liver
Cervical Spine
Kidney   Spleen
Stomach
Hip Joint   Kidney
Pancreas
Ascending Colon   Hip Joint
Duodenum
Appendix   Descending Colon
Bladder
                                                       Rectum
                                   Prostate   Ureter   Prostate
Ovaries   Lower   Sciatic   Small   /Uterus   /Uterus   Small   Sciatic   Lower   Ovaries
/Testes   Back   Nerve   Intestine   /Penis   /Penis   Intestine   Nerve   Back   /Testes

Figure 4.1   Hand Reflexology Chart

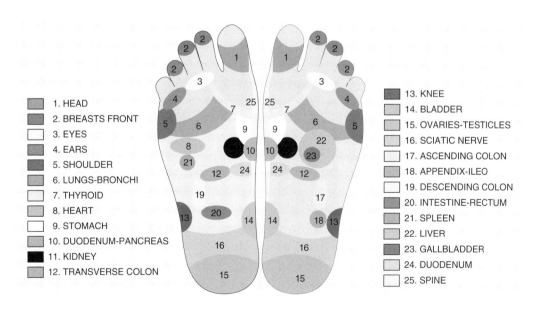

1. HEAD
2. BREASTS FRONT
3. EYES
4. EARS
5. SHOULDER
6. LUNGS-BRONCHI
7. THYROID
8. HEART
9. STOMACH
10. DUODENUM-PANCREAS
11. KIDNEY
12. TRANSVERSE COLON

13. KNEE
14. BLADDER
15. OVARIES-TESTICLES
16. SCIATIC NERVE
17. ASCENDING COLON
18. APPENDIX-ILEO
19. DESCENDING COLON
20. INTESTINE-RECTUM
21. SPLEEN
22. LIVER
23. GALLBLADDER
24. DUODENUM
25. SPINE

Figure 4.2   Foot Reflexology Chart

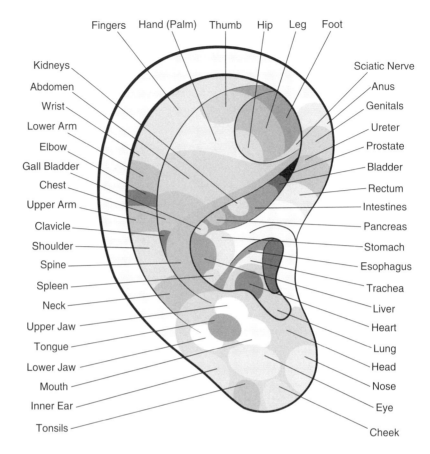

Figure 4.3   Ear Reflexology Chart

Reflexology differs from acupressure, which involves the entire body, as it limits treatment to feet, hands, and ears. However, both therapies believe that there are pressure points on the body that can affect or *reflect* each gland, internal organ, and body part. Reflexology therapists believe pressure on specific points on these areas will increase energy to a specific part of the body, thus prompt healing and increasing the effectiveness of the patient's immune system (Field, 2009). Therapists apply pressure gently and firmly with rocking movements either with their hands, stones, or tools, such as a wooden dowel (Field, 2009; Synovitz & Larson, 2013).

A research study by Degan et al. in 2000 revealed the effectiveness of reflexology in reducing patients' pain. Participants in the study who received three 30-minute reflexology treatments over a period of one week reported a decrease in their lower back pain. In the United States, reflexology therapists are required to complete 110 didactic and 90 clinical hours prior to certification by the American Reflexology Certification Board (2013).

Rolfing or Structural Integration

Rolfing therapy was developed by Ida P. Rolf as a form of hands-on manipulation and client education of the body's movement of muscles. This therapy focuses on the connective tissues, the fascia. The fascia is stretched to release tension and rigidity in order to balance or return the body to alignment. Therapists use their fingers, knuckles, and elbows to stretch the fascia, which becomes tight due to injury, bad posture, emotional problems, or genetic weakness (Fontaine, 2011; Kohatsu, 2002). Rolf practitioners are trained to work on restoring balance to the structure of the entire body. Rolfing therapy differs from other deep-tissue massage therapies, such as myofascial, that focus on relieving tension only in specific areas of the body (Kaye et al., 2011).

Sports Massage

Sports massage is applied to athletes to help them train and perform free of pain and injuries (Fontaine, 2011). This type of specialty massage utilizes classic Swedish massage with other methods, such as compression, pressure-point therapy, cross-fiber friction, joint mobilization, hydrotherapy, and cryotherapy (R. Calvert, 2002; Fontaine, 2011). The different massage techniques are applied to coincide with the athletes' training and competition schedules. For example, on the day of a competition, light massage with long strokes is performed to warm up the muscle fibers, and deep-tissue massage is avoided. After a training session or a competition, cross-fiber friction is used to stimulate blood flow to the muscle tissues followed by cyrotherapy, to decrease inflammation (R. Calvert, 2002). Research studies have identified that the increased blood flow to muscle tissue following massage is effective in reducing muscle pain and stiffness and in promoting healing (Brookes, Woodruff, Wright, & Donatelli, 2005; Hilbert, Sforzo, & Swenson, 2003; Zainuddin, Newton, Sacco, & Nosaka, 2005).

Swedish Massage

Per-Henrik Ling is considered the father of Swedish massage (R. Calvert, 2002). His technique was developed from massage therapies used in China, Egypt, Greece, and Rome. This type of massage is the most common form used in the United States (Fontaine, 2011). Swedish massage uses five types of techniques, including *effleurage* (long strokes), *petrissage* (kneading), *tapotement* (percussion), vibration, and friction of the muscles (Herring & Roberts, 2002). This therapy applies these different techniques to promote relaxation, ease muscle tension, and promote increased circulation to the primary muscle groups of the entire body (Brown, 2010). Massage oil or lotion is used to ensure the smoothness of the strokes. Swedish massage techniques are the basis for other types of massages, such as pregnancy massage and sports massage (Brown, 2010).

Thai Massage

This type of massage, developed in Thailand, is sometimes referred to as passive yoga (R. Calvert, 2002; Fontaine, 2011). The therapist uses his or her whole body to provide treatment, while the receiver of treatment is fully clothed and lies on a futon or mat (Kohatsu, 2002). Thai massage is an ancient bodywork system with a theoretical foundation centered on the invisible energy pathways that run through the body (Pritchard, 1999). The belief is that trapped energy can cause illness, so the therapist works to unblock trapped energy by stroking and applying pressure along energy pathways. Thai massage uses slow, often meditative and rhythmic pressure by fingers, thumbs, hands, forearms, elbows, and feet. It also incorporates yoga-like stretches coupled with gentle rocking motions (Pritchard, 1999).

Trigger Point Massage

Trigger point therapy is a type of deep-tissue massage from Western medicine. It is sometimes referred to as shiatsu massage, which is a light touch therapy from Japan. Trigger point massage is a type of deep-tissue massage that focuses on the tissue structures of the muscles and fascia (the connective tissue) (Synovitz & Larson, 2013). The therapist works to release chronic muscle tension or knots (or adhesions). Trigger point massage helps with chronic muscular pain, spasms, and injury to muscle tissue (Kaye et al., 2009). It is specifically beneficial for chronic muscle tension and contracted areas, such as stiff necks, low back pain, and sore shoulders. It is typically used in conjunction with other massage techniques (Fontaine, 2011).

Massage and Culture

Despite the long history of the use of massage therapy to promote health and wellness, it is not currently seen as an integral part of healthcare in the United States (R. Calvert, 2002). Several studies have identified cross-cultural differences in acceptance of therapeutic touch. The United States continually rates the lowest in the use of therapeutic and healing touch, with most Mediterranean cultures rating as the highest (Shut et al., 2013). The use of therapeutic touch is slowly gaining momentum in the United

States, as shown by statistics from the NHIS in 2007, which identified massage as the third most used complementary treatment in the country (Barnes et al., 2008). The results of the 2012 NHIS indicated that 6.8% of adults use massage; the 2007 NHIS showed that 8.3% used it, and the 2002 NHIS revealed that 5.0% used massage (NCCIH, 2015i). The decrease in massage use between 2007 and 2012 was inconsistent with projections made by researchers who expected an increased rate of touch therapies in the United States (Stussman, Bethall, Gray, & Nahin, 2013).

Risks and Benefits of Massage

Research on massage reveals essentially very little risk, especially when performed by a trained, licensed massage therapist; however, there are some documented side effects, which include allergic reaction or sensitivity to the products used, such as oil or creams (Fontaine, 2011). Some bruising, pain, and discomfort for a brief period of time after a massage have also been reported. There are also some precautions to be aware of when considering which massage therapy to use. People who are on anticoagulation therapy (blood thinning) or those with bleeding disorders should avoid vigorous massage due the increased risk of bleeding or bruising (Fontaine, 2011). Areas of the body that have an infection or open wound should be avoided, as well as areas of tumors, weakened bones, or recent fractures (Herring & Roberts, 2002). Documentation supports the use of massage therapy in patients with cancer and in pregnant women; however, consultation with the oncologist or primary medical provider before using massage therapy is necessary (Hughes et al., 2008; Fontaine, 2011; Walters, 2002).

Research supports the use of massage therapy to help reduce stress, anxiety, blood pressure, and edema, especially in the lower extremities (Sharpe, Williams-Granner, & Hussy, 2007). Studies also indicate the effectiveness of massage therapy in reducing musculoskeletal back pain and potentiating weight gain in premature infants (Beider, Mahrer, & Gold, 2007; Burr, 2005).

Recent studies have focused on the effectiveness of massage therapy as a complementary treatment for specific diseases. Buckle et al. (2008) identified increased cerebral blood flow with light massage in stroke patients. Massage was also noted to help increase the immune function and to decrease stress levels in women undergoing treatment for breast cancer (Billhult, Lindholm, Gunnarsson, & Stener-Victorin, 2009). Another study documented the effect of deep-tissue massage in temporarily reducing heart rate and blood pressure (Kaye et al., 2008).

Acupuncture

History and Overview of Acupuncture

Traditional Chinese medicine (TCM) originated in China several thousand years ago and includes mind and body practices such as acupuncture, moxibustion (burning an herb above the skin over acupuncture points), cupping (heated glass cups applied to the skin along meridians), tui na (Chinese therapeutic massage), qi gong, and tai chi (combining movements and breathing with mental focus) as well as the use of herbal medicines to treat or prevent health problems (NCCIH, 2015d). TCM is rooted in the Eastern philosophy of Taoism. Traditional medicine systems developed in other Asians countries, such as Japan and Korea, utilize similar concepts as TCM with their own variations (NCCIH, 2013f). According to classic Chinese medical books, the first acupuncture needles were made of stone and then bronze. Over the years, the needles became more refined and were made of different types of metal that contributed to the expansion of the field of acupuncture (Cheng, 1999).

Acupuncture and TCM have been practiced in the United States ever since the first immigrants came from China. However, it was not until 1972 when President Nixon visited China that Chinese medicine and acupuncture were brought to public awareness. As interest in and awareness of acupuncture increased in the United States, accredited schools of acupuncture/TCM formed, states began to legalize and regulate the practice of acupuncture, and many classic Chinese texts were published in English (Scarlet, 2015). According to the 2012 NHIS, 1.5% of adults used this form of CAM (NCCIH, 2015i). The 2007 NHIS revealed that an estimated 3.1 million US adults and 150,000 US children had used acupuncture the previous year (NCCIH, 2013f).

Acupuncture is the insertion of needles into specific energy points on the body called *acupoints* along pathways called *meridians* (Kendall, 2002). Meridians are pathways in which the body's qi and blood circulate. Thin filiform needles, often made of stainless steel, are inserted into various acupuncture points on the body. Combinations of points are chosen depending on what health condition is being treated. Although treatment plans are individualized and vary per patient, weekly treatments are generally given until benefit is seen; then the time between treatments gradually lengthens (Pendick, 2013).

The approximately 2,000 acupuncture points on the human body are located on 12 main meridians and eight secondary pathways. Similar to a highway system, the meridians flow along the head, arms, legs, and trunk. Each meridian is connected to an internal organ and carries the energy of that organ's functioning. The 12 main meridians, or channel pathways, on the human body include the lung, large intestine, stomach, spleen, heart, small intestine, bladder, kidney, pericardium, *san jiao* or Triple Burner, gall bladder, and liver (Maciocia, 2000) (see Table 4.1 and Figure 4.4).

TCM theorizes that when there is a blockage in a meridian, pain and illness can result. Acupuncture is considered a technique to balance energy, or qi, to restore the flow of energy in the meridians (Mayo Clinic, 2015). Chinese medicine does not look for causes of disease but rather patterns based on the different principles including imbalances in meridians, yin-yang theory, patterns according to the Five Elements, and pathogenic factors (Maciocia, 2000).

The concept of *qi* is important to understand as the underlying basis of TCM and acupuncture. Qi is most often described as energy and is the foundation of acupuncture philosophy. According to Maciocia (2000), qi is defined as life force, vital power, matter, or vital force. Qi is considered fluid in nature and can assume different manifestations.

Yin-yang theory is another important concept for understanding the foundation of acupuncture and Chinese medical theory. The underlying principle of the theory is that a part can be understood only as member of a whole (Kaptchuk, 2000). Yin and yang can be considered opposite forces that are interconnected, such as day and night, hot and cold, or fire and water (Maciocia, 2000) (see Table 4.2).

The Five Elements of TCM are water, fire, wood, metal, and earth (see Table 4.3). Practitioners can look for patterns based on the Five Elements in order to make a differential diagnosis. Different acupuncture points are selected for a treatment based on what is out of balance (Kaptchuk, 2000).

Table 4.1   12 Meridians Categorized as Yin or Yang with Their Paired Organ

Yin Organ	Yang Organ
Liver	Gall bladder
Lung	Large intestine
Spleen	Stomach
Heart	Small intestine
Kidney	Urinary bladder
Pericardium	*San jiao* or Triple Burner

Source: Maciocia (2000).

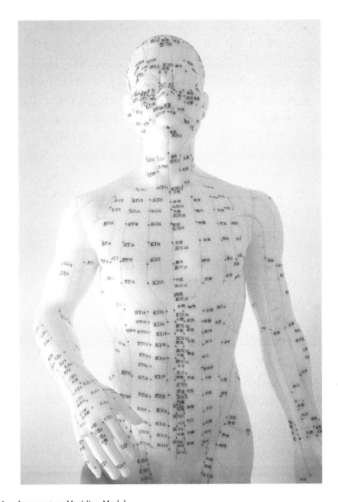

Figure 4.4   Acupuncture Meridian Model

Table 4.2   Characteristics of Yin and Yang

Yang	Yin
Day	Night
Heat	Cold
Dry	Wet
Rapid	Slow
Acute disease	Chronic disease
Full	Empty
Fire	Water

Source: Maciocia (2000).

Table 4.3   The Five Elements

Element	Characteristics Associated with Each of the Five Elements
Fire	Red, summer, bitter taste, growth, joy, and laughing
Earth	Yellow, sweet taste, transformation, pensiveness, and singing
Metal	White, autumn, pungent taste, harvest, sadness, and crying
Water	Black, winter, salty taste, storage, fear, and groaning
Wood	Green, spring, sour taste, birth, anger, and shouting

Source: Maciocia (2000).

Practitioners take a history and examine the patient to determine an acupuncture treatment protocol. In addition to questions pertaining to the patient's chief complaint and health history, Chinese pulse and tongue diagnoses are completed. Chinese pulse diagnosis looks for specific qualities as the blood flows through the body, while the Western approach is centered on the number of pulsations per minute. Tongue diagnosis involves a visual inspection of the tongue for size, color, coating, cracks, and other markings. Using all of the information gathered during the history and examination, practitioners make a differential diagnosis that will assist them in choosing the most appropriate acupuncture points (Kaptchuk, 2000).

Benefits of Acupuncture

In the United States, acupuncture is often associated with treating pain and other health conditions (NCCIH, 2014). In general, acupuncture promotes a sense of relaxation and well-being. According to many studies, acupuncture activates endogenous opioid mechanisms for pain relief. Functional magnetic resonance imaging techniques have shown that acupuncture points affect specific regions of the brain (Kaptchuk, 2002). Viewed from a Western perspective, acupuncture points are thought to stimulate nerves, muscles, and connective tissue in order to release the body's natural painkillers and increase blood flow (Mayo Clinic, 2015).

According to the NCCIH (2014), acupuncture is effective at reducing chronic pain, such as low back pain, neck pain, and osteoarthritis/knee pain. Studies have also shown that acupuncture helps reduce the frequency of tension headaches and prevents migraines. Many studies are being sponsored by the National Institutes of Health, the World Health Organization, and universities worldwide to further investigate what other therapeutic effects acupuncture may have.

Side Effects and Risks of Acupuncture

Acupuncture is generally a safe method of treatment, but there are precautions and possible side effects. Some side effects may include bruising and numbness or tingling at the site of needle insertion. After an acupuncture treatment, some patients may have some dizziness or fainting. Unusual risks of acupuncture include nerve damage, and pneumothorax and other organ puncture. An acupuncture needle could break subcutaneously in the patient, requiring immediate medical attention (California Acupuncture Board, 2015).

There are additional precautions for pregnant women. Safety guidelines recommend avoiding acupuncture points in the lower abdomen and lumbosacral region during the first trimester. After the first trimester, needle points in the upper abdomen and lumbosacral area, as well as other specific acupuncture points that cause strong sensation, are contraindicated (Cheng, 1999). Safety guidelines recommend avoiding acupuncture points in the abdomen, lumbar area, and other specific points that descend energy or create a downward-bearing movement, such as at the top of the shoulders. Spontaneous miscarriage or early labor may be possible risks associated with inappropriate acupuncture points during pregnancy (NCCIH, 2014).

There are standards of practice during treatment protocols. Where needles are to be inserted, the acupuncture points are to be cleaned with an appropriate antiseptic, such as alcohol, prior to insertion. In Title 16, Article 5, of its Standards of Practice, the California Acupuncture Board (2015) requires use of sterile disposable acupuncture needles. Receiving acupuncture from someone who is properly trained and licensed is important for reducing complications and risks.

Acupressure

History and Overview of Acupressure

Rooted in TCM, acupressure incorporates the philosophy of yin and yang, qi, Five Elements, and the meridian system (Robinson, 2011). Acupressure is defined as a form of touch therapy that involves placing pressure on areas of the body to treat pain or other health conditions (NCCIH, 2014). Acupressure is used to promote relaxation and treat disease but without acupuncture needles. Instead, pressure is applied with fingers, hands, elbows, or feet to acupuncture points along the meridians to restore balance (Robinson, 2011). Various amounts of pressure can be applied, and sometimes acupressure involves stretching or using noninvasive massage tools on the acupoints. Acupressure may be an appropriate alternative to acupuncture for persons who are afraid of needles or in children and elderly persons who may not tolerate acupuncture needles.

Research on Acupressure

Acupressure is used to treat a variety of illnesses and symptoms. Evidence-based research shows the effectiveness of acupressure for nausea and vomiting related to pregnancy. When comparing a randomized control group utilizing the acupressure point Pericardium 6 (P6), located between two large tendons on the inside of the wrist, to that of a placebo group not utilizing this point, the degree of nausea and vomiting was significantly lower in the group using the acupressure point. This point was found to help relieve symptoms related to morning sickness (Shin, Song, & Sep, 2007). Special wristbands are sold over the counter that press on this acupressure point to help relieve nausea related to motion sickness, morning sickness, and chemotherapy (National Institutes of Health, 2013).

Shiatsu, a specific type of acupressure, has been studied to determine the effects on lower back pain. Individuals in the study were measured on their anxiety and pain levels before and after a series of four shiatsu treatments. The study demonstrated that both pain and anxiety levels were significantly decreased (Brady, 2001).

Types of Acupressure

Shiatsu

Shiatsu is considered the most common type of acupressure. It originated in Japan, where the word *shiatsu* means "light touch." The shiatsu therapist applies pressure with fingers or palms in a continuous rhythmic motion. This style of acupressure is usually performed on a low table or on the floor. Typically no oils or lotions are applied to the skin, unlike many other styles of massage. Several different types of shiatsu currently are practiced that focus on balancing energy flow (Shiatsu Society UK, 2013). The most common conditions people seek shiatsu for is to treat musculoskeletal pain and psychological problems (Robinson, 2011).

Tui Na

Tui na is a Chinese form of acupressure or manual therapy that is often used in combination with acupuncture and other TCM therapies. The practitioner may knead, roll, brush, or massage acupuncture points to move qi, or energy, to unblock meridians and relax muscles, allowing the body to heal itself naturally. External herbal compresses on the skin may also be used to enhance the treatment. Tui na is often used to treat joint injuries and muscle sprains rather than for general relaxation since the techniques utilized are more focused on a particular area of the body (Pentland, 2005).

Jin Shin Do

Jin Shin Do acupressure is a unique combination of the Japanese style of gentle touch with Chinese acupressure theory and points. The phrase *Jin Shin Do* translates into English as "the Way of the Compassionate Spirit," and the method was developed by Iona Teegaurden (1997). The Jin Shin Do style uses two or more acupressure points, using both hands to apply pressure. This type of acupressure is often used to treat physical or emotional conditions. This technique can be applied by a professional or performed on oneself.

Ohashiatsu

Similar to other types of acupressure, Ohashiatsu combines touch therapy, gentle exercises, and stretches. It also incorporates meditation into the movements of the limbs with stretches. The main difference between Ohashiatsu and other types of acupressure is that it emphasizes the well-being of both the giver and the receiver of the treatment. It is thought that if the treatment givers are relaxed and healthy, they will be able to give a more effective treatment (Ohashiatsu Institute, 2013).

Watsu

Watsu is a gentle form of shiatsu performed in warm water that was developed in the 1980s in California by a shiatsu teacher name Harold Dull. The persons receiving the treatment are supported while they float in water. It is thought that the warm water helps relax the muscles in conjunction with the massage, while taking pressure off the vertebrae to allow the body to be manipulated more easily. This type of therapy is used for spinal cord injuries, stroke, and arthritic conditions. Patients with fever, temperature instability, and conditions that prohibit floating in water for long periods of time should avoid Watsu (Weil, 2013).

Benefits of Acupressure

While most people seek acupressure for a specific ailment, others are looking for relaxation. Although each person's response to treatment varies, some of the benefits include decreased pain, improved blood flow, release of tension, muscle relaxation, and reduction in anxiety and stress levels (Weil, 2015a).

Cautions and Contraindications of Acupressure

There are cautions and special considerations that practitioners should follow when performing acupressure, such as avoiding working directly on burns, ulcerations, and infections. During the first month after an operation, people should not receive applied pressure in the affected site. Caution should be used to avoid pressing deeply in areas containing lymph nodes or working directly on a recently formed scar. In general, caution should be taken during pregnancy, and the abdominal area should be avoided. Acupressure is contraindicated in persons with intestinal cancer, tuberculosis, leukemia, and serious cardiac conditions (Gach, 2004).

Chiropractic

History and Overview of Chiropractic

Chiropractic is a type of CAM that focuses primarily on musculoskeletal system disorders and their relationship to the overall health of the individual. Chiropractic care is a hands-on approach that uses spinal manipulation to treat a variety of complaints, such as back pain, neck pain, pain in the joints of the arms or legs, and headaches (Huebscher & Shuler, 2004). The purpose of manipulation is to restore joint mobility by manually applying a controlled force into joints to reestablish proper alignment. The theory of chiropractic medicine is based on the understanding that alignment of the spinal vertebrae is needed to maintain or improve the body's organs and systems' functioning (American Chiropractic Association, 2013).

The practice of body manipulation for treatment of illnesses can be traced back to as early as 2700 BCE in China and to 1500 BCE in Ancient Greece. The Greek physician Hippocrates is known to have practiced body manipulations and documented the use of manipulation or reduction as an essential form of treatment for many diseases (Whorton, 2002).

Daniel David Palmer is credited as the founder of chiropractic practice in the United States. Palmer created the term *chiropractic* by linking two Greek words, *cheiros*, meaning "hand," and *prakikos*, meaning "practice." In 1897, he opened the Palmer School of Chiropractic based on the *Palmer Method* of treatment. The Palmer Method is based on the belief that all disease results from a disruption of flow of innate intelligence, caused by spinal subluxations that compress the spinal nerves. To correct the subluxations of the spine, the *Hole-in-One* manipulation of the first vertebra is done to restore proper alignment and energy flow of the body (Whorton, 2002).

By 1906, several graduates of the Palmer School of Chiropractic opened competing schools of chiropractic medicine, including the American School of Chiropractic & Nature Cure and the Carver-Denny School of Chiropractic. These schools strayed from the Palmer Method by teaching their students about naturopathic remedies, such as stretching machines and herbal remedies. This was the beginning of the division in the profession, which still exists, between the straight providers, who practice only spinal manipulations, and the *mixers*, who combine other methods with their practice (Keeting, Cleveland, & Menke, 2004). Providers who follow the straight philosophy believe that spinal manipulation alone can treat and cure diseases (Synovitz & Larson, 2013). While chiropractic care remains focused on the function of the spine and its relationship to health, most providers are now becoming mixers, believing that diseases are caused by pathogens that require the incorporation of other treatment modalities into the plan of care (Field, 2009; Synovitz & Larson, 2013). These modalities include the use of massage, ultrasound, and electric muscle stimulation, as well as preventive health practices such as nutrition and exercise (Huebscher & Shuler, 2004; Kohatsu, 2002).

Types of Chiropractic Treatment

Chiropractic treatment has two goals: to relieve pain and to correct subluxations. Different types of chiropractic techniques are applied to accomplish these goals, depending on the patient's diagnosis. Chiropractors make a diagnosis after completing a physical exam and often by obtaining X-rays (Field, 2009). The most common symptoms seen by chiropractors include headaches, back pain, muscle spasms, and sports-related injuries (Synovitz & Larson, 2013). Most chiropractic therapy involves some type of spinal manipulation (Kohatsu, 2002).

Spinal Manipulation

Spinal manipulation is an all-encompassing term that refers to treatment in which the chiropractor moves the client into different positions while applying gentle pressure to specific areas on the spinal facets and the sacroiliac joints (Kohatsu, 2002; Synovitz & Larson, 2013). This is done to reduce subluxation, or misaligned vertebrae, and to reestablish correct vertebral alignment (Fontaine, 2011). Spinal manipulation is performed on patients with neuromusculoskeletal complaints, such as headaches, neck pain, and back pain (Fontaine, 2011).

High-Velocity, Low-Amplitude Thrust Adjustment

In chiropractic medicine, high-velocity, low-amplitude thrust adjustment is the most common form of body manipulation. It is done by moving a joint to the farthest point of its range of motion and then applying a quick, forceful pressure to the spinal facets. This action will emanate a loud cracking noise, or pop, as the facets are forced apart (Lenarz, 2003). The popping sound is caused by the release of carbon dioxide that has accumulated in the synovial fluid in the joint. Studies have indicated that the release of carbon dioxide increases the joint's ranges of motion for a short period of time (Kohatsu, 2002).

Network Chiropractic

Network Spinal Analysis, also known as *Network chiropractic*, was developed by Dr. Donald Epstein (Epstein & Altman, 1994). This type of treatment uses two approaches to therapy: manual adjustment to subluxations of joint facets and treatment of the soft tissue supporting these structures. Prior to an adjustment to the spine, energy techniques, referred to as low-force touches, are applied to relieve the tension in the muscles and soft tissue surrounding the joints (Epstein & Altman, 1994).

Craniosacral Therapy

Developed by Dr. John Upledger, craniosacral therapy (CST) focuses on manipulating the synarthrodial joints of the skull and pelvis to increase the flow of cerebrospinal fluid (CSF). The disruption in the flow of CSF is thought to be the cause of patients' pain and illness. CST therapy is accomplished by applying light touches to a patient's skull, face, spine, and pelvis to restricted soft tissues surrounding the central nervous system (Upledger, 1983).

Benefits and Risks of Chiropractic

Data from the 2002 and 2007 NHIS found that chiropractic therapy was the most commonly used CAM. The 2012 NHIS showed that 8.4% of adults and 3.3% of children use chiropractic care (NCCIH, 2015i). Typically, patients who seek chiropractic care are suffering from musculoskeletal pain, headaches, or problems related to their hands or feet. The majority of patients who receive chiropractic therapy report the treatment they received was beneficial (Wolsko et al., 2003).

There is some controversy regarding the efficacy of spinal manipulation to relieve pain. Some research supports spinal manipulation as a preferred form of treatment for low back pain and for acute as well as chronic headaches (Brontfort, Assendelft, Evan, Hass, & Bouter, 2001; Haldeman & Dagenais, 2001). However, additional studies report a lack of sufficient evidence to support the efficacy of spinal manipulation to relieve pain, especially related to tension headaches (Brontfort, Hass, Evans, Leininger, & Triano, 2010; Fernandez-de-Las-Peñas et al., 2006).

There is also controversy regarding some of the risks associated with chiropractic care. While spinal manipulation is safe when performed by trained and licensed providers, there have been reports of rare serious complications from spinal and cervical manipulations. One of these complications is vertebrobasilar artery stroke (VBA). The National Chiropractic Mutual Insurance Company published a report in 1996 disputing the association of VBA stroke after spinal manipulations (Terrett, 1996). However, since 1996, many published articles have found a direct correlation to the adverse outcome of VBA and cervical adjustment (Ernest, 2007; Haldeman, Carey, Townsend, & Papadopoulos, 2001; Hurwitz et al., 2005; Malone et al., 2002).

Another rare but documented serious complication from spinal manipulation is cauda equina syndrome (CES), which can occur when the bundle of spinal nerves called the *cauda equina* get compressed and are damaged. This damage causes a loss of neurological function to the lower part of the body (Tamburrelli, Genitiempo, & Logroscino, 2011).

Despite the controversy regarding the efficacy and risks associated with chiropractic care, most providers agree on some contraindications to cervical and spinal manipulation. Contraindications include late stages of pregnancy, any history of abnormal bleeding, anticoagulant therapy, advanced osteoporosis, history of spinal malignancies, tumor, and inflammatory disease (NCCAM, 2013d).

Consumer Issues

The California Massage Therapy Council (CAMTC) regulates the practice of massage therapists. At the national level, the American Medical Massage Association provides practice guidelines for practitioners (AMMA, n.d.). Licensed therapists are required to abide by the professional code of conduct and regulations of practice. If clients feel a therapist has not maintained professional standards, they have the right to file a complaint. For further information or to file a complaint about a licensed massage therapist, visit https://www.camtc.org/Complaints.aspx.

For acupuncture, anyone who believes that an acupuncturist has engaged in illegal or unethical activities related to professional practice should file a complaint, in writing. The California Acupuncture Board will review each complaint. In California, the acupuncture board can be contacted at: http://www.acupuncture.ca.gov. For other states where acupuncturists are licensed through the National Certification Commission of Acupuncture and Oriental Medicine (NCCAOM), complaints can be filed at http://www.nccaom.org/. Complaints for professional or ethics violations for physicians practicing acupuncture should be directed to their respective medical boards.

Many regulatory bodies oversee acupressure practitioners, depending on the type of acupressure they are practicing. For example, for therapists practicing Asian body therapies who are licensed through NCCAOM, complaints can be filed at http://nccaom.org.

The Board of Chiropractic Examiners maintains the integrity of the profession by ensuring that practitioners abide by regulations of the California Chiropractic Initiative Act, Business and Professions Code, and the California Code of Regulations relating to the practice of chiropractic. Patients who feel that a practitioner of chiropractic medicine has not maintained professional standards may file a written complaint with the Board of Chiropractic Examiners. A complaint form can be retrieved from: http://www.chiro.ca.gov/forms_pubs/consumer_complaint.pdf.

Consumers also need to become informed on the appropriateness of CAIH use according to their health and disease conditions. The NCCIH emphasizes the importance of becoming informed consumers. This implies taking care of their health by strengthening the communication lines with healthcare providers. Communication between consumers and healthcare providers is essential in CAIH. Consumers need to become knowledgeable about the scientific studies related to the safety and effectiveness of CAIH products and practices and discuss this information with their healthcare providers before making a decision on a particular treatment or therapy (NCCIH, 2015b).

The NCCIH has also called on consumers to increase their health literacy regarding CAM. According to the Centers for Disease Control and Prevention (2015), health literacy is defined in the Patient Protection and Affordable Care Act of 2010, Title V, as "the degree to which an individual has the capacity to obtain, communicate, process, and understand basic health information and services to make appropriate health decisions."

The NCCIH emphasizes that healthcare providers must help consumers strengthen their health literacy so they can understand complementary health approaches in the news, identify missing information from CAM stories, understand scientific information, recognize important details in research studies, understand information related to side effects of CAM approaches, identify the accuracy of the consulted source of information, and know what to do when there are conflicting health news stories (NCCIH, 2015c). These components of health literacy are of special relevance in CAM consumer education. Box 4.1 lists recommendations from the NCCIH for consumers to determine the value of research studies presented in health stories.

Implications for Health Professionals

Massage therapy, acupuncture, acupressure, and chiropractic care are emerging fields of health practice that pose multiple challenges and opportunities for consumers and health professionals. The NCCIH (2015) has

---

BOX 4.1   QUESTIONS CHECKLIST FOR UNDERSTANDING HEALTH NEWS STORIES

- Was the product, procedure, or device tested on people? Findings from animal or laboratory research may not be immediately meaningful to your health.

- Are there alternatives to the approach being discussed? You will want to know what is already available, so you can compare your options.

- Were enough people studied? When the number of people in a study is small, the results aren't as strong.

- Were the results big enough to be meaningful to you? A small difference between two approaches might interest scientists but be of little importance to your health or quality of life.

- Did the researchers consider the many things that can influence results, such as participants' general health or health habits, or discuss the limitations of their results?

- Were the study participants similar to you in ways that may matter, such as age, race, or gender?

- Was the study lengthy enough to show long-term benefits or risks? Natural products may take time before they show benefits; some side effects may take months or years to show up.

- Have other researchers had similar results? One study rarely proves anything.

- Was the study funded by a group that would profit financially from the study findings? If so, you should be wary of the results.

Source: National Center for Complementary and Integrative Health (2015c).

pointed out the current growing trend for *integrative medicine* and *integrative health care*. This trend is happening because of greater evidence-based data on the benefits and risks associated with CAM practices and the inclusion of training modules on CAM for students in the health field (NCCAM, 2013a). The 2014 change in the name of the NCCAM to the National Center for Complementary and Integrative Health reflects this trend (NCCIH, 2015d).

The NHIS conducted by the National Center for Health Statistics in the Centers for Disease Control and Prevention are a major source of information on CAM use in the United States. These surveys are conducted annually, but every five years include questions on CAM use. The 2002, 2007, and 2012 surveys provided information on adults surveys and the 2007 and 2012 surveys included data for children (NCCIH, 2015a). They also provided information on CAM use and socioeconomic status, educational attainment, and insurance coverage. This information is very important for health professionals as it helps identify the populations with major consumer education needs.

The 2012 NHIS revealed that regarding poverty status, the majority of CAM consumers are not poor (38,4%) (as labeled in the survey), have an educational level of a college degree or higher (42.6%), and have private insurance (38.0%) (Clarke et al., 2015). These results pose challenges for healthcare professionals since the need for consumer education is evident not only for the segments with high use of CAM, but also for the populations with low educational levels, underserved populations, economically challenged populations, and those who are uninsured.

The National Advisory Council for Complementary and Alternative Medicine, in its 2010 meeting, presented data on the need for a budget that responded to the growing research and CAM-related training needs for health professionals. According to this council, the budget for the NCCAM in 2010 was close to $129 million and for the year 2011 was $132 million, which shows a growing financial commitment for CAM in the United States (DHHS, 2010). The lack of evidence-based research indicates a need for further studies on the benefits of manipulative and body-based practices such as massage therapy, acupuncture, acupressure, and chiropractic care.

The Patient Protection and Affordable Care Act, also known as the Affordable Care Act (ACA), was signed into law by President Barack Obama. Public Law 111-148 of March 23, 2010, 124 Statute 123, Part I, establishes guidelines to ensure beneficiary access to physician care and other services (US Government, 2010), which directly affect access to CAIH modalities. This part of the law opens various opportunities for CAM practitioners, such as acupuncturists and chiropractic practitioners. With the increasing number of Americans having health insurance with acupuncture and chiropractic benefits, more people can access these services, creating a greater demand for providers of these modalities. Rao (2013) mentioned that alternative medical treatments could be widely accepted now as a result of the ACA since Section 2706 of this law states that insurance providers shall not discriminate against any state-licensed health provider.

Rao (2013) added that CAM practitioners who have gone through certification and licensing procedures should be covered under this part of the law and could be integrated into the healthcare system. Rao illustrated this by providing an example of how a licensed chiropractor should be reimbursed with the same protections as medical doctors. Although this is the ideal, the reality shows that there are still reservations among both consumers and medical providers regarding widely accepting CAIH practice. Since under the ACA each state defines its essential basic services plan, there is a need for advocates of CAIH practices. For instance, some states, such as California, Oregon, and Utah, initially excluded coverage for chiropractic care in their basic benefits plan. Colorado and Oregon are in the process of modifying this clause to allow coverage of chiropractic services (Rao, 2013).

The ACA also hinted at the value of CAIH in its sections on wellness, prevention, and research (Rao, 2013). The Patient-Centered Outcomes Research Institute (2013), strengthened by the health law, is increasing its investment in CAIH research effectiveness. Health professionals and consumers are called to participate in these efforts and provide evidence on the effectiveness and risks associated with CAIH practices.

Consumers also have a right and a responsibility to become knowledgeable on CAIH practices prior to their use. The website of the NCCIH provides guidelines in an effort to increase the knowledge of consumers regarding services. These guidelines include tips for use, safety information, and issues to consider when selecting a CAIH practice and guidelines to follow when choosing a CAM practitioner (NCCAM, 2013c).

Caveat Emptor

Regulatory and Practical Realities: Massage Therapy

According to the CMTC (2015), 43 states in the United States have implemented specific requirements for certification and regulation of massage therapy. Previously, individual towns and counties in each state regulated the practice; currently only a few continue licensure in this way. In 2012,

California passed a state law requiring mandatory certification to practice; previously, certification was just voluntary. The law requires a minimum of 500 education and practice hours from an accredited institution. In addition, the law authorized the regulation and governing of massage therapy in California by CAMTC.

In addition to state licensure, the National Certification Board for Therapeutic Massage and Body Work (NCBTMB) offers a national examination. The criteria for sitting for the exam are the same as for state licensure requirements. These regulations have been implemented in the last few years in order to maintain the credibility of the profession and to ensure client safety (NCBTMB, n.d.).

Regulatory and Practical Realities: Acupuncture

Acupuncture is one of the fastest-growing modalities of TCM (NCCIH, 2015h). While most states require the NCCAOM examination or certification for licensure, the requirements of each state regulatory board differ (NCCAOM, 2015). Comprehensive training is required at an accredited acupuncture school with a minimum of three to four academic years. In additional to graduation from an acupuncture program, the acupuncturist must pass a certification examination administered by NCCAOM. Once licensed, acupuncturists are required to complete continuing education hours to renew their licenses and certifications in topics such as the Health Insurance Portability and Accountability Act, Occupational Safety and Health Administration regulations, and needle safety. The Food and Drug Administration regulates acupuncture needles as medical devices. It requires that the needles comply with safety guidelines, such as being sterile, nontoxic, and labeled for single use (NCCIH, 2014).

The State of California has more acupuncturists than any other state and requires its own examination for licensure and certification. In New York, to practice acupuncture or use the title "licensed acupuncturist," a licensee much be of good moral character, at least 21 years of age, meet education and examination requirements, and be proficient in English (New York State Education Department, 2014). Texas has similar requirements to practice acupuncture as New York, but it also requires an additional ethics exam, graduation from an accredited acupuncture school, completion of the Clean Needle Technique Course, and passing of the practical examination (Texas Medical Board, 2015). Other healthcare professionals, such as medical doctors, can be certified to practice acupuncture. Medical acupuncture is a type of acupuncture performed by physicians (medical doctors and doctors of osteopathy) that is incorporated into Western medical practice. The American Academy of Medical Acupuncture (Helms, 2015) offers training courses and certification in medical acupuncture for physicians.

Regulatory and Practical Realities: Acupressure

It is important to choose an acupressure practitioner who has appropriate training and credentialing. The NCCAOM issues credentials for Asian bodywork therapy, including tui na and other acupressure therapies based on Chinese medical principles. Training includes 500 hours of practical and theoretical education and a certification exam. The Worldwide Aquatic Bodywork Association oversees the training programs and certification for Watsu practitioners. Additional questions to ask acupressure practitioners are how many years of experience they have and if they have experience in the disease or condition that the patient is seeking treatment for.

Regulatory and Practical Realities: Chiropractic

Chiropractic medicine is practiced in many countries and internationally regulated by the Federation of Chiropractic Licensing Boards. In the United States, doctors of chiropractic medicine must obtain state licensure and pass a national certification examination. Prior to sitting for the national examination, the applicant must complete a minimum of 4,200 hours of classroom, laboratory, and clinical experience, with a course of study approved by an accredited agency. The extensive education prepares doctors of chiropractic to diagnose healthcare problems, treat problems within their scope of practice, and refer patients to other healthcare practitioners when appropriate (American Chiropractic Association, 2013).

Conclusion

The Academic Consortium for Complementary and Alternative Health Care (ACCAHC) has been engaged in various policy initiatives, such as defining integrative medicine in 2005, participating in the 2008 Institute of Medicine summit in which CAM was discussed, actively participating in the 2009 NCCAM Strategic Plan, and delineating guidelines for CAM training in the ACCAHC *Meeting the Nation's Primary Care Needs* document (ACCAHC, 2013). Health professionals and consumers should look at these initiatives and become critical agents in these efforts. Health practitioners should also be knowledgeable in CAIH, so they can exercise critical judgment in the selection of the most appropriate modality of care and offer integrative health in their professional roles. In addition, this information will allow them to exercise their health education role and provide consumers with the evidence needed to make informed decisions.

Summary

- The Center for Complementary and Integrative Health from the National Institutes of Health is a reliable source for consumers to make informed decisions when seeking CAIH treatments.
- Manipulative and body-based practices, such as massage therapy, acupuncture, acupressure, and chiropractic medicine, have benefits and risks that need to be considered by consumers.
- When seeking alternative medicine treatment, consumers should seek only licensed providers who are certified in their CAM field.
- Consumers should be aware of the governing bodies of CAM practices and know how to file a complaint if needed.
- Research studies document the effectiveness of massage therapy, acupuncture, acupressure, and chiropractic medicine in the treatment of many disease entities.
- Manipulative and body-based modalities need to be seen as CAIH practices. There must be further exploration of their roles in health maintenance and wellness restoration.

Case Study

Description

A 38-year-old female patient presented with neck pain for the past three months after being rear-ended in a car accident. The pain was worse on the left side, and there was intermittent pain down the left arm. The neck pain was worse at the end of the day and with activities such as lifting and carrying heavy objects. Cervical range of motion was limited when turning her head to the right. X rays of the cervical spine showed a reverse curvature of the neck.

Diagnosis

From a Western medicine perspective, the diagnosis is a cervical sprain strain. The TCM view categorizes this injury as qi and blood stagnation obstructing the meridians.

Treatment

Several distal and local acupuncture points were selected as part of the treatment protocol. Acupuncture treatments were given twice a week for three weeks. Needles were inserted in the body for 30 minutes each visit, and the points were stimulated once during the session after 10 minutes.

Results

After six acupuncture treatments, improvement was observed. The neck pain decreased, and there was no radiating pain down the left arm. Cervical range of motion was now within normal limits.

Questions

1. What is the difference between the Western medicine and the CAM views of the diagnosis?

2. What strengths and weaknesses do you see in the treatment protocol received by this patient?

3. What are some of the risks consumers should be aware of utilizing this type of CAIH practice?

KEY TERMS

Acupressure. A form of touch therapy that involves placing pressure on areas of the body to treat pain or other health conditions (Weil, 2015a).

Acupuncture. The insertion of needles into specific areas of the body called acupoints along pathways called meridians (Kendall, 2002).

Chiropractic. A hands-on approach that uses spinal manipulation to treat a variety of complaints, such as back pain, neck pain, pain in the joints of the arms or legs, and headaches (Huebscher & Shuler, 2004).

Massage therapy. A systematic or scientific manipulation of muscle and other soft tissues through techniques such as rubbing and pressure done by a trained practitioner who uses fingers, forearms, elbows, or feet (NCCIH, 2015e).

Reflexology. A type of massage therapy that focuses on the pressure points of the innervation areas of the feet, hands, and ears, which correspond to organs or muscles, in order to promote relaxation, circulation, and effective body functions (Weil, 2015b).

References

Academic Consortium for Complementary and Alternative Health Care. (2013). Policy Working Group. Retrieved from http://www.accahc.org/policy-working-group

American Chiropractic Association. (2013). *What is chiropractic?* Retrieved from http://www.acatoday.org/Patients/Why-Choose-Chiropractic/What-is-Chiropractic

American Massage Therapy Association. (2013). *History of massage.* Retrieved from https://www.amtamassage.org/articles/3/MTJ/detail/3285

American Reflexology Certification Board. (2013). *National foot reflexology certification brochure.* Retrieved from https://arcb.net/take-the-arcb-exam/

Barnes, P. M., Bloom, B., & Nahin, R. L. (2008). Complementary and alternative medicine use among adults and children: United States, 2007. *National Health Statistics Reports, 12.* Retrieved from https://www.researchgate.net/publication/5786045_Pediatric_Massage_Therapy_An_Overview_for_Clinicians

Beider, S., Mahrer, N. E., & Gold J. I. (2007). Pediatric massage therapy: An overview for clinicians. *Pediatric Clinics of North America, 54*(6), 1025–1041 doi: 10.1016/j.pcl.2007.10.001

Billhult, A., Lindholm, C., Gunnarsson, R., & Stener-Victorin, E. (2009). The effect of massage on immune function and stress in women with breast cancer—a randomized controlled trial. *Journal of Autonomic Neuroscience: Basic and Clinical, 150*(1–2), 111–115. doi: 10.1016/j.autneu.2009.03.010

Brady, L., Henry, K., Luth, J., & Casper-Bruett, K. (2001). The effects of shiatsu on lower back pain. *Journal of Holistic Nursing, 1,* 57–70.

Braun, M., & Simonson, S. (2008*). Introduction to massage therapy* (2nd ed.). Baltimore, MD: Lippincott Williams & Wilkins.

Bronfort, G., Assendelft, W., Evans, R., Hass, M., & Bouter, L. (2001). Efficacy of spinal manipulation for chronic headache: A systematic review. *Journal of Manipulative and Physiological Therapeutics, 24*(7), 457–466.

Bronfort, G., Hass, M., Evan, R., Leininger, B., & Trianon, J. (2010). Effectiveness of manual therapies: The UK evidence report. *Chiropractice & Osteopathy Journal, 18,* 3. doi: 10.1186/1746-1340-18-3

Brooks, C. P., Woodruff, L. D., Wright, L. L., & Donatelli, R. (2005). The immediate effects of manual massage on power-grip performance after maximal exercise in healthy adults. *Journal of Alternative and Complementary Medicine, 11,* 1093–1101.

Brown, A. (2010). *Swedish massage: Enjoying the most popular Western massage.* Retrieved from http://spas.about.com/od/swedishmassage/a/Swedish.htm

Buckle, J., Newberg, A., Wintering, N., Hutton, E., Lido, C., & Farrar, J. T. (2008). Measurement of regional cerebral blood flow associated with the M technique—light massage therapy: A case series and longitudinal study using SPECT. *Journal of Alternative and Complementary Medicine, 4*(8), 903–910. doi: 10.1089/acm.2007.0613

Burr, J. (2005). Jayne's story: Healing touch as a complementary treatment for trauma recovery. *Holistic Nursing Practice, 19*(5), 211–216.

California Acupuncture Board. (2015). *Title 16, Article 4. Examinations & Demonstrations of Competency.* Retrieved from http://www.acupuncture.ca.gov/pubs_forms/laws_regs/art5.shtml

California Massage Therapy Council. (2015). *Frequently asked questions: About CAMTC.* Retrieved from https://www.camtc.org/faq.aspx

Calvert, J. (2011). Nursing and massage from our past. *Massage Today, 11*(12). Retrieved from http://www.massagetoday.com/mpacms/mt/article.php?id=14507

Calvert, R. (2002). *History of massage: An illustrated survey from around the world.* Rochester, VA: Healing Art Press.

Castro-Sánchez, A. M., Matarán-Peñarrocha, G. A., Granero-Molina, J., Aguilera-Manrique, G., Quesada-Rubio, J. M., & Moreno-Lorenzo, C. (2011). Benefits of massage—myofascial release therapy on pain, anxiety, quality of sleep, depression, and quality of life in patients with fibromyalgia. *Evidence-Based Complementary and Alternative Medicine, 2011.* Article ID 561753. doi: org/10.1155/2011/561753

Centers for Disease Control and Prevention. (2015). *Learn about health literacy. What is health literacy?* Retrieved from http://www.cdc.gov/healthliteracy/learn/index.html

Cheng, X. (1999). *Chinese acupuncture and moxibustion.* Beijing, China: Foreign Languages Press.

Clarke, T. C., Black, L. I., Stussman, B. J., Barnes, P. M., & Nahim, R. L. (2015). Trends in the use of complementary health approaches among adults: United States 2002–2012. *National Health Statistics Reports No. 79.* Hyattsville, MD: National Center for Health Statistics.

Coughlin, P. (2002). *Principles and practice of manual therapies.* New York, NY: Churchill Livingstone.

Department of Health and Human Services. (2010). National Advisory Council for Complementary and Alternative Medicine. *Minutes of the 39th meeting.* Retrieved from https://nccih.nih.gov/sites/nccam.nih.gov/files/2010junmin.pdf

Degan, M., Fabris, F., Vanin, F. Bevilacqua, M., Genova, V., Mazzucco, M., & Negrisolo, A. (2000). The effectiveness of foot reflexotherapy on chronic pain associated with a herniated disc. *Professioni Infermieristiche, 53*(2), 80–87.

Epstein, D., & Altman, N. (1994). *Twelve stages of healing: A network approach to healing.* Novato, CA: New World Library.

Ernst, E. (2007). Adverse effect of spinal manipulation: A systematic review. *Journal of the Royal Society of Medicine, 100*(7), 330–338.

Fernandez-de-Las-Penas, C., Alonso-Blanco, C., Cuadrado, M., Miangolarra, J., Barriga, F., & Pareja, J. (2006). Are manual therapies effective in reducing pain from tension-type headache? A systematic review. *Clinical Journal of Pain, 22*(3), 278–285.

Field, T. (2009). *Complementary and alternative therapies research.* Washington, DC: American Psychological Association.

Field, T., Diego, M., Hernandez-Reif, M., Schanberg, S., & Kuhn, C. (2004). Massage therapy effects on depressed pregnant women. *Journal of Psychosomatic Obstetrics & Gynecology, 25,* 155–122. Retrieved from http://www.ncbi.nlm.nih.gov/pubmed/15715034

Fontaine, K. (2005). *Complementary & alternative therapies for nursing practice* (2nd ed.). Upper Saddle River, NJ: Pearson Hall.

Gach, M. R. (2004). *Acupressure precautions: Professional practice procedures and breathing guidelines.* Retrieved from http://www.acupressure.com/articles/acupressure_precautions_guidelines.htm

Haldeman, S., Carey, P., Townsend, M., & Papadopoulos, C. (2001). Arterial dissections following cervical manipulation: The chiropractic experience. *Journal of the Canadian Medical Association, 165*(7), 905–906.

Haldeman, S., & Dagenais, S. (2001). Cervicogenic headaches: A critical review. *Spine Journal 1*(1), 31–46.

Helms, J. M. (2015). *An overview of medical acupuncture.* Retrieved from http://www.medicalacupuncture.org/For-Patients/Articles-By-Physicians-About-Acupuncture/An-Overview-Of-Medical-Acupuncture

Herring, M. A., & Roberst, M. M. (2002). *Complementary and alternative medicine fast facts for medical practice.* Malden, MA: Blackwell.

Hilbert, J. E., Sforzo, G. A., & Swenson, T. (2003). The effects of massage on delayed onset muscle soreness. *British Journal of Sport Medicine, 37,* 72–75.

Huebscher, R., & Shuler, S. (2004). *Natural alternative and complementary health care practices.* St. Louis, MO: Mosby.

Hurwitz, E., Morgenstern, H., Harder, P., Kominski, G. F., Yu, F., & Adams, A. H. (2005). A randomized trial of chiropractic manipulation and mobilization for patients with neck pain: Clinical outcomes from the UCLA neck-pain study. *American Journal of Public Health, 92*(10), 1634–1641.

Kaptchuk, T. (2000). *The web that has no weaver: Understanding Chinese medicine.* New York, NY: McGraw-Hill.

Kaptchuk, T. (2002). Acupuncture: Theory, efficacy, and practice. *Annals of Internal Medicine, 5,* 374–383.

Kaye, A. D., Kaye, A. J., Swinford, J., Baluch, A., Bawcom, B. A., Lambert, T. J., & Hoover, J. M. (2009). The effect of deep-tissue massage therapy on blood pressure and heart rate. *Journal of Alternative and Complementary Medicine, 14*(2), 125–128. Retrieved from http://www.multiview.com/briefs/sdss/pci032009.htm

Keating, J., Cleveland, C., & Menke, M. (2004). *Chiropractic history: A primer.* Association for the History of Chiropractic. Retrieved from https://www.researchgate.net/publication/239735121_Chiropractic_History_a_Primer

Kendall, D. (2002). *Dao of Chinese medicine: Understanding an ancient healing art.* Oxford, UK: Oxford University Press.

Kohatsu, W. (2002). *Complementary and alternative medicine secrets*. Philadelphia, PA: Hanley & Belfus.

Lenarz, M. (2003). *The chiropractic way*. New York, NY: Bantam Books.

Maciocia, G. (2000). *The foundations of Chinese medicine*. Bejing, China: Churchill Livingstone.

Malone, D., Baldwin, N., Tomecek, F., Boxell, C., Gaede, S., Covington, C., & Kugler, K. K. (2002). Complications of cervical spine manipulation therapy: 5-year retrospective study in a single-group practice. *Neurosurgical Focus*, *13*(6). Retrieved from http://www.ncbi.nlm.nih.gov/pubmed/15766233

Manheim, C. J. (2008). *The myofascial release manual* (4th ed.). Thorofare, NJ: Slack.

Mayo Clinic. (2015). *Tests and procedures: Acupuncture*. Retrieved from http://www.mayoclinic.org/tests-procedures/acupuncture/basics/definition/prc-20020778

National Center for Complementary and Alternative Medicine. (2013a). *2007 statistics on CAM use in the United States*. Retrieved from https://nccam.nih.gov/news/camstats/2007

National Center for Complementary and Alternative Medicine. (2013b). *Acupuncture: What You Need to Know*. Retrieved from https://nccih.nih.gov/health/acupuncture/introduction

National Center for Complementary and Alternative Medicine. (2013c). *Be an informed consumer*. Retrieved from http://nccam.nih.gov/health/decisions

National Center for Complementary and Alternative Medicine. (2013d). *Chiropractic: An introduction*. Retrieved from http://nccam.nih.gov/health/chiropractic/introduction.htm?nav=gsa

National Center for Complementary and Alternative Medicine. (2013e). *Movement therapies*. Retrieved from https://nccih.nih.gov/health/integrative-health

National Center for Complementary and Alternative Medicine. (2013f). *Traditional Chinese medicine*. Retrieved from https://nccih.nih.gov/health/chinesemed

National Center for Complementary and Integrative Health. (2014). *Acupuncture: What you need to know*. Retrieved from https://nccih.nih.gov/health/acupuncture/introduction

National Center for Complementary and Integrative Health. (2015a). *About the survey*. Retrieved from https://nccih.nih.gov/research/statistics/NHIS/2012/about

National Center for Complementary and Integrative Health. (2015b). *Be an informed consumer*. Retrieved from https://nccih.nih.gov/health/decisions

National Center for Complementary and Integrative Health. (2015c). *Checklist for understanding health news stories*. Retrieved from https://nccih.nih.gov/health/understanding-health-news

National Center for Complementary and Integrative Health. (2015d). *Complementary, alternative, or integrative health: What's in a name?* Retrieved from https://nccih.nih.gov/health/integrative-health

National Center for Complementary and Integrative Health. (2015e). *Massage therapy*. Retrieved from https://nccih.nih.gov/health/massage

National Center for Complementary and Integrative Health. (2015f). *Selected mind and body practices*. Retrieved from https://nccih.nih.gov/research/statistics/NHIS/2012/mind-body

National Center for Complementary and Integrative Health. (2015g). *13-year trends for complementary approaches where questions are very similar across years*. Retrieved from https://nccih.nih.gov/research/statistics/NHIS/2012/mind-body/trends-text-version

National Center for Complementary and Integrative Health. (2015h). *Traditional Chinese medicine*. Retrieved from https://nccih.nih.gov/health/chinesemed

National Center for Complementary and Integrative Health. (2015i). *What complementary and integrative approaches do Americans use?* Retrieved from https://nccih.nih.gov/research/statistics/NHIS/2012/key-findings

National Certification Board for Therapeutic Massage and Body Work. (n.d.). *"I choose board certified."* Retrieved from http://www.ncbtmb.org/

National Certification Commission for Acupuncture and Oriental Medicine. (2015). *License requirements*. Retrieved from http://www.op.nysed.gov/prof/acu/acupunlic.htm

National Institute of Health. (2013). *Complementary, alternative, or integrative health: What's in a name?* Retrieved from https://nccih.nih.gov/health/integrative-health

National Institute of Health, US National Library of Medicine. (2013). *Nausea and acupressure*. Retrieved from http://www.nlm.nih.gov/medlineplus/ency/article/002117.htm

Nelson, M. (2010). *(Don't) Feel the burn—hot stone massage*. American Massage Therapy Association. Retrieved from http://www.amtamassage.org/articles/3/MTJ/detail/2204

New York State Education Department. (2014). *License requirements*. Retrieved from http://www.op.nysed.gov/prof/acu/acupunlic.htm

Nightingale, F. (1890). *Notes on nursing: What it is and what it is not*. Radford, VA: A & D.

Nutting, M. A., & Dock, L. L. (1907). *History of nursing*. Bristol, UK: Thoemmes.

Ohashiatsu Institute. (2013). *What is Ohashiatsu?* Retrieved from http://www.ohashiatsu.org/us/index.php/what-is-ohashiatsu

Palmer, D. (1998). A brief history of massage. *Positive Health, 32*. Retrieved from http://www.positivehealth.com/issue/issue-32-september-1998

Pentland, S., & Funk, R. (2005). *Tui Na (tuina)—Chinese bodywork massage therapy*. Retrieved from http://tcm.health-info.org/tuina/tcm-tuina-massage.htm

Pendick, D. (2013). *Acupuncture is worth a try for chronic pain*. Harvard Health Publications. Retrieved from http://www.health.harvard.edu/blog/acupuncture-is-worth-a-try-for-chronic-pain-201304016042

Pritchard, S. (1999). *Chinese massage manual: The healing art of tui na*. New York, NY: Sterling.

Raby Institute for Integrative Medicine. (2011). *Manipulative and body-based practices*. Retrieved from http://www.rabyintegrativemedicine.com/pages/manipulative_and_body_based_practices/43.php

Riggs, A. (2007). *Deep tissue massage*. Berkeley, CA: North Atlantic Books.

Remvig, L., Ellis, R. M., & Patijn, J. (2008). Myofacial release: An evidence-based treatment approach? *International Musculoskeletal Medicine, 30*, 29–35.

Rao, A. (2013). *Kaiser Health News. Alternative treatments could see wide acceptance thanks to Obamacare*. Retrieved from http://www.pbs.org/newshour/rundown/how-the-health-reform-law-will-impact-alternative-medicine-access/

Robinson, N., Lorenc, A., Liao, X., (2011). The evidence for shiatsu: A systematic review of shiatsu and acupressure. *BMC Complementary and Alternative Medicine, 11*, 88.

Rost, A. (2009). *Natural healing wisdom and know how: Useful practices, recipes, and formulas for a lifetime of health*. Amherst, NY: Black Dog & Leventhal.

Scarlett, Y. (2015). *A history of Chinese medicine in the United States*. Retrieved from http://library.pacificcollege.edu/acupuncture-massage-news/om-essay-contest/om-essay-contest/1080-a-history-of-chinese-medicine-in-the-united-states-by-yvonne-scarlett-.html

Sharpe, P. A., Williams, H. G., Granner, M. L., & Hussey, J. R. (2007). A randomised study of the effects of massage therapy compared to guided relaxation on well-being and stress perception among older adults. *Complementary Therapies in Medicine, 15*(3), 157–153.

Shiatsu Society UK. (2015). *About shiatsu*. Retrieved from http://www.shiatsusociety.org/sites/default/files/shiatsu_systematic_evidence_review_complete.pdf

Shin, H., Song, Y., & Sep, S. (2007). Effect of Nei-Guan points (P6) acupressure on ketonuria levels, nausea and vomiting in women with hyperemesis gravidarum. *Journal of Advanced Nursing, 59*(5), 509–510.

Shulman, K. R., & Jones, G. E. (1996). The effectiveness of massage therapy intervention on reducing anxiety in the workplace. *Journal of Applied Behavioral Science, 32*(2), 160–173.

Shut, C., Linder, D., Brosig, B., Niemeier, V., Ermler, C. Madejski, K., . . . Kupfer, J. (2011). Appraisal of touching behavior, shame and disgust: A cross-cultural study. *International Journal of Culture and Mental Health, 6*(1), 1–15. doi: 10.1080/17542863.2011.602530

Stager, L. (2009). Supporting women during labor and birth. *Midwifery Today with International Midwife, 92*, 12–15.

Stedman, T. L. (2011). *Stedman's medical dictionary for the health professions and nursing*. Baltimore, MD: Williams & Wilkins.

Stussman, B., Bethall, C., Gray, C., & Nahin, R. (2013). Development of the adult and child complementary medicine questionnaires fielded on the National Health Interview Survey. *BioMed Central, 13*, 1–18. doi: 10.1186/1472-6882-13-328

Synovits, L., & Larsno, K. (2013). *Complementary and alternative medicine for health professionals: A holistic approach to consumer health.* Burlington, MA: Jones & Bartlett.

Tamburrelli, F. C., Genitiempo, M., & Logroscino, C. A. (2011). Cauda equina syndrome and spine manipulation: Case report and review of the literature. *European Spine Journal, 20*(1), 128–131.

Teeguarden, I. (1997). *Acupressure way of health, Jin Shin Do.* New York, NY: Oxford University Press.

Terrett, A. G. (1996). *Vertebrobasilar stroke following manipulation.* N.p.: National Chiropractic Mutual Insurance Company.

Texas Medical Board. (2015). *Acupuncturist eligibility checklist.* Retrieved from http://www.tmb.state.tx.us/page/acupuncture-eligibility-checklist

Tozzi, P., Bongiorno, D., & Vitturini, C. (2011). Fascial release effects on patients with non-specific cervical or lumbar pain. *Journal of Bodywork & Movement Therapies, 15*(4), 405–416. doi: 10.1016/j.jbmt.2010.11.003

Upleger, J. (1983). *Craniosacral therapy.* Seattle, WA: Eastland Press.

US Government. (2010). *Public Law 111–148.* Retrieved from http://www.gpo.gov/fdsys/pkg/PLAW-111publ148

US National Institute of Health. (2012). *Chiropractic for hypertension in patients.* Retrieved from https://clinicaltrials.gov/ct2/show/NCT01020435

Walter, L. (2002). *Kind touch massage.* New York, NY: Sterling.

Weil, A. (2013). *Wellness therapies: Watsu.* Retrieved from http://www.drweil.com/drw/u/ART03102/Watsu.html

Weil, A. (2015a). *Acupressure.* Retrieved from http://www.drweil.com/drw/u/ART03230/Acupressure.html#_ga=1.90287450.1525645785.1461708918

Weil, A. (2015b). *Reflexology.* Retrieved from http://www.drweil.com/drw/u/ART00546/Reflexology-Dr-Weil-Wellness-Therapies.html

Whorton, J. C. (2002). *Nature cures: History of alternative medicine in America.* Oxford, UK: Oxford University Press.

Wolsko, P. M., Eisenberg, D. M., Davis, R. B., Kessler, R., & Phillips, R. (2003). Patterns and perceptions of care for treatment of back and neck pain: Results of a national survey. *Spine, 28*(3), 292–297.

Zainuddin, Z., Newton, M., Sacco, P., & Nosaka, K. (2005). Effects of massage on delayed-onset muscle soreness, swelling, and recovery of muscle function. *Journal of Athletic Training, 40*, 174–180.

CHAPTER 5

AYURVEDA AND OTHER COMPLEMENTARY HEALTH APPROACHES

Peter Garcia and Monika Joshi

Complementary, alternative, and integrative health (CAIH) practices are increasingly gaining recognition among the general public. Thus, primary care practitioners have had to acknowledge the appropriate use of such therapies. Although many CAIH therapies, such as yoga and chiropractic care, have gained medical recognition among allopathic practitioners, the spectrum of modalities of many other CAIH therapies remains untested to mainstream Western medical practices, in part due to limited evidence-based research. Another complicating factor is the wide array of CAM therapies, which make it difficult to identify or categorize them. One of the most widely used classification structures, first developed by the National Center for Complementary and Alternative Medicine (NCCAM) in 2000 and updated in 2014, divided CAM modalities into five categories: (1) alternative medical systems, (2) mind-body interventions, (3) biologically based treatments, (4) manipulative and body-based methods, and (5) energy therapies. This classification was revised by the National Center for Complementary and Integrative Health (NCCIH, 2015c), which currently divides complementary health practices into three subgroups: (1) natural products, (2) mind and body practices, and (3) other complementary health approaches.

The more commonly accepted CAM practices of massage, yoga, and relaxation techniques are widely recommended in today's Western medical practices

LEARNING OBJECTIVES

At the completion of this chapter, students will be able to:

- Identify the theoretical and scientific basis of ayurveda, aversion therapy, art therapy, prayer therapy, light therapy, enzyme therapy, cupping, and magnet therapy.

- Explain the benefits and risks of ayurveda and other selected complementary health approaches.

- Discuss the emerging role of ayurveda and other selected complementary, alternative, and integrative health (CAIH) therapies in Western medicine.

- Discuss consumers' issues related to the selection and utilization of ayurveda and other selected CAIH therapies.

- Discuss the role of health professionals in education and advocacy related to ayurveda and other selected CAIH therapies.

(Goldbas, 2012). The purpose of this chapter is to introduce the reader to lesser known, less practiced, and perhaps more controversial therapies. A principal CAM therapy presented and discussed in this chapter is the natural approach of ayurveda (also called ayurvedic medicine), which was initially categorized as an alternative medical system by NCCAM (2011) and is now classified by the NCCIH (2015c) as a complementary health approach.

Ayurvedic medicine may be considered a prime CAIH modality since it is a holistic type of medical practice that promotes health and wellness through various CAM therapies and often avoids traditional Western pharmacotherapy. Its origin is traced to India. Though its aim focuses primarily on health promotion, it is also practiced to treat certain illnesses. In the United States, the modalities of CAM therapies often are used independently or as a sole treatment, but ayurvedic medicine practitioners utilize many forms of CAM modalities that synergistically promote healing and client well-being. The aim of this chapter is to help readers understand the use of sole therapies and also consider the holistic approach of a multi-modalities system such as practiced in ayurveda. This chapter introduces readers to the other categories proposed by the NCCIH with brief examples of therapies for each category.

Theoretical Concepts

Overview

In 1992, the NCCAM was established to govern, regulate, and research the use and application of safe and effective CAM therapies in healthcare practices. In 2005, at the request of the National Institutes of Health (NIH) and the Agency for Healthcare Research and Quality, the Institute of Medicine (IOM) produced the report titled *Complementary and Alternative Medicine in the United States*, which assessed what is known about Americans' reliance on CAM therapies and helped the NIH in developing research methods and setting priorities for evaluating CAM products and approaches. The IOM (2005) found that more than one-third of adults in the United States reported that they have pursued some form of CAM therapies.

The report recommended that healthcare should incorporate both comprehensive and evidence-based practices for conventional medical treatments as well as complementary and alternative therapies. The IOM

(2005) suggested that both treatment modalities should follow the same standards for demonstrating clinical effectiveness as well as the same general evidence-based principles that allow new research methods to test how some therapies may have to be devised and implemented. The IOM stated that the ultimate goal is the provision of client-safe alternative medicine practices that infuse both the science and art of CAM therapies and practices.

As a result of the IOM report, research on various CAM therapies emerged. Evidence-based knowledge is now being promoted for other complementary health approaches, such as ayurveda.

Modalities

Ayurveda

A traditional healthcare model practiced in India, *Ayurveda* is a Sanskrit term made up of two words *Ayus* and *Veda*, which translates to "science of life." Ayurveda, a 5000-years-old system, is visualized as the umbrella to holistic natural modalities of CAM (Brar et al., 2012). Practitioners of ayurveda follow a model of natural healing that originated in the Vedic culture of India. The teachings of ayurvedic practices stem from three primary textbooks: the *Charaka Samhita, Sushruta Samhita*, and the *Ashtanga Hridyayam*. Various adaptations and continuous practices of all ayurvedic teachings are based on the combined teaching of these texts (NCCIH, 2015b; Rioux, 2012). Just as there are various branches of Western medicine, there are branches of ayurveda. For example, general medicine is called *kaya chikitsa*, psychiatry is called *bhut vidya*, pediatrics is called *baala* or *kaumara chikitsa*, and surgery is referred to as *shalya chikitsa* (Halpern, 2009).

Ayurveda approaches health in a holistic manner that addresses the physical, psychological, and spiritual aspects of the individual. All variables of a person's well-being are assessed when rendering a plan of therapy. These elements make ayurveda a prime CAIH practice since it is focused on restoring health and maintaining wellness. Ayurveda also includes the woven tapestry of offering wisdom for living vibrantly and realizing one's full potential. According to the NCCIH (2015b):

> Key concepts of Ayurvedic medicine include universal interconnect-edness (among people, their health, and the universe), the body's constitution (*prakriti*), and life forces (*dosha*), which are often compared to the biologic humors of the ancient Greek system. Using

these concepts, Ayurvedic clinicians render individualized treatments, including compounds of herbs or proprietary ingredients, [and] advise on diet, exercise, and lifestyle recommendations.

An ayurvedic treatment plan usually includes dietary considerations, lifestyle modifications, use of natural or organic herbs, massage or touch therapy, and cleansing techniques. Ayurveda utilizes therapies that incorporate the five senses: taste, smell, sight, touch, and sound (Halpern, 2009). Teaching preventive guidelines and managing illnesses are incorporated into all treatment plans as well.

The basic principles of ayurveda originate in the theoretical framework of the five elements of air, ether, fire, water, and earth. Based on these elements, people are categorized into three basic constitutional (body) types, or *doshas*, known as *vata (motion), pitta (metabolism), kapha (structure)*, with many different subcategories or subtypes (Halpern, 2009). This complex categorization is determined by the ayurvedic clinician after an extensive and comprehensive assessment.

Ayurvedic principles view illness or negative stressors as an imbalance, which is called *vikruti*. Once the cause of an imbalance is determined, its reversal becomes part of the treatment plan. Unlike Westernized medical models, the treatment of the same illness in two individuals may be different based on the individuals' constitutional types, which have been determined by the ayurvedic physician (NCCIH, 2015b).

The five elements and their qualities of 10 pairs of opposites govern the three distinct body humors. Table 5.1 lists the qualities of the elements and governing actions.

Each person is born with the basic framework of these three *doshas*, which determines the physical, mental temperament, and characteristics

Table 5.1   Ayurveda *Doshas*

Doshas	Pairing	Qualities	Governing Action
Vata	Air and ether	Cold, dry, mobile, light, subtle, flowing, sharp, rough, and clear	Motion
Pitta	Fire and water	Hot, moist, light, subtle, flowing, mobile, sharp, hard, rough, and clear	Digestion and metabolism
Kapha	Earth and water	Cold, moist, heavy, gross, dense, static, dull, soft, smooth, and cloudy	Lubrication, structure, growth stability, and immune strength

Source: Halpern (2009).

innate within us. Ayurvedic practices synthesize the application of living harmoniously with one's natural body type. Disharmony with one's *dosha* coupled with external factors will result in disease if natural healing of the five senses is not utilized to attempt to restore a harmonious continuum. The three *doshas* and their parings play a critical part in identifying and then treating via the five-sense therapy, which includes the sense of taste, sound, smell, sight, and touch, designed to return a person to a more innate balance of their *doshas* (Brar et al., 2012).

According to ayurvedic practitioners, our health and well-being depends on what we consume. This consumption also includes environmental exposures. When we consume inappropriate proportions (too much or too little) or are exposed to environmental factors that are incongruent with what our bodies require, illness or an imbalance occurs. An imbalance can stem from any of the five senses; thus, treatments include pacifying the senses based on their imbalance.

Ayurveda and the Sense of Taste

Ayurvedic practitioners believe that all of nature, including food, is made up of five elements and possesses its own unique qualities. Ayurveda talks about six tastes: sweet, sour, salty, pungent, bitter, and astringent. Each taste is made up of a unique combination of elements and their qualities. The ayurvedic practitioner must understand the qualities in the food and tastes and then match them with a person's *dosha*. Good health is the result of harmony of the individual's mind, body, and spirit with the universe (WebMD, 2015a). Practitioners provide guidance to enhance health positively and holistically. Table 5.2 summarizes the sense of taste with examples of foods, as well as the effects on the three *doshas*.

Ayurvedic practitioners must possess complex knowledge and apply the principles of the sense of taste and the appropriate foods to balance a client's holistic health. For example, sweet taste is made up of earth and water and has heavy, moist, and cool qualities, which are similar to individuals of *kapha dosha*. Excess intake of sweet foods may aggravate *kapha dosha*, whereas *vata* and *pitta doshas* may benefit from sweet tastes because of the qualities of heaviness and moisture needed for their body type (Brar et al., 2012).

According to ayurvedic principles, the salty taste is thought of as hot or "fire taste" as it contains fire and water elements. This is beneficial for *vata dosha* and provides balance. It may aggravate the *pitta dosha* even though it is not as hot as the sour taste. *Kapha dosha* is aggravated by kapha's moist quality. The taste of salt is uniquely important for people with anxiety and is thought to reduce the intensity of panic attacks when taken as a salt lick during the attack (Brar et al., 2012).

The bitter taste has air and ether elements with cool, dry, and light qualities and thus is best for balancing *pitta dosha* and *kapha dosha*. The bitter taste is best known for its *pitta*-reducing functions of purifying the blood. Most bitter tastes strengthen the purifying functions of the liver. The bitter taste also reduces blood sugar levels, and large amounts of bitters may result in weight loss. Each ayurveda practitioner must apply the complex principles of the sense of taste to balance a person's health.

As in many schools of health, ayurvedic principles are too complex to summarize in a chapter. However, the focus on the senses and their primary role on a person's well-being is unique to this practice model.

Ayurveda and the Other Senses: Smell, Sound, Sight, and Touch

In addition to food, ayurvedic practitioners believe that all senses interact within the body as a whole; therefore, all five senses are also addressed in the other senses, which interact within the body. Table 5.3 presents interactions based on the senses and their corresponding methods of treatment.

Sense of Smell   Aromatherapy is the use of essential oils from plants, flowers, herbs, or trees as a complementary health approach. Various

Table 5.2   Taste and Ayurvedic Qualities

Taste	Element	Main Qualities	Example
Sweet	Earth and water	Heavy, stable, moist, cool, soft, and smooth	Nuts (including peanuts, almonds, and cashews)
			All dairy products
Sour	Earth Earth with some water	Heavy, stable, moist, and hot	Fermented foods (e.g., yogurt and tempeh)
Salty	Water and fire	Hot and moist	Shellfish, most seafood, and salts
Pungent	Fire and air	Light, hot, dry, and mobile	Chili peppers and the stronger spices
Astringent	Earth and air	Cool, dry, stable, and hard	Beans, cranberries, and pomegranate
Bitter	Air and ether	Light, cool, dry, and mobile	Leafy greens; some herbs, such as goldenseal

Source: Halpern (2009).

Table 5.3   Ayurveda and Use of the Senses

Sense	Method of Treatment	Mode of Treatment	Ayurveda Application
Smell	Aromatherapy	Natural oils, secretions, and smells from flowers and plants	*Vata* imbalance is pacified with warming oil and sweet and spicy blends, such as aroma of sandalwood and cinnamon. *Pitta* imbalances are pacified with cooling oils, such as rose and sandalwood. *Kapha*'s health may benefit from stimulating oils, such as cinnamon and patchouli.
Sound	Music	Music, sounds of nature	Mantras, meditation, and healing sounds are used as indicated by the clinician.
Sight	Color therapy or chromotherapy	Use of colors in daily life and home environment	Colors affect mind and mood. *Vata* may benefit from warm, soft, moist colors, such as orange, yellow, green, brown, and purple. *Pitta* may benefit from cool and calming colors, such as blue, white, gold, and brown. *Kapha* may benefit from warming and light colors, such as red, orange, yellow, gold, purple, and violet.
Touch	Massage	Oils	*Vata* and *Pitta* imbalances can benefit from gentle massage. *Kapha* imbalances may benefit from moderate to deep massage.

Source: Halpern (2009).

aromas come from different parts of plants; for instance, rose oil comes from the flower, frankincense comes from a resin, and cinnamon comes from bark (NCCIH, 2015a).

Aromas work more directly on the mind but also have subtle effects on the body. In ayurvedic medicine, the sense of smell is a very important aspect in the treatment of some psychological disorders. There are various ways to experience the odors and smells of oils. Mist bottles, incense sticks, and scented candles are examples. Aromatic herbs are also used in steam therapies called *svedana* (Rastogi & Chiapelli, 2013).

Aromatic oils are often very strong and need to be diluted appropriately under the direction of the ayurvedic practitioner (Halpern, 2009; Rastogi & Chiapelli, 2013). The ayurvedic practitioner needs to work closely with a client to select which aromas and oils are conducive to enhancing harmony and equilibrium within the body. Failure to do so can result in burning irritation of specific mucous membranes of the body or potential allergy-induced reactions.

Sense of Sound   Sounds in our environment can be harmonious or disharmonious. In ayurvedic healing, the most important sound therapies are *mantras*, which are specially energized words or sounds. They may be simple single sounds or special phrases sung in various ways. All spoken words that condition humans are in the form of a mantra. When we repeat an angry thought toward a person or situation outwardly or quietly in our mind, it becomes a dark mantra.

As important as sound is for healing, if used properly, silence can also be a healing tool. When inner silence is achieved, the mind becomes clear and is at peace, making space for deeper healing. People may start with just a few minutes of silence surrounding them to develop a less active mind for relaxation. Then they may slowly increase the time in silence to an hour a day without any internal dialogue or external sounds. As time passes, greater stillness is achieved and benefits are attained.

Quality of communication can be hot/cold, moist/dry, heavy/light, sharp/dull, soft/hard, and smooth/rough. A person with a *vata* imbalance may speak quickly, with frequent change of subject (mobile), without much passion (cold), and may lack compassion (dry). Consciously choosing to speak or be spoken to with balancing elements can restore equilibrium. A friendly (warming), caring and compassionate (moist), sincere and stable (heavy), kind (soft) conversation will support this healing pattern. A person with *pitta* imbalances may speak with judgment and passion (hot), to the point (sharp), aggressive (rough), and without compassion (dry). Communication that is less intense (cool) and more compassionate (moist) can control the fire of the individual. Choice of kind words with a pleasant voice can also balance the *pitta dosha*. The various tones and sounds and their associations are complex ideologies that require ayurveda practitioner guidance (Brar et. al., 2012; Halpern, 2009; NCCIH, 2015a; WebMD, 2015a).

Sense of Sight   The conscious use of color can alter thoughts, feelings, perceptions, and imagination. A tremendous amount of information is taken in through sight, and that information affects our minds and emotions. Color is a vibrational energy that enters the eyes and goes directly to the brain.

In order to understand healing through color, one must know the elements and qualities in colors and how they can affect each *dosha*. For example, the color red is considered powerful and can be perceived as intimidating. The color black is also powerful and portrays supreme confidence. Depending on the constitution and nature of an imbalance, colors may support well-being or contribute to making it difficult for the healing process to occur. An uncommon therapy used in ayurveda involves the ingestion of natural color infused into water. Color can be infused and applied to an individual's treatment plan in various ways. A knowledgeable and experienced clinician is necessary for the process (Halpern, 2009).

Sense of Touch   Touch can be used for healing or to cause harm. The ayurvedic art of touch therapy involves matching the type of touch to the specific person. Some people thrive on increased amounts of touching, and some require only a small amount of touch to achieve optimal health. Some flourish from strong, deep touch; others, a gentle touch. By understanding the qualities inherent in each specific type of touch, the ayurvedic practitioner can prescribe the type that a person needs to achieve healing and harmony (Brar et. al., 2012; Halpern, 2009; NCCIH, 2015c; WebMD, 2015a).

According to the 2007 National Health Interview Survey, more than 200,000 US adults had used ayurveda in the previous year (NIH, n.d.). Ayurveda has not gained full mainstream incorporation into current Western medicine. But the general philosophies of ayurvedic medicine and various sense and body therapies separately under different modalities of CAM therapies continue to gain favor in public awareness and thus have gained momentum among healthcare clinicians and practitioners.

The following remaining categories have Western relevance and have a research-based clinical foundation. The abundance of numerous therapies for each CAIH category needs to be acknowledged.

Light Therapy

Light therapy, also known as bright light therapy or phototherapy, is a CAIH therapy that has been used to treat specific mental health disorders, such as seasonal affective disorder (SAD). SAD is a type of depression that occurs typically in fall or winter, when there is less natural daylight or sun. Flaskerud (2012) found that bright light can affect chemicals in the brain, such as serotonin, and can affect or enhance mood and effectively treat SAD. A study assessing SAD and light therapy in adolescents showed profound results improving mood and depression (Niederhofer & von Klitzing, 2012). Other conditions treated with light therapy include sleep disorders, jet lag, and some forms of dementia. More recently, light therapy has been studied to assess its effects on bipolar disorder, sleep patterns, and cognitive function after brain injury. However, results are inconclusive regarding the benefits and effects on these conditions.

The treatment consists of sitting near a device called a light therapy box, which mimics natural outdoor light, at specific times, typically mornings, for specific durations and intensities. Direct staring into the light is contraindicated as this may cause eye damage (UM Health System, 2005). The therapy should be prescribed by a knowledgeable provider.

Scientific evidence of the efficacy of light therapy has been established for other conditions. For example, light therapy has been utilized to treat skin conditions, such as psoriasis. A very commonly prescribed use of light therapy is to treat neonatal jaundice (Smeltzer, Bare, Hinkle, & Cheever, 2010). These forms of therapy, however, are evidence-based procedures, are widely used, and typically involve ultraviolet light therapy prescribed by a medically trained clinician (Mayo Clinic, 2015).

Other Alternative Medical Therapies

Other forms of CAIH therapy that are categorized as mind and body therapies by the NCCAM (2014) are aversion therapy, art therapy, prayer, reiki, and meditation. Table 5.4 summarizes the theoretical and scientific basis of each of these CAIH modalities.

Enzyme Therapy

Enzyme therapy involves taking enzyme supplements as an alternative medicine practice for some forms of cancer. Enzymes are natural proteins

Table 5.4   Other Mind and Body CAM Therapies

Aversion therapy	Involves exposure to or application of an undesired or negative stimuli while engaged in the specific behavior typically viewed as undesirable or unwanted. Usually associated with alcoholism, smoking, fingernail biting, or excessive eating.
Art therapy	Often used to create or enhance awareness of self or creativity. May also be used to cope with symptoms of stress, traumatic experiences, or depressed mood. Used to enhance cognitive abilities through the practice of creating art. Includes talking about art, viewing art, or actual participation with a trained art therapist.
Prayer therapy	Used in many cultures and religions to empower, provide hope, induce harmony of mind, and ease anxiety or agitation. A universal practice among most religions.
Reiki	An ancient traditional Tibetan practice that uses hand symbols and breathing techniques to manipulate energy forces that are thought to effect balance and harmony. Power source energy travels through the reiki practitioner into the client's body.
Meditation	A relaxation technique and therapy that focuses the mind on specific thoughts. Chants, silence, or sounds often are used in conjunction with meditation.

Source: National Research Council (2005).

that can act as catalysts. Digestive enzymes, mostly made in the pancreas, break down food and help with the absorption of nutritional elements into the blood. Metabolic enzymes help in building new cells and repair damaged ones in the blood, tissues, and organs. Theoretically, this process would also pertain to cancerous or abnormal cells (American Cancer Society, 2013).

A significant amount of discussion has surfaced regarding enzyme therapy and its use for the treatment of multiple illnesses. It is believed that the increased utilization of enzymes via dietary intake, in pill or intravenous therapy form would improve the function of these enzymes. In certain instances, scientific research appears to support this belief. Data from the American Cancer Society (2013) suggest that some pancreatic enzymes may have high cancer-fighting properties. They appear to work similarly to chemotherapy by keeping abnormal cancer cells from proliferating.

Proponents of enzyme therapy believe the use of supplemental oral enzymes may have positive health benefits for numerous health issues. The intake of enzyme supplements is often cited as improving allergies, digestive health, weight loss, circulation, and the immune system. The naturally occurring enzymes in the human body have specific functions; for example, amylase, an enzyme produced by the pancreas, breaks down starch, and it is expected that ingestion of this naturally occurring enzyme can help the human body carry out its functions. Enzyme replacement therapy has gained recognition for specific genetic disorders. For patients with the complex disease called Fabryz disease, an X-linked lyosomal storage disorder, replacement of a deficient enzyme has increased life expectancy and eased manifestations (Salviati, Burlina, & Borsini, 2010).

Controversy exists within the medical field regarding the selling to the general public of enzymes derived from plant and animals to supplement human enzymatic functions. The lack of underlying scientific research and evidence is the reason most often given. In the United States, the Food and Drug Administration (FDA) has classified enzymes as food additives, so a prescription is not needed to purchase them. The FDA (2013) provides a list of enzyme preparations approved as food additives on its webpage, however, conflicting and insufficient data continue to limit their use by mainstream practitioners in the full support of their consumption and prescriptive use.

Cupping

A therapeutic approach, originating in China, in which a cup made either of glass or bamboo is applied to the affected area (skin), and through the application of heat, air is suctioned out so that the skin and superficial muscle layer is drawn into and held in the cup (Dharmananda, 1999).

Cupping practitioners believe that the practice helps move blood throughout the body, hence promoting rapid healing. Research has been conducted to suggest the benefits of cupping with specific pain conditions, skin disorders such as herpes zoster, and respiratory ailments such as dyspnea. When combined with other CAM modalities such as acupuncture or meditation, cupping showed increased efficacy for disorders such as facial paralysis or spondylosis (Cao, Li, & Lui, 2012). Another study found that cupping therapy improved pain levels along with range of motion in patients with lower back pain (Markoowski et al., 2014)

Cupping therapy includes various modalities. Dry cupping is based on suction only. Wet cupping incorporates suction and controlled medicinal bleeding. In both modalities, "a flammable substance such as alcohol, herbs, or paper is placed in a cup and set on fire. As the fire goes out, the cup is placed upside down on the patient's skin. As the air inside the cup cools, it creates a vacuum. This causes the skin to rise and redden as blood vessels expand" (WebMD, 2014).

The cup is left in place for 5 to 10 minutes. Some side effects may include discomfort, burns, bruises, and skin infection. This therapy should not be applied to sites with deep venous thrombosis or ulcers, on an artery, or on a pulse that can be felt. Cupping should be avoided in women who are pregnant or menstruating, and in people with metastatic cancer, bone fractures, or muscle spasms (British Cupping Society, n.d.). Western medicine looks at cupping with skepticism since no scientific studies have been conducted on this CAIH modality.

Magnet Therapy

The use of magnets for specific types of health concerns has long been practiced in Japan. Magnet therapy has gained public awareness in the United States, where initially it was used by athletes to treat sports-related injuries. Traditionally, the term *magnet therapy* refers to the use of static magnets placed directly on the body, generally over regions of pain. Magnet therapy advocates believe that the electromagnetic fields created by the placement of the magnets improve specific human illnesses. One study found that patients experienced less sensory pain when wearing a magnetic bracelet, though objective results showed no efficacy or improvement in functional ability (Richmond et.al., 2009). In another clinical trial looking at fibromyalgia, a chronic pain disorder, results did suggest an improvement in subjects, but results again did not reveal statistical significance suggesting that further research is warranted (Alfano, Taylor, and Foresman, 2001).

Other conditions for which people wear magnets include general pain, pain after surgery, low back pain, foot pain, heel pain, osteoarthritis, rheumatoid arthritis, fibromyalgia, chronic fatigue syndrome, carpal tunnel syndrome, painful menstrual periods, nerve pain caused by diabetes (diabetic neuropathy), sports injuries, and migraine headache (WebMD, 2015c).

Despite the research thus far, there is still no clear answer as to how magnets physiologically work on the body or area of application. Consequently, the effects or benefits of magnet therapy are not clinically proven. Despite this, this form of therapy has gained popularity in United States, often being marketed via trendy bracelets that are magnetized and advertised to promote balance and coordination or to relieve pain. More research is needed on these and other related CAIH modalities (NCCIH, 2015c).

Consumer Issues

The need for research to provide scientific evidence for the efficacy of ayurveda and other complementary health approaches is large. Despite a report by the IOM (2011) that attempted to encourage the establishment of standardized clinical practice guidelines, significant gaps in knowledge still exist for medical practitioners and consumers. With the establishment of required criteria, evidence-based protocols, and practice guidelines, practitioners can review the available literature and decide on appropriate treatments. As CAIH modalities become substantiated through research findings it is likely that CAIH modalities will gain increased acceptance, and CAIH will be more integrated into the US healthcare system.

According to the IOM (2011), when reviewing research that attempts to provide evidence regarding CAM therapies, it is important to note whether it:

1. Provides consistent, systematic review of evidence.

2. Has been developed by multidisciplinary knowledgeable contributors.

3. Provides the evidence and guidelines that are transparent and reproducible.

4. Shows clear and truthful relationships between CAM practices and supplies explicit evidence of benefits of the specific alternative practice.

The NCCIH (2015b) alerted consumers that ayurveda uses products that may contain minerals, metals, or herbs which may be harmful if used improperly or without the supervision of a trained practitioner. According to the NCCIH, ayurvedic products have the potential to be toxic, and some of their active components have not been studied for safety in controlled clinical trials. A study conducted in 2008 examined 193 ayurvedic products and found that 21% contained lead, mercury, and/or arsenic levels higher than the acceptable daily intake guidelines.

One of the ayurvedic texts called *Rasa Shastra* (Vedic alchemy or process of purifying metals for herbal preparations that are used in India) indicates that Ayurveda uses *bhasmas*—metals that go through a purification process, which turns them into ash; They are not able to be used in United States due to questions of their safety and efficacy, and thus have not been approved by the FDA. As ayurvedic products in the United States are regulated as dietary supplements, they are not required to meet the same safety and effectiveness standards as conventional medicines (NCCIH, 2015b).

According to the NCCIH (2015b), consumers should be cautious when using any of the therapies described in this chapter. It recommends not using ayurvedic medicine to replace conventional care, or with pregnant women, nursing mothers, and children without consultation with a healthcare provider. According to the NCCIH, "There are not enough well-controlled clinical trials and systematic research reviews—the gold standard for Western medical research—to prove that the approaches are beneficial."

Consumers of CAIH modalities such as ayurveda, aversion therapy, art therapy, prayer therapy, light therapy, enzyme therapy, cupping, and magnet therapy must communicate with their healthcare providers to ensure coordinated and safe care. In addition, consumers should look for information related to credentialing of their CAIH providers on the NCCIH fact sheet titled "Credentialing: Understanding the Education, Training, Regulation, and Licensing of Complementary Health Practitioners," available at the NCCIH website (NCCIH, 2015b).

Implications for Health Professionals

Today's healthcare providers believe that health is not only the absence of disease. The current definition of health suggests that it is a continuum which impacts the whole individual and extends beyond infirmity and other physical ailments (Smeltzer, Bare, Hinkle, & Cheever, 2010). Nurses, health educators, and other health professionals are trained to recognize that their primary goal is to assist clients in realizing their greatest health potential. They also acknowledge that avoidance of disease is not always possible, but that one of their goals should be to assist individuals to maintain the best possible health in any circumstance. Unconventional healthcare practices, such as ayurveda, are part of a holistic health continuum and should play a role not only in the treatment of disease but in the maintenance of sustained health and harmony.

Practice guidelines follow a standard of care; however, before such standards can be created, evidence must be accumulated to support the standards. Evidence is needed to create healthcare guidelines pertaining to CAM. Licensure and credentialing processes for ayurvedic and other CAM practitioners need to be established in order to protect the consumer. In the United States, "No states license Ayurvedic practitioners, although a few have approved Ayurvedic schools such as California College of Ayurveda since 1995. Many Ayurvedic practitioners are licensed in other health care fields, such as midwifery or massage" (NCCIH, 2015b). This causes problems for practitioners who seek to include CAM therapies, such as ayurveda, into their treatment regimen since no unified national licensing criteria ensure the quality of these practitioners. Therefore, ultimately it is up to individual healthcare providers to identify appropriate CAM practitioners to whom patients needing CAIH modalities can be referred.

Health professionals ought to advocate for more research on ayurveda and other complementary health approaches. According to studies sponsored by the NCCIH, the effectiveness of ayurvedic medicine for schizophrenia and diabetes is inconclusive. Some ayurvedic practitioners use turmeric for inflammatory conditions and other disorders. Evidence from clinical trials indicated that turmeric may help with some digestive disorders and arthritis. Additional research supported by the NCCIH showed that "varieties of boswellia (*Boswellia serrata, Boswellia carterii*, also known as frankincense) produce a resin that has shown anti-inflammatory and immune system effects in laboratory studies. A 2011 preliminary clinical trial found that osteoarthritis patients receiving a compound derived from *B. serrata* gum resin had greater decreases in pain compared to patients receiving a placebo" (NCCIH, 2015b).

Ayurveda practitioners usually have some form of traditional medical or nursing training. In addition, they could receive a certification as a Certified Ayurveda Specialist (CAS) after attending a specialized CAIH school. The National Ayurvedic Medical Association (2015) has been working on credentialing ayurvedic practitioners to standardize its practice in the United States.

Western health educators strive to maintain and instill the concepts of healthy living, health promotion, and optimal disease management for targeted audiences or the general public. These basic foundations are inherent to the principles of ayurveda and other complementary health approaches. Often ayurveda, like most CAM therapies, is used as a complement to the Western management of disease. The vast array of

CAIH options can be overwhelming for consumers, but with research, guidance, and legitimate information from health professionals, individuals can use therapies that are appropriate to their needs and in accordance with healthcare practitioners' standards and protocols for practice.

Caveat Emptor

The gold standard in allopathic, or Western, medicine is the scientific method and evidence-based practices. Treatment modalities are accepted once they have been scientifically proven to be effective and show that benefits exceed the harm they may cause. Practices are further redefined and implemented into standards of care accepted by allopathic practitioners. Healthcare systems must adhere to practice guidelines and standards of care. This fact has caused some practitioners to hesitate about using certain CAM practices. Although some CAM therapies, such as chiropractic care, have become common in Western medical practice, most other CAIH therapies lack the evidence-based research necessary to show their scientific benefits and proof of effectiveness.

Brar et al. (2012) completed a comprehensive meta-analysis focused on ayurvedic interventions and treatment regimens based on diagnostic identification. The authors reviewed evidence of effectiveness in over 44 ayurveda clinical trials that were published from 1980 to 2009. They determined that there was rarely full use of diagnostic criteria and treatment plans for ayurveda, which is in contrast to Western evidence-based medicine. In the United States, diagnostic tests are used to assess and may confirm a diagnosis, which is then treated by evidence-based treatment plans. Over 24% of the research reviewed did not utilize any ayurvedic diagnostic criteria. The authors concluded that until specific regulatory practices are established, consumers should exercise caution with the prescribed practice intervention of ayurveda. Similarly, in an article on ayurveda by Rioux (2012), a consensus statement suggested that until relevant research on ayurvedic benefits and risks is completed, it is unethical for medical practitioners to incorporate these modalities into their practice. Although ayurvedic practitioners may receive a certification after attending a specialized school of CAM and although their basic principles of health maintenance are congruent with Western philosophies, they still remain at a disadvantage in occidental practice due to lack of reliable research or evidence-based information.

In addition, mainstream practice generally does not incorporate practices that are not held accountable by a form of licensure or certification.

Still, the use of non-Westernized healthcare or nonconventional practices as complementary approaches to health and illness has received significant attention recently. Increasingly, Western medical clinicians are recommending and referring patients for CAM therapies, such as yoga, chiropractic therapy, acupuncture, and massage, in conjunction with traditional treatment modalities. However, the use of non-Westernized healthcare practices on their own, as alternative, not complementary, approaches, has received far less acceptance in the United States. To achieve a level of appropriate scientific knowledge, health professionals must educate themselves on CAIH therapies and look for opportunities for continuing education provided by science-based entities, such as the NCCIH, among others.

Clients depend on healthcare providers to ensure that their practice methods are safe, effective, and scientifically proven. Evidence-based therapies, treatments, and medicines remain the hallmark and gold standard for current practice protocols. To date, although there has been a dramatic increase in interest and utilization of CAM practices, unfortunately, researchers have not formulated a significant amount of evidence. Therefore, a gap between practice, research, and acceptance of practice by Western medical practitioners has ensued. Health professionals and consumers should advocate for increasing research on CAIH practices. The generation of evidence and scientific knowledge on CAIH therapies is essential for the integration of these practices into Western care.

Conclusion

The public, health educators, and practicing healthcare clinicians are observing an increasing awareness and an integration of various complementary health approaches with conventional medical practice regimes. However, because standards of care in the healthcare system are based on research findings supporting the efficacy of any treatment, the lack of evidence-based practice research for many CAIH therapies has created a dilemma on their use or the formal implementation of such therapies. Intuitively, most medical practitioners adhere to the holistic approaches of most CAIH therapies, but due to the lack of scientific efficacy, continued skepticism currently exists and thus implementation into treatment regimens remains minimal at best.

Scientific evidence provided by the IOM and NCCIH through their funded research continues to examine, establish, and advance standardized plans of care that could integrate CAIH practices into the training and practice of today's healthcare providers. As healthcare continues to advance and evolve, once a strong body of evidence is generated regarding their efficacy, CAIH therapies will gradually be incorporated into mainstream medical treatment plans.

Summary

- Utilization of CAIH therapies and practices has become more common in the United States as their therapeutic benefits have gained some validation in the medical profession. The lack of evidence-based outcomes on most therapies, however, contributes to the tepid reception of CAIH therapies in the medical profession.

- Health professionals, patients, consumers, and health-conscious advocates continue to explore and incorporate CAIH therapies as an alternative form of health maintenance or in conjunction with traditional medical therapies for existing illnesses. Increasingly, Western medical practitioners and healthcare insurance companies are heavily promoting heath maintenance and disease prevention.

- The general public's demand for low-cost, noninvasive medical therapies and wary views of medicines continues to grow. Thus, the holistic and naturalistic principles of ayurveda and other CAIH therapies are becoming more common in all realms of healthcare. Only with continued research and scientific-based outcomes will their true benefit and use be realized.

- Ayurveda, aversion therapy, art therapy, prayer therapy, light therapy, enzyme therapy, cupping, and magnet therapy are CAIH approaches that need to be researched further. Health professionals and consumers need to be cognizant of the benefits and risks of these therapies.

- Consumers need to communicate with their healthcare practitioners about their use of CAIH therapies to maximize safety and ensure coordinated care.

Case Study

Description

A six-year-old female with a history of mild and stable allergen asthma with chronic hives all over the body and severe itching for a year is brought in by her mother for consultation with a Clinical Ayurvedic Specialist (CAS).

At the time of consultation, the girl's pediatrician and an allergist specialist had rendered extensive assessment and treatment. She was on asthma medication. Although extensive pediatric and adult allergy blood tests were done, she tested negative for all allergens. However, increased levels of immunoglobulin were discovered. Several of these tests were reported as traumatic for the patient. She had no known food or drug allergies and was negative for other medical conditions.

The mother stated that the hives first appeared after red ants in the yard bit the girl a year ago. The family was working with an allergy clinic and did not want to continue with so many medicines for long-term use. The mother reported that the allergist was aware of alternative therapy consultation and also was frustrated by the lack of therapeutic response to traditional therapies. Initially, the family elected to proceed with acupuncture, but due to the child's fear of needles, that treatment was not pursued. The mother then heard about ayurveda through word of mouth at a local yoga studio and wanted to try a holistic and natural approach to whole-body balance for her child.

Ayurvedic History

The patient presented as a pleasant and curious child. After a thorough and comprehensive assessment, she was found to have *pitta* and *vata* imbalances. The *pitta* imbalance was evidenced by the hives, itching, and her strong personality with intensity. The *vata* imbalance was evidenced by a dry cough, and she was found to have chronic constipation. This was also supported by physical assessment.

The dietary assessment revealed routine consumption of peanut butter and jelly sandwiches, yogurt, instant oatmeal, bagels, dry toast, cheese, crackers, fruit cups, marinated garlic, hot dogs, lots of garlic in pesto and bread, as well as citrus juice in the mornings.

Ayurvedic Treatment Plan

Treatment was planned in order to pacify *vata* and *pitta dosha* without aggravating *kapha*. Chronic constipation was addressed with the mother, and the patient was taught to pay close attention to bowel movements to ensure easy and complete daily evacuation. To ease the digestive system, the patient was taken off dairy products such as cheese, pizza, and yogurt.

Almond butter was substituted for peanut butter. Dietary recommendations, such as warm oatmeal with ghee or clarified butter, were given to help with the internal moisture. Garlic was completely eliminated. Licorice tea was introduced for internal lubrication as well.

One teaspoon of fresh organic homemade cilantro juice was given as needed to work as a natural antihistamine to help with the hives. The leftover green pulp was used on the skin for external relief from itching. Neem oil was used on the skin to remove the hot qualities of *pitta* and rejuvenate the tissue. Some herbal extracts mixed in a large bottle of water were taken daily to support the liver and reduce overall *pitta* in the body. No pharmaceutical medications were used.

In two weeks, the patient still had small red bumps, almost like a heat rash. At that point, she was asked to keep a food journal with a daily account of bowel movements and details about the skin rash. After about a month of using the ayurveda therapies, there was significant improvement with the rash and the hives were almost gone. After several months of ayurvedic counseling and use of therapy, the rash and hives resolved. Based on food journal experience, the mother thought that the use of commercial yogurt (with a color additive) may have been a trigger for the hives in her child and has since stayed away from it. Over this course, the ayurveda practitioner assessed all senses and stressors, and got to know the child and her own perceptions and personality. The practitioner specifically chose all of the therapies for this specific patient and her ailments. All therapies were natural and nontoxic to the body. At no time did the ayurveda practitioner discredit or recommend cessation of her medications without the consent of her pediatrician. The ayurveda practitioner encouraged the patient and her family to inform her pediatrician, allergist, and other healthcare providers about the ayurvedic treatment being received in order to coordinate care and maximize safety.

Questions

1. How is an ayurvedic assessment different from a Western medical assessment?

2. How is an ayurvedic treatment different from a Western medical treatment?

3. What are the benefits and risks of ayurveda?

4. What research studies could be consulted to determine the appropriateness of ayurveda treatment in this case study?

5. What consumer issues should be raised by health professionals when educating the family in this case study?

KEY TERMS

Ayurveda. A complementary health approach that originated in India and that incorporates herbs, massage, specialized diets, exercise, and lifestyle recommendations (NCCIH, 2015b).

Dosha. A life force, humor, or body type (NCCIH, 2015b).

Kapha. An ayurvedic body type, or *dosha*, that governs structure and lubrication and consists of earth and water elements (WebMD, 2015a).

Light therapy. Treatment method that involves exposure to light brighter than indoor light but not as bright as direct sunlight. It is suggested for the treatment of seasonal affective disorder and some sleep disorders (WebMd, 2015b).

Magnet therapy. Use of magnets for health concerns such as pain, osteoarthritis, rheumatoid arthritis, fibromyalgia, and chronic fatigue syndrome, among others (WebMD, 2015c).

Pitta. An ayurvedic body type, or *dosha*, that governs digestion and metabolism and consists of fire and some water elements (WebMD, 2015a).

Vata. An ayurvedic body type, or *dosha*, that governs movement and consists of space and air (WebMd, 2015a).

Vikruti. State of imbalance in an individual's *doshas* (Chopra Center, 2015).

References

Alfano, A. P., Taylor, A. G., & Foresman, P. A. (2001). Static magnetic fields for treatment of fibromyalgia: A randomized controlled trial. *Journal of Alternative and Complementary Medicine, 7*, 53–64.

American Cancer Society. (2013). *Targeted therapy.* Retrieved from http://www .cancer.org/acs/groups/cid/documents/webcontent/003024-pdf.pdf

Brar, B., Chhibar, R., Murthy, V., Srinivasa, V., Dearing, B., McGowen, R., & Katz, R. (2012). Use of ayurvedic diagnostic criteria in ayurvedic clinical trials: A literature review focused on research methods. *Journal of Alternative and Complementary Medicine, 18*(1), 20–28.

British Cupping Society. (n.d.). *Welcome to BCS.* Retrieved from http://www .britishcuppingsociety.org/

Cao, H., Li, X., and Liu, J. (2012). An updated review of the efficacy of cupping therapy. *PLos ONE, 7(2).*

Chopra Center. (2015). *Prakruti and vikruti.* Retrieved from http://www.chopra .com/prakruti-and-vikruti

Dharmananda, S. (1999). *Cupping.* Retrieved from http://www.itmonline.org/arts/ cupping.htm

Flaskerud, J. H. (2012). Seasonal affective disorders. *Issues in Mental Health Nursing,* *33*(4), 266–268. doi: 10.3109/01612840.2011.617028

Food and Drug Administration. (2013). *Enzyme preparations used in food (partial list).* Retrieved from http://www.fda.gov/Food/IngredientsPackagingLabeling/GRAS/EnzymePreparations/default.htm

Flynn, L. L., Bush, T. R., Sikorski, A., Mukherjee, R., & Wyatt, G. (2011). Understanding the role of stimulation of reflexology: Development and testing of a robotic device. *European Journal of Cancer Care, 20*(5), 686–696.

Goldbas, A. (2012). An introduction to complementary and alternative medicine (CAM). *International Journal of Childbirth Education, 27*(3), 16–20.

Halpern, M. (2009). *Principles of ayurvedic medicine* (10th ed.). Grass Valley, CA: Halpern.

Institute of Medicine of the National Academies. (2005). *Complementary and alternative medicine in the United States.* Washington, DC: National Academies Press. Available at http://www.nap.edu/catalog/11182/complementary-and-alternative-medicine-in-the-united-states

Markowski, A., Sanford, S., Pikowski, J., Fauvell, D., Cimino, D., & Caplan, S. (2014). A pilot study analyzing the effects of Chinese cupping as an adjunct treatment for patients with subacute low back pain, improving range of motion, and improving function. *Journal of Alternative and Complementary Medicine,* pp. 113–117.

Mayo Clinic. (2015). *Phototherapy/ultraviolet light treatment.* Retrieved from http://www.mayoclinic.org/departments-centers/dermatology/arizona/services/phototherapy-ultravioet-light-treatment

National Ayurvedic Medical Association. (2015). *Welcome to our community.* Retrieved from http://www.ayurvedanama.org/

National Center for Complementary and Alternative Medicine. (2014). *NCCAM facts-at-a-glance and mission.* Retrieved from http://nccam.nih.gov/about/ataglance

National Center for Complementary and Integrative Health. (2015a). *Complementary, alternative, or integrative health: What's in a name?* Retrieved from https://nccih.nih.gov/health/integrative-health

National Center for Complementary and Integrative Health. (2015b). *Ayurvedic medicine: An introduction.* Retrieved from https://nccih.nih.gov/health/ayurveda/introduction.htm

National Center for Complementary and Integrative Health. (2015c). *Aromatherapy.* Retrieved from https://nccih.nih.gov/health/aromatherapy

National Research Council. (2005). *Complementary and alternative medicine in the United States.* Washington, DC: National Academies Press.

Niederhofer, H., & von Klitzing, K. (2012). Bright light therapy as monotherapy of non-seasonal depression for 28 adolescents. *International Journal of Psychiatry in Clinical Practice, 16*(3), 233–237.

Rastogi, S., & Chiapelli, F. (2013). *Hemodynamic effects of* Sarvanga Swedana *(ayurvedic passive heat therapy): A pilot observational study*. Retrieved from http://www.ncbi.nlm.nih.gov/pmc/articles/PMC3821243/

Richmond, S. J., Brown, S. R., Campion, P. D., Porter, A. J., Moffett, J. A. K., Jackson, D. A., . . . & Taylor, A. J. (2009). Therapeutic effects of magnetic and copper bracelets in osteoarthritis: A randomised placebo-controlled crossover trial. *Complementary Therapies in Medicine, 17*(5), 249–256.

Rioux, J. (2012). A complex, non-linear dynamic systems perspective on ayurveda and ayurvedic research. *Journal of Alternative and Complementary Medicine, 18*(7), 709–718.

Salviati, A., Burlina, A. P., & Borsini, W. (2010). Nervous system and Fabry disease, from symptoms to diagnosis: Damage evaluation and follow-up in adult patients, enzyme replacement, and support therapy. *Neurological Sciences, 31*(3), 299–306.

Smeltzer, S., Bare, B., Hinkle, J., and Cheever, K. (2010). *Brunner and Suddarth's Textbook of Medical-Surgical Nursing* (12th ed.). Philadelphia: Wolters Kluwer Health/Lippincott Williams and Wilkins.

UM Health Service Newborn Care Committee. (2005). *Your baby, jaundice, and phototherapy*. Retrieved from http://www.med.umich.edu/1libr/pa/umphototherapy.htm

WebMD. (2014). *Cupping therapy*. Retrieved from http://www.webmd.com/balance/guide/cupping-therapy

WebMD. (2015a). *Ayurvedic medicine*. Retrieved from http://www.webmd.com/balance/guide/ayurvedic-treatments

WebMD. (2015b). *Light therapy—Topic overview*. Retrieved from http://www.webmd.com/depression/tc/light-therapy-topic-overview

WebMD. (2015c). *Magnet therapy*. Retrieved from http://www.webmd.com/vitamins-supplements/ingredientmono-1177-magnet%20therapy.aspx?activeingredientid=1177&activeingredientname=magnet%20therapy

CHAPTER 6

THE ROLE OF SPIRITUALITY IN HEALING

Dominick L. Sturz

According to Kosmin and Keysar (2009), approximately 80% of Americans have a religious affiliation. The Pew Forum's US Religious Landscape Survey has supported this claim, whereas a representative sample of more than 35,000 individuals suggested that almost 78% of the US population claim a religious affiliation. Additionally, of the roughly 23% who did not claim religious affiliation, only 4% identified themselves as either atheist or agnostic respectively, while 15.8% reported "nothing in particular," although they may have religious or spiritual beliefs (Pew Forum on Religion & Public Life, 2015). Similar reports are found worldwide, although analyses of over 2,500 global surveys and censuses representing more than 230 countries revealed that more than 8 in 10 people around the world identify with a religious group, with many considering themselves unaffiliated with a particular faith and reporting spiritual beliefs such as belief in a universal spirit (Pew Forum on Religion & Public Life, 2012). So seemingly universal is the importance of spirituality that it is included as a dimension of wellness by the National Wellness Institute (and many other organizations)—albeit a dimension that is commonly overlooked or ignored in favor of focus on other dimensions (i.e., physical, emotional, mental, social, and occupational).

Research on religiosity, spirituality, and aging suggest that religiosity and spirituality are important to many throughout their life span and that importance steadily increases throughout the life cycle (Atchley, 2008; Moberg, 2005; Peacock & Poloma, 1999). However, when facing

LEARNING OBJECTIVES
At the completion of this chapter, students will be able to:

- Identify the theoretical and scientific basis of prayer, meditation, healing touch, shamanism, traditional Chinese medicine spiritual practices, traditional Indian medicine spiritual practices, and African and Latin American spiritual practices such as *Santería*, *Espiritismo*, and *curanderismo*.

- Describe the difference between religiosity and spirituality.

- Identify spiritual/religious methods of healing utilized in a historical perspective.

- Describe current spiritual and religious practices used to address health concerns.

- Identify practical realities facing health educators and other health professionals when addressing their patients' spiritual needs.

(continued)

LEARNING OBJECTIVES
(*continued*)

- Describe methods and strategies of integrating spirituality within treatment plans.

- Discuss the value of spiritual healing modalities as complementary, alternative, and integrative health practices.

mortality, patients often struggle with their spirituality, which makes it crucial to integrate the spiritual domain into healing techniques, including empathy and care (Seccareccia & Brown, 2009). This is true regardless of the many different religions and philosophical belief systems that utilize spiritual practices of healing. Whether through shamans, soothsayers, mediums, religious leaders, or spiritual healers, spirituality has been practiced as a form of healing for thousands of years. Though specific beliefs and practices differ, the basic premise that faith, spirituality, and/or religion could affect a person's healing process is shared across cultures, languages, and ethnic groups (Torosian & Biddle, 2005).

This chapter presents various forms of spiritual healing, such as prayer, meditation, healing touch, traditional Chinese medicine (TCM) spiritual practices, traditional Indian medicine (TIM) spiritual practices, shamanism, and African and Latin American spiritual practices such as *Santería*, *Espiritismo*, and *curanderismo*. These practices are discussed as complementary, alternative, and integrative health (CAIH) modalities that emphasize individuals' well-being and health maintenance.

Theoretical Concepts

Overview

Pargament (1997) defined the term *religiosity* as the practices and beliefs related to organized religious affiliations or specified divine powers. Generally, religiosity can be segmented into two basic dimensions—extrinsic and intrinsic. Extrinsic religious motivation involves the use of religion as a means to an end, such as improved social status through church attendance or justification of certain individually held beliefs. Intrinsic religious motivation, however, moves beyond simple church attendance and involves religion as a central motivation in life. People who have high intrinsic religious motivation believe sincerely in the teachings of their religion and attempt to live their lives in accordance with its teachings.

Somewhat different from religiosity, the term *spirituality* implies the presence of a personal system of beliefs, often giving purpose and meaning in life (Grant, 2012;

Post, Puchalski, & Larson, 2000). In fact, spirituality is described by the National Center for Complementary and Integrative Health (NCCIH, 2015a) as a sense of meaning and purpose in life, beyond mere materialistic value. A characteristic of this definition is that it encompasses the feeling of connection to something larger than self while also allowing for the inclusion of religiosity. A weakness of the definition may be that it is too vague and allowance of the large degree of overlap with religiosity can be confusing when attempting to differentiate the terms (Levin, 2009).

In spirituality, beliefs are internalized on an individual basis; in religiosity, there is a sense of belonging to a community that shares similar beliefs and values (Hsiao et al., 2008; Koenig, 2004). In spirituality, there is a sense of something intangible in relation to the soul, a feeling of relationship to a higher power of one's choice (Gockel, 2009; Williams-Orlando, 2012). This higher power is identified by many names, depending on individuals' traditions, religious beliefs, or spiritual views. For example, Christians often refer to God; Muslims to Allah; and Hindus to Vishnu and his incarnations, Shakti and her manifestations, and Shiva (Ridenour, 2001).

Moxy, McEvoy, Bowe, and Attia (2011) summarized the terms nicely by stating that spirituality is a feeling of connectedness one has with a higher power, while religions are organized systems that share certain beliefs, rituals, and worship. Considering these descriptions, spirituality may play an important role in a person's religiosity, although many who consider themselves spiritual may not necessarily identify with a specific religion or particular doctrine. Further, spirituality may be the driving force behind participation in religious activities, or participation in religious activities may foster and enhance a person's sense of spirituality. Alternatively, people may fully participate in religious activities absent any feeling of connectedness to a higher power. It is safe to regard both spirituality and religiosity as multidimensional constructs with both overlapping and unique traits (Levin, 2009).

Historical Considerations

Historically, traditional healers and physicians often were monks, priests, shamans, and others and utilized places of worship, such as temples, shrines, and churches, to combine religious and/or spiritual practices with prayer and incantations to help heal the sick. Some of the earliest places of worship were considered responsible for nursing the poor and ill back to health (Friedlander, Kark, & Stein, 1986; Torosian & Biddle, 2005). Similar to the spiritual practices found in Eastern traditions (e.g., TCM, ayurveda, etc., many of which are discussed at length throughout this and other chapters of this text), Western societies were also looking toward their spiritual connections and faith to understand infirmities. For example, while the Church of Rome was influential in the government of early Western Europe (from the fifth century through the Middle Ages), Christian healing began to combine spirituality and religious healing in the belief that living by the "laws of nature" was God's will. Illness was a sign that an individual was not adhering to these laws and therefore was immoral. Early physicians formed associations, both formal and informal, to share the body of knowledge concerning religious practices in healing, which were subsequently taught and applied in universities and hospitals alike (Aldridge, 1991; Lucchetti, Lucchetti, & Puchalski, 2012; Sheldrake, 2007).

As scientific discovery and medical advances improved, medical communities slowly embraced the "science of healing" and seemingly became less reliant on spiritually based methods. Particularly important was the discovery of cells in the mid-19th century, which led to cell and germ theories. During that time, Louis Pasteur and Robert Koch, among others, were instrumental in leading the germ theory forward by demonstrating that disease could be linked to specific microorganisms, or germs. This ultimately led to the development of diagnostic procedures, treatments, and disease prevention techniques based on microorganisms (Association of the British Pharmaceutical Industry, 2015). Of course, this is not to say that spirituality-based medicine disappeared; most certainly it did not. Thousands of years of belief and practice have carried traditional methods into modern-day approaches.

Modalities

Certain Eastern philosophies/traditions, such as Buddhism and Taoism (Daoism), do not rely on an identified deity as a source of their spirituality yet believe healing is a derivative of the spiritual harmony/balance between mind and body. Through the removal of distortions, distractions, and delusions, the mind is purified and healing can occur. Purification of the mind through meditation and compassion can lead to a state of calmness, thus preparing a person for higher levels of consciousness. Once the mind has been purified, the body must also undergo purification for balance. Different types of yoga are commonly utilized to help achieve this purpose (Kakar, 2003). In Buddhism, Taosim, and Hinduism, this purification process becomes a cycle of spiritual progression, not only benefiting a person's current life through enhanced physical, spiritual, and emotional health and balance, but also laying the groundwork for continued progression in the person's reincarnated life as he or she moves toward higher consciousness (Kumar, 2002).

Meditation, prayer, church attendance, and yoga are examples of spiritually based mind-body therapies that are frequently used (in addition to herbs and supplements) by individuals in modern times to assist in coping with their illnesses and to promote healing (Ellison, Bradshaw, & Roberts, 2012). Others turn to God, speak with clergy, and/or immerse themselves in religious texts and individual prayer to cope (Hart, 2008). Each practice has its own merits in the healing process. While some spiritual practices help with coping and recovery, others provide individuals with a sense of inner peace and tranquility. Among the many different belief systems that utilize spiritual practices of healing, meditation and prayer are two of the most commonly shared.

Meditation

Found throughout many cultures and traditions, meditation is utilized to calm the mind, increase awareness, and reduce stress through self-regulation. There are many types of meditation. Three of the more commonly utilized categories of meditation include: (1) focused attention, where an individual focuses all attention on a mantra, sound, or word; (2) open monitoring, where an individual focuses attention on observation and monitoring of both internal and external events over a period of time; and (3) devotional, where an individual focuses attention on a deity. To think of meditation as an emptying of one's mind for clarity would be a mistake. While some meditations involve focusing the mind for awareness and calm, other techniques involve guided imagery and visualization wherein there is consistent stimulation, which promotes relaxation and healing (Ornish et al., 2002).

The National Health Interview Surveys revealed that meditation was used by 7.6% of adults in 2002, 9.4% in 2007, and 8.0% in 2012. These three surveys found meditation to be among the five most commonly used CAM therapies (Clarke et al., 2015). Research has suggested that meditation can improve one's immune system and brain function, increase relaxation, decrease anxiety, pain, and insomnia, and help recovering addicts avoid relapse (Hart, 2008; Williams-Orlando, 2012).

Prayer

A popular approach to healing in Christian, Judaic, and Islamic tradition, prayer is one of the most popular CAM techniques used by individuals from various belief systems around the world. According to research, 60% of the population surveyed in the United States indicated that they use prayer for improved health, making it the most popular of all CAM techniques

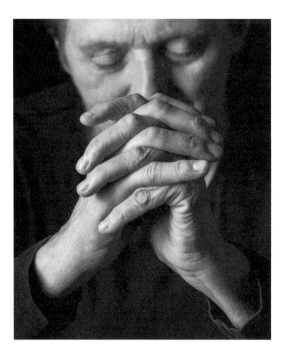

Figure 6.1   Prayer

utilized (Hart, 2008). Prayer (Figure 6.1) often takes the form of nonverbal or verbal worship, with or without requests for guidance or intervention through spiritual means.

Among those who pray, there exists a spiritual relationship between the devotee and some higher power. There is a feeling of connectedness between one's soul/energy source and something free of physical boundaries that has the ability to transcend physical life and spiritual afterlife alike (Stanley, 2009). Prayer in healing is based on faith in divine or supernatural intervention by God, Jesus Christ, Allah, or some higher power/deity to alleviate sickness in the infirm, change circumstances in times of challenge, and give hope to those in need (Zeiders & Pekala, 1995). Believers in the power of prayer have utilized it in various forms, with hopes of improving either their own health or the health of others. Allaboutprayer .org defines intercessory prayer as that in which an individual or group prays on behalf of others—for instance, praying for the healing of those who are ill. Intercessory prayer is a common practice in many religious organizations, and although it is faithfully practiced, has shown little benefit in the majority of methodologically rigorous studies. However, some well-controlled studies have shown small but significant effects.

Research on the effects of nonintercessory types of prayer has shown that prayer can be associated with feelings of comfort, encouragement, connectedness, acceptance, and unconditional love. Prayer can also be an effective method of coping with various illnesses, ailments, and diseases (Baverstock & Finlay, 2012; Williams-Orlando, 2012).

The National Health Interview Surveys in 2002, 2007, and 2012 comprise the most comprehensive, nationally represented data sets in the United States regarding complementary medicine (Stussman, Bethell, Gray, & Nahin, 2013). Analysis of the 2002 and 2007 surveys suggests that approximately 47% of the respondents (representing a weighted 179 million individuals) prayed in 2002 and roughly 53% of respondents (representing a weighted 194 million individuals) prayed in 2007 (Wachholtz & Sambamthoori, 2013). In addition, prayer specifically utilized as a method of dealing with health concerns (e.g., depression) is increasing, regardless of whether one has health insurance or not. Preliminary analyses of the 2012 data appear to support similar observations, although published results specific to prayer remain forthcoming.

Healing Touch

In Christian traditions, prayer for the sick would sometimes accompany the "laying on of hands" on an infirm individual in the belief that the Holy Spirit would provide healing through prayer and physical touch. In hospice/palliative care settings, a similar practice—healing touch—has been gaining popularity with both healthcare practitioners and volunteers alike. Healing touch may have its origins in the practice of laying on of hands, although it differs in that healing touch is an energy-based, therapeutic approach that utilizes the practitioner's hands to influence the energy field surrounding the client's body in order to energize and balance his or her personal energy field, thereby affecting the client's mental, physical, emotional, and spiritual health (see Figure 6.2).

Healing touch (Figure 6.2) has been reported to support wound healing, spiritual development, and an array of life's transitions (e.g., moving, job changes, relationship changes, birth, living with health conditions, death). (Van Aken & Taylor, 2010; Wang & Hermann, 2006). Van Aken and Taylor (2010) explored healing touch in treatment of those with moderate depression. Healing touch sessions were given in four stages to individuals reporting moderate depression. Analysis uncovered the psychosocial problem and the stages and strategies that are utilized in the process of coping with depression. The four stages were identified as: (1) belief in practitioner, (2) self and future self, (3) integrating all aspects of self,

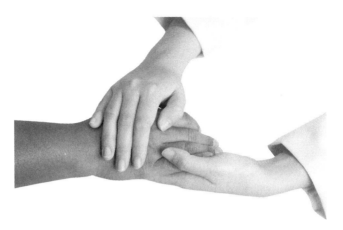

Figure 6.2   Healing Touch

and (4) accessing inner strength and resources and engaging with life. The researchers encouraged patients to learn healing touch techniques for self-utilization in times of anxiety or depression. Healing touch has also been utilized with noncommunicative hospice patients, as human touch is something everyone inherently needs. Families of those in hospice care often reported loved ones appearing more relaxed and peaceful, even with simple hand and arm massages (Van Aken & Taylor, 2010).

Values such as trust, honesty, tolerance, hope, service, faith, and compassion are often associated with spirituality (Williams-Orlando, 2012). In addition to helping individuals cope with illness, these values help healthcare practitioners form positive relationships with their patients. Williams-Orlando (2012) suggested that only 20% of physicians actually question their patients about their spirituality; however, many patients report the desire to have their physician pray with them (Williams, Meltzer, Arora, Chung, & Curlin, 2011). Although some patients wish to utilize their spirituality as a method of healing, many healthcare practitioners are not comfortable with the topic. This fact should concern health educators and health professionals, considering that data from the National Health Interview Surveys on Complementary and Alternative Medicine in 2002, 2002, and 2012 suggest that patients are increasingly utilizing spiritual practices, such as prayer, as a means of coping with health concerns (Clarke et al., 2015; Wachholtz & Sambamthoori, 2013).

When patients face life-threatening illness and disease, difficult questions pertaining to the meaning of their suffering or applicability of their faith often arise. They often question why the circumstance is happening to them (e.g., what happens when they die), and many turn to their faith to find answers at these difficult times. When answers potentially involve individuals' personal beliefs or systems of faith, these types of questions can be difficult for healthcare practitioners to address. Unfortunately, many physicians and healthcare practitioners are uncomfortable communicating with their patients about issues of spirituality and faith, due to either lack of education about the topic or fear of making nonspiritual clients uncomfortable (Williams-Orlando, 2012).

It is becoming increasingly clear that educating healthcare practitioners on matters of spirituality and faith plays an integral role in holistic health and healing. Medical colleges have started taking notice of this need and have begun implementing spirituality courses within their curricula (Puchalski, 2001). Reports show that in the early 1990s, only a few medical colleges offered spirituality courses, yet now the majority make these courses available to their medical students (Koenig, Hooten, Lindsay-Calkins, & Meador, 2010). Although these courses generally are not compulsory, they do offer hope that future classes of graduating medical students will be able to communicate at some level about their patients' spirituality and beliefs, perhaps even incorporating these factors into their medical treatment plans.

Winkelman et al. (2011) suggested that healthcare practitioners may consider utilizing a spirituality screening tool, such as Puchalski's Faith, Importance and Influence, Community, and Address (FICA) spiritual history and assessment tool (Pulchalski & Romer, 2000) to guide spiritual care practices. Similar tools include HOPE, FACT, and the Berg Cultural/ Spiritual Assessment. Healthcare practitioners can include such tools as part of a comprehensive initial medical assessment to characterize patient religiosity and/or spirituality and inform the practitioner regarding specific spiritual concerns and patient preferences for spiritual care and treatment plans. Inclusion of various spiritual practices, such as meditation, herbs, and yoga, in treatment plans has been shown to have positive effects on coping with illness, improved recovery measures, and improvements in quality of life (Ano & Vasconcelles, 2005; Puchalski, 2001). Meanwhile, the religious practices of church attendance and prayer have each been associated with improvements in morbidity and mortality (Gunderson, 2000; Idler, McLaughlin, & Kasl, 2009).

CAM modalities utilizing spiritual beliefs and religious practices have been successful in helping individuals cope with chronic conditions, such as cancer, asthma, and multiple sclerosis (Singh, Raidoo, & Harries, 2004). Centering on their faith allows many to focus on something other than the physical condition of their body and the pain they are feeling. This focus can help protect against deepening anguish and may provide a glimmer of happiness during challenging times (Molassiotis, Potrata, & Cheng, 2009). The sense of peace that comes with spiritual focus during times of illness can also extend to family members, providing them with the strength and ability to cope with their loved one's struggles.

Gockel (2009) conducted a qualitative study of 12 participants utilizing spirituality as a method of healing, in hopes of describing the process of spiritual coping. Eleven participants described themselves as spiritual but not religious, while one participant described himself as a practicing Buddhist, being both spiritual and religious. Interviewed participants were videotaped in 90-minute sessions as they described their experiences with spirituality and healing. Study participants described a sense of "openness" during the early stages of healing; they disregarded boundaries and were more open to different healing methods. Another common theme was the shift to a "spiritual perspective." As participants utilized spiritual methods, they felt a stronger connection to their own spirituality. They reported that relying on their spirituality lead to a greater sense of meaning. Last, participants reported feeling a "sacred" connection through utilization of spiritual healing methods. This narrative study described how spirituality could be an effective form of healing—both physically and mentally. Participants described facing adversity and turning it into an opportunity for spiritual growth and development as well as greater self-awareness, which benefited them during the healing process.

Shamanism

A shaman is a "traditional healer who is said to act as a medium between the invisible spiritual world and the physical world. Most gain knowledge through contact with the spiritual world and use the information to perform tasks such as divination, influencing natural events, and healing the sick or injured" (NCCIH, 2015b).

The word *shaman* is a Siberian tribal word that refers to the journey a man or woman goes through during an altered state of consciousness. The "shamanic journey" is precipitated by drumming and other percussion instruments, such as rattles. During this journey, the healer is able to diagnose and treat diseases as well as interact with spirits, power animals, angels, and spiritual teachers. Shamans are selected by the spirits, and teachings are passed on through oral tradition from generation to generation. Shamans extend their body energy to the patient in the process of healing by placing their hands on the client (Shamanic Healing Institute, 2015).

Traditional Chinese Medicine and Spirituality

Involvement of one's spirit is a common practice in many Eastern traditional medicines, including TCM. TCM is based on these principles:

> The human body is a miniature version of the larger, surrounding universe; harmony between two opposing yet complementary forces, called *yin* and *yang*, supports health, and disease results from an imbalance between these forces; five elements—fire, earth, wood, metal, and water—symbolically represent all phenomena, including the stages of human life, and explain the functioning of the body and how it changes during disease; Qi, a vital energy that flows through the body, performs multiple functions in maintaining health. (NCCIH, 2015c)

Based on thousands of years of philosophy, medicine, and reflection, TCM has two primary foundations—the mind and body are inseparable, and one must have and cultivate good spirit in order to have good health (Shi & Zhang, 2012). In TCM, the spirit is commonly referred to as *qi* or *chi*, and it represents the energy of one's life force, which can be a source of healing (Mok, Wong, & Wong, 2010).

TCM has been highly influenced by the teachings of Buddhism, Taoism, and Confucianism, with each contributing toward the development of spiritual beliefs regarding the healing power of Chinese medicine (Mok et al., 2010; Shi & Zang, 2012). Confucian ethics have been influential in Chinese beliefs regarding the importance of helping others, maintaining strong relationships, obligation, and death (Mok et al., 2010; Woo, 1999). Similarly, Taoist teachings have influenced the Chinese belief in the importance of living in harmony with nature, while Buddhism teaches that doing wrong unto others can ultimately result in illness and disease. For example, it is believed that if someone treats an innocent person cruelly or devalues life, he or she will inevitably fall ill; meanwhile, following the tenets of harmony and doing no harm will act to prevent illness (Shi & Zhang, 2012).

In regard to healing, the Chinese believe in strong relationships that lead to familial bonds and spirituality, which are viewed as instrumental resources for treatment of chronic conditions. In addition to the use of TCM, some rely on the teachings of Chinese philosophies (i.e., Buddhism, Taoism, and Confucianism) when facing terminal illness. For instance, once people are able to face the severity of their illness and are accepting of the eventuality of sickness or death, they increasingly begin to look beyond themselves for methods of coping. Research tells us this stage of acceptance is frequently when individuals turn toward their g/God, faith, beliefs, and philosophies in order to find meaning in life and potentially in their suffering (Mok et al., 2010).

Zang Fu is a theory that explains relationships, pathological changes, and physiological functioning of different organs within the human body. In TCM, *zang* and *fu* organs represent generalized pathophysiology and are responsible for creating, storing, or directing one's qi, which can be used to explain infirmities/disease and create a plan for treatment. Zang Fu, which utilizes herbs, acupuncture, and qi gong (i.e., a method of aligning breath, movement, and awareness in order to guide qi throughout the body, which in turn promotes healing and balance), continues to be a widely accepted practice within TCM. TCM also includes other forms of CAIH practices, such as "acupuncture, moxibustion (burning an herb above the skin to apply heat to acupuncture points), Chinese herbal medicine, tui na (Chinese therapeutic massage), dietary therapy, and tai chi and qi gong (practices that combine specific movements or postures, coordinated breathing, and mental focus)" (NCCIH, 2015c).

Traditional Indian Medicine and Spirituality

Western societies are also turning to TIM to help them through various illnesses and chronic conditions. Indian healing traditions are some of the oldest in the world (Kakar, 2003), with deeply spiritual beliefs rooted in Hinduism guiding vital holistic assessments and healing practices (Bhagwan, 2012). Ayurveda is one such form of TIM rapidly growing throughout much of Europe and elsewhere (Kessler, Wischnewsky, Michalsen, Eisenmann, & Melzer, 2013). The traditional practice of ayurveda is rooted in spirituality and dates back more than 5,000 years to its origins in India (Bautista, Moehler, & Joubert, 2011; Patwardhan, 2010). Ayurveda is part of the *upaveda* (i.e., auxiliary knowledge) and is considered a supplement to the sacred Hindu *vedas* (i.e., scriptures), which were traditionally passed from one generation to the next via oral tradition.

The traditional origins of ayurveda hold that Brahma passed down the science to Dhanvantari, physician of the gods. In ayurvedic practice, the body is dominated by three elements—*vata* (air), *pitta* (fire), and *kapha* (water). These three elements work in tandem to keep the body functioning properly. When these elements are in balance, an individual retains health; when the elements are imbalanced, however, sickness arises (Narayan, 1998). It is the balance and harmony between mind, body, and spirit that prevents illness and contributes to a healthy life. Treatments to heal illness can involve consumption of warm foods; spices, such as

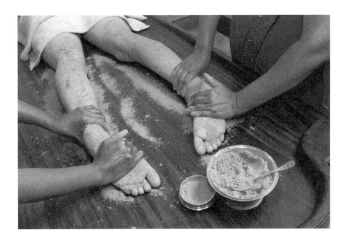

Figure 6.3   Ayurvedic Foot Massage

cinnamon and cardamom; herbs combined with certain minerals, such as sulfur and gold; proper hygiene; exercise; meditation; massage (Figure 6.3); and yoga. Spiritual healing in ayurveda (e.g., *Daiva-Vyapasraya*) requires self-evaluation of spiritual harmony, which often results in utilization of *yogasanas* (chanting of mantras and meditations) to restore balance and harmony with the universe in order to facilitate healing.

Many people around the world utilize meditation and yoga as spiritual methods of healing. In TIM meditation, practitioners utilize visualizations and narratives in order to focus attention on an ailment and bring it back into balance and good health. This meditation has been considered an effective therapy for Hindus and non-Hindus alike, as every major world religion has traditions of meditation (Bhagwan, 2012; Haber, 2013). Similarly, yoga is an ancient healing practice that unites the mind, body, and spirit (Pankhaniam, 2005). Some consider spirituality to be the heart of yoga—via self-awareness, discovery, and actualization. Empirical evidence suggests that meditation and yoga can each relieve symptoms of depression and anxiety through increased relaxation. They have also been found to be beneficial coping methods, helping individuals confront addictive behaviors (Hanna & Green, 2004; Marlatt & Kristeller, 1999; Oman & Thorsesen, 2005).

When yoga is combined with psychotherapy—which focuses on resources, wisdom, and guidance to aid in coping—Eastern and Western philosophies work together harmoniously (Sing Kiat Ting, 2012). Hindu shamanic healers have utilized yoga psychotherapy to reduce stress and improve self-esteem. Generations of Hindus have embraced this integrative approach, partly due to how easily the approach can be integrated into one's work and social and personal life at any age (Bhagwan, 2012).

African and Latin American Spiritual Practices and Health

Traditional medicine throughout the African continent, as in the cultures discussed previously, is widely based on spiritual beliefs and practices. It also shares the belief that one's body is inseparable from mind and spirit. For example, Ethiopian tradition holds that good health is the balance between spiritual, social, mental, and physical aspects, which make a person whole. More than half of the population of Ethiopia currently relies on traditional healers and practices (Bihran, Giday, & Teklehaymanot, 2011). Healers are called on to treat everything from childbirth to toothaches and often use herbs and combine various plants, animals, and minerals to form traditional medications. Traditional healers often seek the guidance of ancestral spirits through dream interpretation, channeling, or throwing of bones. Traditional dancing, drumming, and chanting are common spiritual interventions to help cure illness and disease, especially when witchcraft is a suspected cause (Kassaye, Amberbir, Getachew, & Mussema, 2006). Church attendance and prayer are also common healing practices in Ethiopa and other African countries. Of note, some African practices have influenced certain religious and spiritual practices throughout Latin America and beyond.

Santería   *Santería* originates from the merging of the Yoruba religion of West Africa with Roman Catholicism, as slaves were transported to the Caribbean and Americas. Primarily practiced in the Caribbean (i.e., Cuba, Haiti, Puerto Rico, Trinidad) and Brazil, *Santería* holds the tradition that spiritual energy comprises every living thing, and its purpose is to move one forward toward the divine. It is believed that illness in a believer can be due to the activity of spirits, which may be remedied through rituals and ceremonies that often include animal sacrifice, drumming, chanting, the burning of candles, ritual bathing, and use of herbs.

Orishas (Figure 6.4), similar to saints in the Catholic faith, are viewed as demigods in the *Santería* faith. Traditionally, they are believed to look after the earth and all the affairs of humankind, with each holding dominion over a specific form of nature. Additionally, they are tasked with delivering the prayers of the faithful to God (Beetlestone, 2009; Blanchard, 2009). The *orishas* are often called upon for healing through use of a *santero*, or practitioner, who is consulted to relieve or solve problems that are difficult for clients to solve on their own (Baez & Hernandez, 2001). Prayers to *orishas* and consultations with *santeros* are thought to be helpful because of the clients' belief in the power of spirits and the process of healing through their faith.

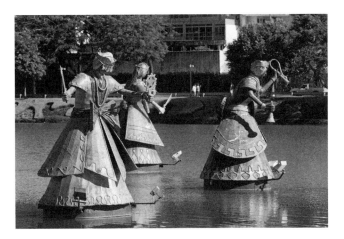

Figure 6.4   Orishas fountain in Bahia, Brazil.

Espiritismo   *Espiritismo*, which is practiced in the Caribbean and Latin America, also believes in the presence and activity of spirits among the living world. It is believed that illness and health can be explained by encounters with spirits, which either cause harm or provide protection. Mediums are utilized to communicate with spirits, and rituals are necessary to strengthen the presence of good spirits and banish evil ones. It is believed that the material, the spiritual, or a combination thereof causes all negative issues in life. Rituals are utilized to restore balance and harmony between spirit and body, thus promoting healing. These typically include herbal bathing, group healing sessions, and prayer (Baez & Hernandez, 2001).

Espiritismo is intertwined with the religious practices of Catholicism (and other faiths), and its rituals are viewed as harmonious with Latin American culture (especially in Puerto Rico), thus increasing acceptance and belief in its effectiveness (Rivera, 2005). The rituals are an important source of emotional support for *Espiritismo* participants, who believe they are empowered by the interaction of humans, spirits, and God, which allows them to feel a sense of independence and freedom from the negative influence of "ignorant spirits" that are viewed as responsible for all illnesses, major and minor (Rivera, 2005).

Curanderismo   Another traditional Latin American medical practice connecting the physical and the spiritual is *curanderismo* (to heal), which was developed within pre-Colombian and Aztec civilizations in order to connect with the spirit world as a method of healing. One of the major tenets in *curanderismo* is that there should be a high level of spirituality in one's balance with nature. Healing is facilitated by a *curandero/a* (native healer), who utilizes a holistic approach toward the individual in need, with therapies that include herbs, acupressure, massage, diet, prayer, and the wearing of amulets (e.g., spiritual and religious portrayals of the Sacred Heart of Jesus or the Virgin Mary) for protection against magic. *Curanderos* also use holy objects and sacred words in situations that require interventional channeling of spirits for the purpose of healing (Applewhite, 1995; Lopez, 2005; Tafur, Crowe, & Torres, 2009). Faith is instrumentally important in this culture, with practitioners feeling they are both protected and healed through the power of their faith.

Consumer Issues

Many patients want to discuss their spirituality and religious beliefs with their healthcare practitioners. Although some practitioners are uneducated about the topic and thus may feel uncomfortable, patients often indicate wanting the practitioner to engage in the subject. Discussions about one's spiritual practices can benefit decision making, understanding or acceptance of the illness/disease, and improved coping. A majority of medical colleges in the United States have acknowledged the importance of these practices through the addition of CAM courses within their curricula. Whether the client's practices are consistent with a practitioner's own is not of primary importance. What is important is for the practitioner to have knowledge, acceptance, and respect for different viewpoints, traditions, and beliefs about healing (Williams-Orlando, 2012).

Although spiritual/religious practices used in healing may have potential ethical concerns, research shows positive associative effects in coping, recovery, and mortality. Correlational research suggests that those who practice their religion on a daily basis are likely to live longer than those who do not practice a religion. Spiritual practices have been shown to improve coping skills during times of challenge such that stress is reduced, inner strength is increased, and the general outlook on life is improved—resulting in stronger relationships and increased enjoyment in life (Puchalski, 2001). Improved recovery outcomes may be one of the most important implications of spiritual practice in CAM. For example, multiple studies have found that heart surgery patients who expressed their spiritual beliefs and maintained regular spiritual practices had better postoperative physical function and outcomes, compared to those who did not (Ai, Park, Huang, Rodgers, & Tice, 2007; Casar-Harris et al., 1995; Contrada et al., 2004; Oxman, Freeman, & Manheimer, 1995).

Meraviglia (2006) conducted a study of women suffering from breast cancer to explore the effects of spiritual practices on their quality of life. Participants were 21 and older, had breast cancer, and resided in both urban and rural areas in Texas. Results indicated a positive correlation between meaning in life and psychological wellness and a negative correlation with physical responses. Meaning in life was found to be a mediator of breast cancer effects on physical and psychological well-being. Overall, the author concluded the practice of spirituality supports physical and psychological well-being.

Further research has suggested that discussions regarding spiritual practices lead to improved measures of patient acceptance of their condition and may benefit patient care outcomes. For example, discussion between a healthcare practitioner and patient about spirituality may strengthen the relationship bonds, allowing for increased trust and comfort discussing matters of mortality, which ultimately helps patients understand or accept their disease. Discussions regarding spirituality also affect patients' health decisions, as they may openly take the time to involve their spiritual/religious beliefs in medical decisions. Because research has repeatedly suggested that patients utilize their spirituality as a coping mechanism, discussing spirituality with patients provides healthcare professionals the opportunity

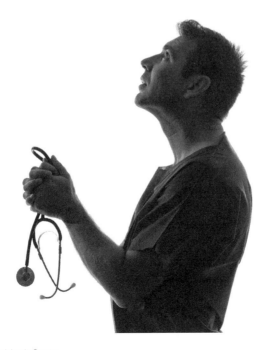

Figure 6.5   Physician in Prayer

to allow them to cope, to understand their methods, and potentially to address their spiritual needs.

Many physicians and other healthcare practitioners report their own spirituality likely affects their approach to healing (Figure 6.5), especially when working in hospice care or palliative care for the terminally ill (Seccareccia & Brown, 2009). Unfortunately, during the course of such care, practitioners and family place great attention on the physical domain of health treatment, while frequently the spiritual domain is not attended to. During these times, it is common for patients to spiritually struggle; for this reason, it is imperative that the spiritual domain is integrated within healing techniques (Seccareccia & Brown, 2009). Some believe that the foundation of a healing relationship between physician (and likely treatment teams and volunteers) and the dying patient is the embracing of spirituality. Interestingly, Kozak et al. (2009) found that physicians who consider themselves spiritual receive better patient reviews compared to those who do not. Regardless of the personal spiritual beliefs of healthcare professionals, respect and compassion should be at the forefront of all patient interaction. It does not matter whether patient and care provider share similar beliefs; what matters are that patient beliefs are respected and considered an elemental aspect of their care.

Commonly, spiritual healing practices are used by consumers in the United States as complementary forms of care. They are often combined with Western treatment modalities (NCCIH, 2015a). Whether spiritual healing practices are used as complementary, alternative, or integrative health modalities, consultation with a healthcare professional is always advised in order to avoid undesirable side effects and to improve quality of care.

Implications for Health Professionals

Healthcare professionals, including health educators, should not impose their personal views regarding spiritual/religious-based CAM practices, but should provide their clients with fair and balanced (i.e., describing benefits and risks) information based on empirical knowledge. In order to provide proper care and respect, it is helpful for healthcare educators and practitioners to have baseline knowledge regarding their clients' spiritual or religious traditions. Trust should be established during the initial and subsequent meetings. This trust can be gained in part through use of empathetic listening and nonjudgmental tolerance for belief systems that may be different from one's own. Utilization of a spiritual assessment tool can help healthcare practitioners ensure that their patients' needs are being met (Ai & McCormick, 2009; Borneman, Ferrell, & Puchalski, 2010).

When discussing or educating patients about the use of spirituality in healing, it is imperative to be accepting of patients' beliefs, even when they contradict those of the healthcare professional or educator. After educators and providers gain an understanding of patient beliefs and traditions, they should organize their teaching and treatment methods in a manner that is consistent with those beliefs and traditions. Healthcare practitioners and educators must develop an adequate knowledge of various spiritual/religious-based CAM practices in order to have accurate conversations with patients from different cultures and traditions (Johnson, Priestley, & Johnson, 2008). Essentially, a healthcare professional should be educated first, before educating others.

When healthcare practitioners (e.g., physicians, nurses, and educators) are made aware of spiritual methods of healing employed by their patients, they should help to identify and potentially recommend reputable CAM practitioners. They should schedule follow-up appointments to monitor patient response to spiritual therapies (e.g., use of herbs, faith healing, or intercessory or affirmative prayer) and modify treatment plans as necessary. Medical records should be noted detailing the CAM therapies initiated, which helps treatment teams maintain effective communication and continuity of care.

It is important to highlight that any notation within a patient's medical records falls under the protection of the Health Information Privacy Rule of the Health Insurance Portability and Accountability Act (HIPAA) of 1996 and should remain confidential and accessible only to authorized healthcare professionals and staff. The preamble to the Privacy Rule of the Department of Health and Human Services (HHS) explains that healing methods that are solely spiritual are not considered healthcare, and those religious practitioners and/or clergy who offer healing services that are solely spiritual are not considered healthcare providers under the rule (Tovino, 2005). Thus, if patients want medical records to be shared with religious practitioners outside of their medical treatment team, they must explicitly authorize such action.

In addition to ensuring patient safety, following these recommendations allows health educators and other health professionals to engage in shared decision making with their patients and demonstrates respect for their values, beliefs, and spiritual needs (Cady, 2009). Discussing spiritually based treatment options during admission or initial meetings can alleviate potential surprises and allow both healthcare professionals and patients to remain on the same page.

Healthcare administrators should consider implementing policies and procedures for handling spiritual/religious-based healing methods that are patient-centered—especially for the use of herbs, which may alter the effectiveness or safety of conventional treatment regimens. Quality control, risk management, and nurse managers should have distinct responsibilities, yet overlapping supervision during the use of these therapies in order to ensure close monitoring for safety and efficacy.

Health professionals should advise patients of the benefits and risks of utilizing complementary and alternative techniques separately or in combination with conventional methods. Healthcare practitioners and educators should also convey an inclusive, nonjudgmental, nonthreatening attitude and work diligently to accommodate patients' spiritual treatment requests based on current empirical evidence, when available.

Caveat Emptor

The topic of spiritual and religious practices as methods of healing is not without controversy (Polzer, Casarez, & Engebretson, 2012). Many people following traditional spiritual-based practices fail to inform their conventional healthcare professionals about their complementary and alternative treatments for fear of criticism or belief that these methods are without potentially negative effects. This can be an important issue, especially when people forgo medical treatments and instead attempt to heal themselves solely through reliance on religious faith and prayer. Some feel that responsible health educators and other healthcare practitioners should proactively discuss holistic methods, such as spirituality, with their patients (Cohen, Wheeler, Scott, & Anglican Working Group, 2001; Chattopadhyay, 2007; Pesut, 2006; Pesut & Thorne, 2007) while others feel uncomfortable approaching the topic and feel that healthcare practitioners should not discuss it (Polzer, Casarez, & Engebretson, 2012). Those who choose to discuss holistic methods of healing, including spiritual/faith-based practices, should be aware of possible ethical and legal implications when referring their clients to CAM practitioners or when utilizing spiritual/faith-based practices as adjunctive therapy.

There is the potential for laws to regulate the ability of healthcare providers to utilize (or recommend) certain traditional therapies alongside or in place of conventional practices (Cady, 2009). For example, many states, but not all, provide legal protection for those who utilize only faith healing practices (Grant, 2012). Although the US Constitution guarantees freedom of religion, the HHS does not recognize solely spiritual healing methods as healthcare, nor does it recognize as healthcare providers clergy or religious practitioners who are solely spiritual leaders (Tovino, 2005). Obviously, this presents an opportunity for confusion and controversy. It is highly recommended that health educators and other healthcare practitioners familiarize themselves with local laws and regulations pertinent to their practice and that they ensure that their clients are fully informed and consent to applied techniques.

A true dilemma exists concerning prayer and the patient–healthcare provider relationship. A conscientious healthcare practitioner may desire to fulfill patient wishes concerning prayer, yet may not want to cross a spiritual/religious boundary unintentionally through active participation. Alternatively, a healthcare practitioner who declines a patient/client request for prayer runs the risk of damaging their professional relationship and trust, which may ultimately negatively affect the healing process (Williams-Orlando, 2012). Although it is certainly ethical to pray with or for patients/clients at their request, it is important to discuss these actions prior to doing so, as some people may consider praying on their behalf without their knowledge to be unethical.

Another concern with physicians and spiritual practices, such as prayer, is their lack of spiritual/religious education or experience in medical school. Even when a healthcare educator or practitioner is familiar with certain practices (and might also utilize them personally), there is a fear of saying something wrong, choosing incorrect words, or not being able to fully answer patient questions when they have not been trained to handle such topics in an environment of professional care (Hart, 2008).

One example of spiritual practices being utilized successfully in an environment of professional care can be found at Mercy Medical Center in Merced County, California. The hospital caters to a large Hmong population, who often rely on traditional practices for healing; and the hospital was prompted to formally acknowledge and address this important issue within its own system of care by establishing the first Hmong shaman hospital policy in the nation (Brown, 2009). The hospital approved nine traditional ceremonies, including soul calling and soft chanting. This policy was established to bridge the divide between Western medicine and immigrant beliefs, allowing patients to utilize spiritual practices of healing in hospital settings.

Conclusion

Although people around the globe have utilized spiritual and religious-based practices for thousands of years, difficulty remains when attempting to differentiate between the two and their role in the care of patients. Part of the challenge resides in the shifting paradigms of acceptance and usage of the terms in published literature. Spirituality and religiosity can be defined differently, depending on how a particular society or culture perceives them within its own traditions (Hart, 2008). Regardless, the lines between the two (although distinct) sometimes are blurry, resulting in the current use of the term *spirituality* as a catchall of sorts—referring to those who are secularly spiritual, religiously spiritual, or some combination thereof.

Spiritual practices are some of the oldest forms of healing, and their popularity has risen and fallen over the centuries. Spiritual and religious practices for healing have been frequent choices for stand-alone or adjunctive therapy for a variety of illnesses and chronic conditions and as a way to cope with terminal illness. Many view the combination of conventional Western medicine with traditional healing practices as patient-centered holistic approaches that allow for healing, compassion, and cultural respect (Aldridge, 1991; Hsiao et al., 2008). In order for clients to benefit from this balanced approach, healthcare practitioners should be made aware of any complementary or alternative treatments individuals are considering. Healthcare practitioners should seek to increase their knowledge about various spiritual/religious-based practices for healing, their effects, and potential safety concerns. Cultural competence has become a major focus in healthcare and education. Being knowledgeable and tolerant of spiritual practices as acceptable forms of healing can be an effective way for a culturally competent practitioner to interact with people of various cultures, traditions, and beliefs.

Summary

- *Religiosity* and *spirituality* are distinct terms. *Religiosity* relates to the practices and beliefs related to organized religious affiliations or specified divine powers (Pargament, 1997). *Spirituality* implies the presence of a personal system of beliefs, often giving purpose and meaning to life (Grant, 2012; Post et al., 2000).

- Prayer, meditation, church attendance, and yoga are examples of spiritually based mind-body therapies that are frequently used (in addition to herbs and supplements) by individuals to assist in coping with illness and to promote healing.

- Spiritual and religious practices for healing have been frequent choices for stand-alone or adjunctive therapy for a variety of illnesses and chronic conditions and as a way to cope with terminal illness.

- Although some healthcare practitioners lack knowledge of and may feel uncomfortable with the topic of spirituality, many consumers express the desire to communicate with them about their spirituality; some report the desire to have their healthcare practitioner pray with them.

- One of the largest complaints in regard to spiritual methods of healing is the lack of awareness regarding established guidelines and standards of care (e.g., Federation of State Medical Boards' Guidelines on physician practices involving CAM). This is most noticeable in the lack of adequate regulation of herbs and herbal supplements, which, when taken in combination with prescription medications, can result in serious side effects.

- Spiritual healing modalities are prime examples of complementary, alternative, and integrative health since they are aimed to restore health and wellness.

- Health professionals, including health educators, should not impose their personal views regarding spiritual/religious-based practices but rather should provide their clients with fair and balanced (i.e., describing benefits and risks) information based on empirical knowledge.

Case Study

Description

Isaac is a 53-year-old former professional athlete who has been diagnosed with an inoperable brain lesion. Isaac's treatment team informed him that no treatment was available, and there was no hope for recovery or remission. Isaac began experiencing depressive episodes, highlighted by suicidal ideation. He lost all interest in the sport he previously loved, felt empty inside, could no longer concentrate, experienced sleep disturbances, and expressed thoughts of suicide. When a nurse visited Isaac for home care, he continually focused their discussions on his religious beliefs. He indicated that he was born and raised Catholic but did not regularly attend church, nor had he explored or engaged in spiritual practices other than prayer. Isaac explained to his nurse his feelings about religious teachings that consider suicide a sin and his desire to go to heaven. Isaac's struggle with his religious beliefs were making his already depressed mood worse.

Diagnosis

Based on the history of the presenting illness and depressive symptomology, in addition to the inoperable brain lesion, a diagnosis of mild/moderate major depressive disorder, subtype melancholic depression, was given. Additionally, conversations between Isaac and his treatment team suggested that he was experiencing a spiritual crisis.

Treatment

As there was no hope for remission from the brain lesion, the treatment team focused their efforts on Isaac's depression. He was prescribed a selective serotonin reuptake inhibitor, and cognitive-behavioral therapy sessions were recommended. Isaac's treatment plan was inclusive of his spirituality and allowed him to discuss his religious beliefs as a way to assist in coping with his diagnosis.

Results

During this time of crisis, Isaac's beliefs were not helping him cope with his disease. His religious beliefs were a source of fear and guilt, as he was conflicted between his desire to end his life while he still had control and choice and using his spirituality as a source of strength. In addition to the helplessness he was already feeling, his religious conflict exacerbated his depression. Through use of medication and self-reflection and the help of his treatment team, Isaac eventually let go of his feelings of helplessness. Although he still felt hopeless about his chances for recovery, Isaac was able to discuss these issues as a way to help him foster spiritual awareness. Isaac found hope through his faith. Eventually, he talked less of suicide and more about feeling a sense of control over finding peace before he died. He felt secure in his religious beliefs and continued to work on his spiritual practices of daily prayer, reading of inspirational materials, listening to tapes, and discussing his feelings and philosophy of life.

Reflection

This case study demonstrates ways in which our sense of spirituality, which is different for each individual, affects our philosophy of life. This case showed how nurses and other healthcare practitioners can educate patients without exposing personal bias. Through exploration and reflection, both the nurse and the patient worked toward further understanding of Isaac's spirituality and his personal meaning of healing. This case showed how a spiritual crisis changed an individual's perspective, and how spiritual reflection helped him cope with the crisis as a part of his healing process.

Questions

1. What ethical considerations are appropriate to this case?

2. What lessons for your professional practice can you learn from this case?

3. How can health educators and other health professionals decide whether patients' spirituality should be considered in their treatment?

4. What consumer issues are relevant in this case?

KEY TERMS

Curandero/curandera. Traditional healer of the Latin American tradition of *curanderismo*, often utilizing herbs, acupressure, massage, diet, prayer, and the wearing of amulets for protection against magic or the purpose of healing (Applewhite, 1995; Lopez, 2005; Tafur et al., 2009).

Qi. Also referred to as *chi* and popular in Chinese culture, qi is described as one's vital force or natural/spiritual energy (NCCIH, 2015c).

Religion. Organized systems that share certain beliefs, rituals, and worship (Pargament, 1997).

Shaman. Traditional healer who acts as a medium between the invisible spiritual world and the physical world. A shaman contacts the spiritual world in order to perform tasks such as divination, influencing natural events, and healing the sick (NCCIH, 2015b).

Spirituality. A feeling of connectedness with a higher power (Grant, 2012; Post et al., 2000).

Traditional Chinese Medicine (TCM). A healing system that encompasses multiple practices, such as acupuncture, moxibustion, Chinese herbal medicine, tui na, dietary therapy, tai chi, and qi gong (NCCIH, 2015c)

Traditional Indian Medicine (TIM). Healing traditions with deeply spiritual beliefs rooted in Hinduism guiding vital holistic assessments and healing practices (Bhagwan, 2012).

References

Ai, A. L., & McCormick, T. R. (2009). Increasing diversity of Americans' faiths alongside Baby Boomers' aging: Implications for chaplain intervention in health settings. *Journal of Healthcare Chaplaincy*, *16*(1–2), 24–41. doi: 10.1080/08854720903496126

Ai, A. L., Park, C., Huang, B., Rodgers, W., & Tice, T. N. (2007). Psychosocial mediation of religious coping: A prospective study of short-term psychological distress after cardiac surgery. *Personality and Social Psychology Bulletin, 33,* 867–882.

Aldridge, D. (1991). Spirituality, healing and medicine. *British Journal of General Practice, 41,* 425–427.

Ano, G. G., & Vasconcelles, E. B. (2005). Religious coping and psychological adjustment to stress: A meta-analysis. *Journal of Clinical Psychology, 61*(4), 461–480. doi: 10.1002/jclp.20049

Applewhite, S. L. (1995). Curandersimo: Demystifying the health beliefs and practices of elderly Mexican Americans. *Health & Social Work, 20*(4), 247–253.

Association of the British Pharmaceutical Industry. *Louis Pasteur and the germ theory of disease.* Retrieved from http://www.abpischools.org.uk/page/modules/ infectiousdiseases_timeline/timeline4.cfm?coSiteNavigation_allTopic=1

Atchley, R. C. (2008). Spirituality, meaning, and the experience of aging. *Generations, 32*(2), 12–16.

Baez, A., & Hernandez, D. (2001). Complementary spiritual beliefs in the Latino community: The interface with psychotherapy. *American Journal of Orthopsychiatry, 71*(4), 408–415. doi: 10.1037/0002-9432.71.4.408

Baverstock, A., & Finlay, F. (2012). Faith healing in paediatrics: What do we know about its relevance to clinical practice? *Child Care Health and Development, 38*(3), 316–320. doi: 10.1111/j.1365-2214.2011.01284.x

Bautista, C., Moehler, T., & Joubert, R. (2011). CAM use in Asia-Pacific. *Applied Clinical Trials, 6.* Retrieved from http://www.appliedclinicaltrialsonline.com/ cam-use-asia-pacific

Beetlestone, M. (2009). *To Santeria and back.* Bloomington, IN: Trafford.

Bhagwan, R. (2012). Glimpses of ancient Hindu spirituality: Areas for integrative therapeutic intervention. *Journal of Social Work Practice, 26*(2), 233–244. doi: 10.1080/02650533.2011.610500

Bihran, W., Giday, M., & Teklehaymanot, T. (2011). The contribution of traditional healers' clinics to public healthcare system in Addis Ababa, Ethiopia: A cross-sectional study. *Journal of Ethnobiology and Biomedicine, 7*(39), 39–39. doi: 10.1186/1746-4269-7-39

Blanchard, M. (2009). From Cuba with saints. *Critical Inquiry, 35*(3), 383–416. Retrieved from http://www.jstor.org/stable/10.1086/598813

Borneman, T., Ferrell, B., & Puchalski, C. M. (2010). Evaluation of the FICA tool for spiritual assessment. *Journal of Pain Symptom Management, 40*(2), 163–173. doi: 10.1016/j.jpainsymman.2009.12.019

Brown, P. L. (2009, September 20). A doctor for disease, a shaman for the soul. *New York Times.* Retrieved from http://www.nytimes.com/2009/09/20/us/20shaman .html?_r=1

Cady, R. F. (2009). Legal issues related to complementary and alternative medicine. *JONA's Healthcare Law, Ethics, and Regulation, 11*(2), 46–51. doi: 10.1097/NHL.0b013e3181adbc9b

Casar Harris, R., Amanda Dew, M., Lee, A., Amaya, M., Buches, L., Reetz, D., & Coleman, G. (1995). The role of religion in heart-transplant recipients' long-term health and well-being. *Journal of Religion and Health*, *34*(1), 17–32. doi: 10.1007/bf02248635

Chattopadhyay, S. (2007). Religion, spirituality, health and medicine: Why should Indian physicians care? *Journal of Postgraduate Medicine*, *53*(4), 262–266.

Clarke, T. C., Black, L. I., Stussman, B. J., Barnes, P. M., & Nahin, R. L. (2015). Trends in the use of complementary health approaches among adults: United States, 2002–2012. *National Health Statistics Reports, 79.*

Cohen, C. B., Wheeler, S. E., Scott, D. A., & Anglican Working Group. (2001). Walking a fine line—physician inquiries into patients' religious and spiritual beliefs. *Hastings Center Report*, *31*(5), 29–39. Retrieved from http://www.ncbi .nlm.nih.gov/pubmed/12974116

Contrada, R. J., Goyal, T. M., Cather, C., Rafalson, L., Idler, E. L., & Krause, T. J. (2004). Psychosocial factors in outcomes of heart surgery: The impact of religious involvement and depressive symptoms. *Health Psychology*, *23*(3), 227–238. doi: 10.1037/0278-6133.23.3.227

Ellison, C. G., Bradshaw, M., & Roberts, C. A. (2012). Spiritual and religious identities predict the use of complementary and alternative medicine among US adults. *Preventive Medicine: An International Journal Devoted to Practice and Theory*, *54*(1), 9–12. doi: 10.1016/j.ypmed.2011.08.029

Friedlander, Y., Kark, J. D., & Stein, Y. (1986). Religious orthodoxy and myocardial infarction in Jerusalem—a case control study. *International Journal of Cardiology*, *10*(1), 33–41. doi: 10.1016/0167-5273(86)90163-4

Gockel, A. (2009). Spirituality and the process of healing: A narrative study. *International Journal for the Psychology of Religion*, *19*(4), 217–230. doi: 10.1080/10508610903143248

Grant, A. (2012). Incorporating spirituality into the work of the holistic practitioner. *Journal of the Australian Traditional-Medicine Society*, *18*(2), 101–103.

Gundersen, L. (2000). Faith and healing. *Annals of Internal Medicine*, *132*(2), 169–172.

Haber, D. (2013). *Health promotion and aging: Practical applications for health professionals*. New York, NY: Springer.

Hanna, F., & Green, A. (2004). Asian shades of spirituality: Implications for multicultural school counseling. *Professional School Counseling*, *7*(5), 326–333

Hart, J. (2008). Spirituality and health. *Alternative and Complementary Therapies*, *14*(4), 189–193. doi : 10.1089/act.2008.14406

Hsiao, A., Wong, M. D., Miller, M. F., Ambs, H., Goldstein, M. S., Smith, A., . . . Wenger, N. S. (2008). Role of religiosity and spirituality in complementary and alternative medicine use among cancer survivors in California. *Integrative Cancer Therapies*, *7*(3), 139–146. doi : 10.1177/1534735408322847

Idler, E., McLaughlin, J. , & Kasl, S. (2009). Religion and the quality of life in the last year of life. *Journals of Gerontology: Series B: Psychological Sciences and Social Sciences*, *64B*(4), 528–537. doi: 10.1093/geronb/gbp028

Johnson, P., Priestley, J., & Johnson, R. D. (2008). A survey of complementary and alternative medicine knowledge among health educators in the United States. *American Journal of Health Education*, *39*(2), 66–79.

Kakar, S. (2003). Psychoanalysis and Eastern spiritual healing traditions. *Journal of Analytical Psychology*, *48*(5), 659–678. doi: 10.1111/1465-5922.00426

Kassaye, K. D., Amberbir, A., Getachew, B., & Mussema, Y. (2006). A historical overview of traditional practices and policy in Ethiopia. *Ethiopian Journal of Health Development*, *20*(2), 127–134. doi: 10.4314/ejhd.v20i2.10023

Kessler, C., Wischnewsky, M., Michalsen, A., Eisenmann, C., & Melzer, J. (2013). Ayurveda: Between religion, spirituality, and medicine. *Evidence-Based Complementary and Alternative Medicine, 2013*. Article ID 952432. doi: 10.1155/2013/952432

Koenig, H. G. (2004). Religion, spirituality, and medicine: Research findings and implications for clinical practice. *Southern Medical Journal*, *97*(12), 1194–1200. doi: 10.1097/01.smj.0000146489.21837.ce

Koenig, H. G., Hooten, E. G., Lindsay-Calkins, E., & Meador, K. G. (2010). Spirituality in medical school curricula: Findings from a national survey. *International Journal of Psychiatry Medicine*, *40*(4), 391–398. doi: 10.2190/PM.40.4.c

Kosmin, B. A., & Keysar, A. (2009). *American Religious Identification Survey (ARIS2008)*. Hartford, CT: Trinity College.

Kozak, L. E., Kayes, L., McCarthy, R., Walkinshaw, C., Congdon, S., Kleinberger, J., . . . Standish, L. J. (2009). Use of complementary and alternative medicine (CAM) by Washington state hospices. *American Journal of Hospice and Palliative Medicine*, *25*, 463–468. doi: 10.1177/1049909108322292

Kumar, S. M. (2002). An introduction to Buddhism for the cognitive-behavioral therapist. *Cognitive and Behavioral Practice*, *9*(1), 40–43. doi: 10.1016/S1077-7229(02)80038-4

Levin, J. (2009). "And let us make us a name": Reflections on the future of the religion and health field. *Journal of Religion & Health*, *48*(2), 125–145. doi: 10.1007/s10943-009-9243-0

Lopez, R. (2005). Use of alternative folk medicine by Mexican American women. *Journal of Immigrant Health*, *7*(1), 23–31

Lucchetti, G., Lucchetti, A. L. G., & Puchalski, C. M. (2012). Spirituality in medical education: Global reality? *Journal of Religious Health*, *51*, 3–19. doi: 10.1007/s10943-011-9557-6

Marlatt, G. A., & Kristeller, J. L. (1999). Mindfulness and meditation. In W. R. Miller (Ed.), *Integrating spirituality in treatment* (pp. 67–84). Washington, DC: American Psychological Association Books.

Meraviglia, M. (2006). Effects of spirituality in breast cancer survivors. *Oncology Nursing Forum*, *33*(1), E1–E7. doi: 10.1188/06.ONF.E1-E7

Moberg, D. O. (2005). Research in spirituality, religion, and aging. *Journal of Gerontological Social Work*, *45*(1–2), 11–40. doi: 10.1300/J083v45n01_02

Molassiotis, A., Potrata, B., & Cheng, K. K. F. (2009). A systematic review of the effectiveness of Chinese herbal medication in symptom management and improvement of quality of life in adult cancer patients. *Complementary Therapies in Medicine, 17*(2), 92–120. doi: 10.1016/j.ctim.2008.11.002

Mok, E., Wong, F., & Wong, D. (2010). The meaning of spirituality and spiritual care among the Hong Kong Chinese terminally ill. *Journal of Advanced Nursing, 66*(2), 360–370. doi: 10.1111/j.1365-2648.2009.05193.x

Moxey, A., McEvoy, M., Bowe, S., & Attia, J. (2011). Spirituality, religion, social support and health among older Australian adults. *Australasian Journal on Ageing, 30*(2), 82–88. doi: 10.1111/j.1741-6612.2010.00453.x

Narayan, I. (1998). Basic principles of Ayurveda. *Journal of the Australian Traditional Medicine, 4*(1), 9–11

National Center for Complementary and Alternative Medicine. (2005). *CAM at the NIH: Focus on complementary and alternative medicine.* DHHS Publication No. XII-1. Washington, DC: US Government Printing Office.

National Center for Complementary and Integrative Health. (2015a). *Introduction to health and spirituality.* Retrieved from https://nccih.nih.gov/training/videolectures/8/1

National Center for Complementary and Integrative Health. (2015b). Terms related to complementary and integrative health. Retrieved from https://nccih.nih.gov/health/providers/camterms.htm

National Center for Complementary and Integrative Health. (2015c). *Traditional Chinese medicine: An introduction.* Retrieved from https://nccih.nih.gov/health/whatiscam/chinesemed.htm

Oman, D., & Thoresen, C. E. (2005). Do religion and spirituality influence health? In R. F. Paloutzian & C. L. Park (Eds.), *Handbook of the psychology of religion and spirituality* (pp. 435–459). London, UK: Guilford Press.

Ornish, D., Love, S., Lerner, M., Kushi, L., Remen, R. N., Boon, H., . . . Stronach, K. (2002). *Breast cancer: Beyond convention.* New York, NY: Atria Books.

Oxman, T. E., Freeman, D. H., & Manheimer, E. D. (1995). Lack of social participation or religious strength and comfort as risk factors for death after cardiac surgery in the elderly. *Psychosomatic Medicine, 57*(1), 5–15.

Pankhania, J. (2005). Yoga and its practice in psychological healing. In R. Moodley & W. West (Eds.), *Integrating traditional healing practices into counseling and psychotherapy* (pp. 246–256). Thousand Oaks, CA: Sage.

Pargament, K. I. (1997). *The psychology of religion and coping.* New York, NY: Guilford Press.

Patwardhan, B. (2010). Ayurveda and integrative medicine: Riding a tiger. *Journal of Ayurveda and Integrative Medicine, 1*(1), 13–15. doi: 10.4103/0975-9476.59820

Peacock, J., & Poloma, M. (1999). Religiosity and life satisfaction across the life course. *Social Indicators Research, 48*(3), 321–345.

Pesut, B. (2006). Fundamental or foundational obligations? Problematizing the ethical call to spiritual care in nursing. *Advances in Nursing Science, 29*(2),125–133

Pesut, B., & Thorne, S. (2007). From private to public: Negotiating professional and personal identities in spiritual care. *Journal of Advanced Nursing, 58*(4), 396–403. doi: 10.1111/j.1365-2648.2007.04254.x

Pew Forum on Religion & Public Life. (2012). *The Global Religious Landscape Survey: A report on the size and distribution of the world's major religious groups as of 2010.* Retrieved from http://www.pewforum.org/files/2014/01/global-religion-full.pdf

Pew Forum on Religion & Public Life. (2015). *America's changing religious landscape: Christians decline sharply as share of population; unaffiliated and other faiths continue to grow.* Retrieved from http://www.pewforum.org/files/2015/05/RLS-08-26-full-report.pdf

Polzar Casarez, R. L., & Engebretson, J. C. (2012). Ethical issues of incorporating spiritual care into clinical practice. *Journal of Clinical Nursing, 21*(15–16), 2099–2107. doi: 10.1111/j.1365-2702.2012.04168.x

Post, S. G., Puchalski, C. M. & Larson, D. B. (2000). Physicians and patient spirituality: Professional boundaries, competency and ethics. *Annals of Internal Medicine, 132,* 578–583. Retrieved from http://www.ncbi.nlm.nih.gov/pubmed/10744595

Puchalski, C. M. (2001) The role of spirituality in healthcare. *Proceedings of Baylor University Medical Center, 14*(4), 352–357.

Puchalski, C., & Romer, A. L. (2000), Taking a spiritual history allows clinicians to understand patients more fully. *Journal of Palliative Medicine, 3*(1), 129–137. doi: 10.1089/jpm.2000.3.129

Ridenour, F. (2001). *So what's the difference?: A look at 20 worldviews, faiths and religions and how they compare to Christianity* (3rd ed.). Ventura, CA: Regal Books.

Rivera, E. T. (2005). Espiritismo: The flywheel of the Puerto Rican spiritual traditions. *Interamerican Journal of Psychology, 39*(2), 295–300.

Seccareccia, D., & Brown, J. B. (2009). Impact of spirituality on palliative care physicians: Personally and professionally. *Journal of Palliative Medicine, 12*(9), 805–809. doi: 10.1089/jpm.2009.0038

Shamanic Healing Institute. (2015). *What is shamanism?* Retrieved from http://www.shamanic-healing.org/?page=what_is_shamanism

Sheldrake, P. (2007). *A brief history of spirituality.* Ventura, CA: Regal Books.

Shi, L., & Zhang, C. (2012). Spirituality in traditional Chinese medicine. *Pastoral Psychology, 61*(5–6), 959–974. doi: 10.1007/s11089-012-0480-x

Sing Kiat Ting, R. (2012). The worldviews of healing traditions in the East and West: Implications for psychology of religion. *Pastoral Psychology 61,* 759–782. doi: 10.1007/s11089-012-0439-y

Singh, V., Raidoo, D., & Harries, C. (2004). The prevalence, patterns of usage and people's attitude towards complementary and alternative medicine (CAM)

among the Indian community in Chatsworth, South Africa. *BMC Complementary and Alternative Medicine, 4*(1), 3. doi: 10.1186/1472-6882-4-3

Stanley, R. (2009). Neurobiology of chakras and prayer. *Zygon, 44*(4), 825–846.

Stussman, B. J., Bethell, C. D., Gray, C., & Nahin, R. L. (2013). Development of the adult and child complementary medicine questionnaires fielded on the National Health Interview Survey. *BMC Complementary and Alternative Medicine, 13*, 328. doi: 10.1186/1472-6882-13-328

Tafur, M. M., Crowe, T. K., & Torres, E. (2009). A review of curanderismo and healing practices among Mexicans and Mexican Americans. *Occupational Therapy International, 16*(1), 82–88. doi: 10.1002/oti.265

Torosian, M. H., & Biddle, V. R. (2005). Spirituality and healing. *Seminars in Oncology, 32*, 232–236. doi: 10.1053/j.seminoncol.2004.11.017

Tovino, S. A. (2005). Hospital chaplaincy under the HIPAA Privacy Rule: Health care or "just visiting the sick"? *Scholarly Works*, Paper 392. Retrieved from http://scholars.law.unlv.edu/facpub/392

Van Aken, R., & Taylor, B. (2010) Emerging from depression: The experiential process of healing touch explored through grounded theory and case study. *Complementary Therapies in Clinical Practice, 16*(3), 132–137. http://dx.doi.org/10.1016/j.ctcp.2009.11.001

Wachholtz, A. B., & Sambamthoori, U. (2013). National trends in prayer use as a coping mechanism for depression: Changes from 2002 to 2007. *Journal of Religion and Health, 52*(4), 1356–1368. doi: 10.1007/s10943-012-9649-y

Wang, K. L., & Hermann, C. (2006). Pilot study to test the effectiveness of healing touch on agitation in people with dementia. *Geriatric Nursing, 27*(1), 34–40.

Winkelman, W. D., Lauderdale, K., Balboni, M. J., Phelps, A. C., Peteet, J. R., Block, S. D., . . . Balboni, T. A. (2011). The relationship of spiritual concerns to the quality of life of advanced cancer patients: Preliminary findings. *Journal of Palliative Medicine, 14*(9), 1022–1028. doi: 10.1089/jpm.2010.0536

Williams, J. A., Meltzer, D., Arora, V., Chung, G., & Curlin, F. A. (2011). Attention to inpatients' religious and spiritual concerns: Predictors and association with patient satisfaction. *Journal of General Internal Medicine, 26*(11), 1265–1271. doi: 10.1007/s11606-011-1781-y

Williams-Orlando, C. (2012). Spirituality in integrative medicine. *Integrative Medicine, 11*(4), 34–40.

Woo, K. Y. (1999). Global exchange: Care for Chinese palliative participants. *Journal of Palliative Care, 15*, 70–74.

Zeiders, C. L., & Pekala, R. (1995). A review of the evidence regarding the behavioral medical and psychological efficacy of Christian prayer. *Journal of Christian Healing, 17*(3), 17–28.

COMPLEMENTARY, ALTERNATIVE, AND INTEGRATIVE HEALTH APPROACHES AMONG AMERICAN INDIANS AND ALASKA NATIVES

Vickie D. Krenz and Amber Huhndorf

The term *American Indian* encompasses the vast diversity of indigenous peoples of the Americas, including North America, Central America, and South America (Norris, Vines, & Hoeffel, 2012). Many terms are used to describe the indigenous peoples of North America, including American Indians, Native Americans, First Nations, and Aboriginal people. The US Census Bureau estimates that there are 5.2 million people who identify as American Indians or Alaska Natives, with an estimated 2.9 million people who identify as American Indian or Alaska Native alone and 2.3 million in combination with one or more other races (Norris et al., 2012).

In the United States alone, there are 566 federally recognized American Indian tribes and groups of Alaska Natives, representing an estimated 1.9 million tribal people. In addition, there are an estimated 245 federally nonrecognized tribes in the petition process in the United States (Miller, 2004; US Department of the Interior, 2014). The Canadian government estimates that there are 1.1 million people who self-identify as an Aboriginal person, including 700,000 First Nations, 390,000 Metis, and 50,000 Inuit (Statistics Canada, 2010). Each tribal community represents a unique integration of traditional practices, language, beliefs, and healing practices.

LEARNING OBJECTIVES

At the completion of this chapter, students will be able to:

- Identify the complementary and alternative medicine practices most frequently used by American Indians and Alaska Natives as described in the current literature.

- Understand the unique diversity of American Indian tribes and communities in North America.

- Understand the concepts of health, wellness, and spiritual balance held by American Indians.

- Understand the function and role of American Indian healers.

- Describe the common complementary, alternative, and integrative health healing practices used by American Indian healers.

- Discuss the implications of American Indian healing practices for consumers and health professionals.

This chapter presents the most common complementary, alternative, and integrative health (CAIH) healing practices used by American Indian and Alaska Native healers. It discusses the applications for consumers and health professionals of the various complementary and alternative medicine (CAM) modalities used by American Indians and Alaska Natives. This chapter focuses on selected themes and healing practices across American Indian communities.

Theoretical Concepts

Overview

Traditional healing practices have been an integral part of American Indian culture and were used for generations prior to the introduction of Western medical practices. Traditional healing has been practiced for thousands of years by American Indians. Many American Indians view Western medicine as a CAM that is supplemental to traditional healing practices. Unlike Western medicine, American Indian healing practices focus on the spiritual underlying causes of physical ailments and diseases. In the discussion of CAM practices in this chapter, the term *traditional* will be used for the healing beliefs and practices of the indigenous people of North America.

Traditional healing practices have gained considerable attention among social scientists, anthropologists, and biomedical practitioners. An extensive body of anthropological and ethnological literature has been written with detailed discussions on the cultural perspectives and healing practices of American Indians (Landy, 1977; Moerman, 1998). However, much of this academic literature has been generated by nonnative researchers and pertains to a small number of tribal communities. Furthermore, American Indian healers guard their medicinal and ritual practices from people outside their communities. As their healing practices and ceremonies are considered to be "powerful medicine," they must be used appropriately by skilled healers. Often traditional healing practices are passed on through oral communication, resulting in a lack of written literature (Struthers, Eschiti, & Patchell, 2004). Unfortunately, there remains a dearth of current published data on the prevalence and breadth of traditional healing practices among American Indians (Johnston, 2002; Mackenzie, Taylor, Bloom, Hufford, & Johnson, 2003; Struthers, Eschiti, & Patchell, 2008).

Heterogeneity of Native Americans and Their Approaches to CAM

Western medicine focuses on the physical and mental components of health but lacks the spiritual dimension that is essential for healing among

American Indians. As noted by Lamphere (2000), American Indians often blend Western medicine with traditional healing practices that bring balance and harmony to their spiritual dimensions. Marbella, Harris, Diehr, Ignace, and Ignace (1998) reported that 42% of Milwaukee tribal patients used an herbalist for treatment. Kim and Kwok (1998) reported that there is rarely a perceived conflict between using a native healer and conventional medicine among Navajo patients who utilized an Indian Health Services (IHS) hospital ambulatory care clinic. Mehl-Madrona (1999) reported both health benefits and improved cost-effectiveness in the medical treatment of chronic physical illness using an integrative traditional Native American healing practice treatment. Novins et al. (2011) indicated that biomedical services and traditional healing were important sources of care in American Indian communities.

American Indian CAM practices are as diverse as their communities. It is not possible to cover traditional medicine across all American Indian groups. Many nonnative people assume that all American Indians follow the same healing and spiritual practices (i.e., peyote), which cannot be farther from reality. Furthermore, traditional healing practices rely on the in-depth knowledge of a healer (or medicine man or woman, shaman, etc.), who must tailor treatment to the unique needs of a "patient" or community.

Perceptions of Health and Wellness

The concept of "wellness" has broad meaning and includes the dimensions of physical, mental, social, emotional, and spiritual well-being. Western health perspectives have focused on the physical etiology, symptoms, and treatment of disease. Illness is perceived as a physical dimension that is treated independently to alleviate or cure disease. When people are sick, they consult with a physician to treat their symptoms or illness. Medications are prescribed to address the physical disease and in many cases without concern for the individual's spiritual well-being (Hartman & Gone, 2012; Weaver, 2002).

In contrast, American Indian concepts of health and illness are intimately intertwined with spiritual issues. In general, American Indian perceptions of health and wellness are centered on the integral balance of the mind, heart, spirit, and body. American Indians believe that everything on Earth has a spirit, including people, animals, plants, and the earth itself (i.e., rocks, rivers, formations, etc.). Furthermore, every person or thing is interconnected and balanced with the spirit of nature. This interconnectedness ("the web of life") ties individuals to the community and everything around them (BigFoot & Schmidt, 2010; Farrer, 1991; Hill, 2006; Hodge & Nandy, 2011; McCormick, 1997; Portman & Garrett, 2006;

Wilson, 2003; Yurkovich, Hopkins-Lattergrass, & Rieke, 2012). This concept is reflected in the Navajo belief *Sa'ah Naagháí Bik'eh Hózhó*, which represents harmony and balance in all aspects of the physical and spiritual world (Day, Silva, & Monroe, 2014; Lewton & Bedone, 2000; Schwarz, 2008; Struthers et al., 2004).

The circle has significant symbolism for American Indians as the cycle of life. The North American Plains tribes conceptualized "health" or "living the good life" in the Medicine Wheel, which represents the basic four directions: North, East, South, and West (Four Worlds Development Project, 1984–1989; Gilgun, 2002; Vogel et al., 2013; Warne, 2005). For many American Indians, the Medicine Wheel (or "Sacred Hoop") depicts the interconnectedness of the four elements necessary to support health and balance. As shown in Figure 7.1, the Medicine Wheel incorporates the cycle of life (i.e., baby, youth, adult, and elder), the four directions of human growth or balanced life (i.e., emotional, the heart, yellow; intellect, the mind, white; physical, the body, black; and spiritual, the soul, red) and the four aspects of human society (i.e., individual, family, community, and nation) (Portman & Garrett, 2006). For many American Indians, the colors of the Medicine Wheel reflect the four qualities of a balanced life: red, birth; yellow, growth; black, maturity; and white, death. The four directions can also depict the four peoples of Earth, including South ("red-skinned people"), East ("yellow-skinned people"), West ("black-skinned people"), and South ("white-skinned people"). At the center of the Medicine Wheel

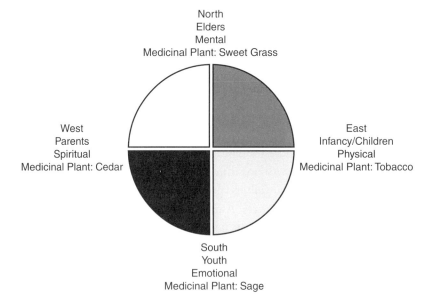

North
Elders
Mental
Medicinal Plant: Sweet Grass

West
Parents
Spiritual
Medicinal Plant: Cedar

East
Infancy/Children
Physical
Medicinal Plant: Tobacco

South
Youth
Emotional
Medicinal Plant: Sage

Figure 7.1   Medicine Wheel

is the Creator from which all life originates and which is the energy central to the rest of the wheel (Garrett, 1999).

This concept of balance and interconnectedness extends beyond an individual to living in harmony with others, community, and the spirit world. Thus, to be "healthy" encompasses a balance between all aspects of life. Spirituality and the spiritual nature of the universe are central to American Indian beliefs of health and well-being. As noted by Portman and Garrett (2006), spiritual practices are so integrated into daily life that many American Indian languages lack a specific word for *religion*. For many American Indians, physical ailments are the result of an imbalance in an individual's mind, heart, or spirit (Carlock, 2006; Locke, 1990; Struthers et al., 2008). Illness is the result of an imbalance of one's spirit or the result of spiritual problems leading to negative thinking, lifestyle, or interference from supernaturals directing malevolent activities toward humans (Coyhis & Simonelli, 2008; Moodley & West, 2005). Thus, healing practices often integrate spiritual and physical treatments to restore balance and spiritual wholeness in a person (Bassett, Tsosie, & Nannauck, 2012; Cohen, 1998; Garrett, 1999; Garrett & Garrett, 1996; Kaufman, Litchfield, Schupman, & Mitchell, 2012).

Causes of Disease

The causes of "disease" vary greatly among American Indian tribes. Diseases can be attributed to internal causes (i.e., negative thinking, including low self-esteem, greed, shame, blame, depression, anger, etc.), external causes (i.e., germs believed to be spirits of deceased humans, environmental poisons, alcohol, some types of food, etc.), imbalances in relationships, loss of soul, witchcraft or spells, or a combination of factors (Bassett et al., 2012; Jimenez, Garroutte, Kundu, Morales, & Buchwald, 2011). In addition, illness may be attributed to spiritual or supernatural causes, including offending a spirit, violation of a taboo (Thomason, 1991), animals, or "soul loss" (Snow & Stans, 2001).

Milne and Howard (2000) and Csordas (2000) noted that many Navajos attribute multiple causes to a wide variety of illnesses, including skin disorders, gastrointestinal problems, arthritis, mental disturbances, deafness, and others. Adams, Garcia, and Lien (2010) reported that the Chumash believe that disease results from an imbalance between the Sun and Sky Coyote, which results in weather conditions that support life (i.e., hot and dry versus cool and wet year). Many tribal communities hold the belief that illness is the result of a curse or evil spirits (Jilek, 1982; Mails, 1996; Portman & Garrett, 2006; Wyman, 1973).

Modalities

Traditional healers are highly respected and represent diverse roles and functions across their tribal communities. These individuals often are known as medicine men or women, shamans, and herbalists. The recognition (path) of a healer varies greatly and can be the result of family lineage, spiritual guidance or teaching from a healer (mentor), a "gift," or a life-changing event (Kinney, 2012; Snow & Stans, 2001; Struthers, 2003; Struthers et al., 2008). Prescriptions and treatments are passed from one generation to the next through oral communication. Most often healers learn traditional healing practices by studying for many years with a recognized tribal healer.

The primary role of healers is to address the sacred or spiritual issues that result in illnesses. Healers may utilize a wide variety of diagnostic methods, including visions, listening, spiritual awareness, and intuition (Cohen, 1998; Snow & Stans, 2001). In addition, traditional healers must possess an extensive knowledge of healing treatments that address the specific needs of the patient. As with Western medical specialties, a wide variety of healers are identified for their unique specialties, including herbalists, chanting healers, seers, ceremonial healers, sweat leaders, and others.

The reasons for seeking native healers for common medical conditions vary among American Indians. Kim and Kwok (1998) reported that Navajo patients consulted with traditional healers for common medical conditions, including arthritis, depression, diabetes, and "bad luck." Marbella et al. (1998) reported that common reasons for using a traditional healer among the Milwaukee tribal communities included spiritual well-being, guidance, truth, balance, reassurance, and cleansing of oneself. Bassett, Tsosle, and Nannauck (2012) reported that American Indians often sought the help of traditional healers to treat traumatic injury, unhealthy home environments, low self-esteem, and cultural identity problems.

In their CAM practices, American Indians are utilizing traditional medicine that they have practiced for thousands of years. American Indian traditional healing practices are the synthesis of culture, healing, and spiritual balance. In general, American Indian traditional healing practices can be classified into two categories: plant-based healing practices and ceremonial healing practices (Greensky et al., 2014; Struthers et al., 2008; Uprety, Asselin, Dhakal, & Julien, 2012). It is important to note that there are considerable variations within the specific healing practices and protocols. These variations are based on the tribal beliefs of the cause of the health condition, the healer's training, and individual diagnoses. Individual patients are considered to have unique symptoms and underlying causes of their disease. Therefore, each medicinal approach must be evaluated and treated appropriately. Every tribal community has unique cultural perspectives and beliefs regarding the causes of imbalance and the resulting illness, and specific treatments are required. Therefore, traditional healers work within their cultural health belief systems to treat the perceived underlying cause of the illness.

Plant-Based Healing Practices

American Indians have used herbs, plants, and roots to maintain wellness and treat a wide array of disorders for thousands of years. For many tribal communities, medicinal plants are a spiritual gift used to maintain wellness or to treat diseases and disorders. Herbal healers possess extensive knowledge of ethnobotanical herbs and plants available in their geographical location. Furthermore, there is considerable variation among healers in the preparation and administration of the medicinal treatment.

The extensive number of medicinal plant species used by American Indians has been well documented. The types and uses of specific medicinal plants are as uniquely tied to individual American Indian tribal communities as the geographical availability of each plant. Moerman (1996, 1998, 2002; Moerman & Estabrook, 2003) documented over 3,660 species of vascular plants (i.e., ferns, club mosses, gingkos and related taxa, gymnosperms or conifers, and angiosperms) used by American Indians for traditional foods and medicines in North America. Uprety et al. (2012) reported a total of 546 medicinal plant taxa used to treat 28 disease and disorder categories by the Aboriginal people of the Canadian boreal forest (e.g., Mi'kmaq, Malecite, Abenaki, Penobscot, Innu/Montagnais, Cree, Atikamekw, Algonquin/Anishinabe, Ojibwa/Anishinabe, and Chippewas). Vandebroek et al. (2004) detailed the use of medicinal plants by indigenous communities in the Bolivian Andes and Amazon.

Medicinal plants may be used individually or in combination with other plants. Villa-Caballero et al. (2010) found that 77.8% of Native American diabetics reported using CAM herbal treatments, including American ginseng (7.9%), garlic (20.6%), green tea (36.5%), multivitamins (34.9%), vitamin E (38.1%), and prickly pear cactus (3.2%). There is a considerable variation in the ways medicinal plants are prepared and used for treatment purposes. Bailey and Day (1989) reported that over 400 traditional plants have been used for the treatment of diabetes mellitus. Yeh, Eisenberg, Kaptchuk, and Phillips (2012) reported that the most commonly used herbs and plant derivatives for glycemic control included ginseng species (American, *P. quiquefolius*), garlic (*Allium sativum*), milk thistle (*Silibum marianum*), aloe (*aloe vera*), trembling aspen (*Populous tremuloides*), and cow parsnip (*Heracleum lanatum*). Similarly, Devil's Club (*Echinopanaxhorridum*) is used by the Athabascan to treat colds, cancer, depression, stomach problems, broken bones, burns, coughs/chest congestion, and inflammation (National Library of Medicine, 2006).

Tobacco is commonly considered to have strong spiritual and healing properties among most American Indian communities with the exception of the Alaska Natives (Unger, Soto, & Baezconde-Garbanati, 2006). It can be chewed, snuffed, or mixed with other substances into a liquid drink. In addition, tobacco (*Nicotiana attenuate, Nicotiana clevelandii, Nicotiana glauca*) is used by the Navajo, Piaute, Shoshoni, Cahuilla, and Hawaiian peoples to treat cuts, bruises, swellings, and other wounds (Bean & Saubell, 1972; Nadeau, Blake, Poupart, Rhodes, & Forster, 2012; Struthers & Hodge, 2004; Train, Henrichs, & Archer, 1941).

Extensive volumes have been written on the use of plant-based medical treatments by American Indians. Table 7.1 displays a sampling of medicinal plants and methods of preparation and tribe used to treat general physical symptoms. A comprehensive Native American ethnobotany database is available through the University of Michigan (http://herb.umd.umich.edu/) (Moerman, 2002; Moreman & Estabrook, 2003).

Spiritual Healing Practices

Spiritual healing practices are as diverse as the American Indian people. As noted, American Indians believe that physical health is deeply intertwined with the mind and spirit. Thus, spiritual healing ceremonies are often used to address the individual's spiritual needs and to restore balance. The wide range of healing practices and ceremonies cannot be adequately expressed in a single chapter. Greensky et al. (2014) described the range of traditional health practices used among American Indians for pain management, including ceremonial tobacco, sweat lodge ceremonies, chanting, pipe ceremonies, crystals, vision quests, healing ceremonies, dance ceremonies, and smudging.

Ceremonial Tobacco

As mentioned, tobacco is widely considered a strong medicine and used for ceremonial purposes. Tobacco is used most often to produce smoke for spiritual purposes to communicate with the spirits. The use of tobacco in ceremonial practices varies greatly among American Indian communities

Table 7.1 Examples of Physical Symptoms and Medicinal Plants Used by Tribal Communities

Disease/Symptom	Medicinal Plant	Preparation (Tribal Community)
Pain	"Chuchupate" (*Lomatium californicum*)	Root chewed for headache, rubbed on body for any sort of pain, scent inhaled for headache (Chumash) (Timbrook, 2007)
	Coastal sagebrush (*Artemisia californica*)	
	Carolina willow (*Salix amphibian*)	Chewed (contains salicylates, a precursor to aspirin) (Seminole) (Snow & Stans, 2001)
	Common yarrow (*Achillea millefolium*)	Leaves and stalks have been widely used among the Plains tribal communities (e.g., Pawnee and Chippewa) for pain relief (Densmore, 1974)
	Willow leaves (*Salix spp.*)	Used in a poultice or bath for skin infections or irritations
		Chewed leaves used for pain from insect bites
		Ash sprinkled on severe burns or cuts to prevent infection (Athabascan) (National Library of Medicine, 2011)
Stomach Pain	Canadian wild ginger (*Asarum candadense L.*)	Stomach ailments and indigestion (by the Cherokee, Ojibwe, Micmac, and Menomini) (Anderson, 2000)
	Sassafras (*Sassafras albidum*)	Roots, bark, new shoots, and leaf pith have been widely used for stomach ailments (i.e., diarrhea, indigestion, constipation, gallstones) by the Cherokee, Chippewa, Choctaw, Creek, Delaware, Oklahoma, Houma, Iroquois, and Seminole (Immel, 2001)
	Spotted ladysthumb (*Polygonum persicaria L.*)	Leaves and flowers have been used by the Chippewa (Densmore, 1928) and Cherokee (Hamel & Chiltoskey, 1975)
Women's Ailments	American red raspberry (*Rubus ideaeus L.*)	Strong infusion of leaves used for childbirth pains and decoction used for menstrual period (Cherokee) (Hamel & Chiltoskey, 1975)
		Decoction of stems and upper part of roots used to help a woman recover after childbirth (Cree) (Leighton, 1985)

(Continued)

Table 7.1 Examples of Physical Symptoms and Medicinal Plants Used by Tribal Communities *(continued)*

Disease/Symptom	Medicinal Plant	Preparation (Tribal Community)
	Ragleaf bahia (*Asteraceae*)	
	Beardlip penstemon (*Penstemon barbatus*)	Leaves, roots, and compound decoctions used to treat menstrual pain (Navajo) (Vestal, 1952)
	Sanicle (*Senicula marilandica L.*)	Roots used to treat menstrual pain and slow parturition (Micmac) (Chandler, Freeman, & Hooper, 1979)
Infectious Diseases	Silver maple (*Acer saccharinum*)	Hot infusion was used to treat measles (Cherokee) (Hamel & Chiltoskey, 1975)
	Bud sagebrush (*Picrothamnus desertorum*)	Used as a wash for influenza (Shoshoni) (Train et al., Henrichs, & Archer, 1941)
	Curlleaf mountain mahogany (*Cercocarpus ledifolus*)	Inner bark used to treat diphtheria (Shoshoni) (Train et al., Henrichs, & Archer, 1941)
	Pale purple coneflower (*Echinacea pallida*)	Used to treat mumps and measles (Cheyenne) (Hart, 1981)
	Sneezeweed (*Helenium puberulum*)	Used to treat influenza (Chumash) (Timbrook, 2007)
	Arroyo willow (*Salix lasiolepis*)	Bark tea used to treat malaria (Chumash)
Cuts	Balsam fir (*Abies balsamea*)	Poultice of pitch applied to cuts (Cree)
		Compound decoction applied to cuts, bruises, sprains, or sores (Iroquois)
		Sap smeared over burns, sores, and cuts (Penobscot) (Moerman, 2002)
	Western yarrow (*Achillea millefolium*)	Infusion of plant used as a wash for cuts and saddle sores (Navajo, Paiute) (Moerman, 2002)
	Big sagebrush (*Artemisia tridentate*)	Decoction of leaves used for antiseptic wash of cuts, wounds, or sores (Paiute, Shoshoni) (Moerman, 2002)
	California barberry (*Mahonia pinnata*)	Liquid from chewed root placed on cuts, wounds, and abrasions to prevent swelling; decoction of root used for cuts and bruises (Miwok) (Moerman, 2002)

Fever	Common yarrow (*Achillea milleforium L.*)	Infusion (Cherokee)
		Infusion of leaves given to babies (Iroquois)
		Florets placed on coals and smoke inhaled to break a fever (Ojibwe) (Moerman, 2002)
	Calamus (*Acorus calamus L.*)	Decoction of plant used (Dakota, Omaha, Pawnee) (Moerman, 2002)
	Hazel alder (*Alnum serrulata*)	Hot infusion of berries used (Cherokee) (Moerman, 2002)
	Stinking chamomile (*Anthemis cotula*)	Cold infusion of dried roots and stems used (Iroquois)
		Cold infusion of leaves (Mohegan) (Moerman, 2002)
	Big sagebrush (*Artemisia tridentate Nutt.*)	Decoction of leaves for malarial fever (Paiute)
		Decoction of leaves for sweating and to break a fever (Shoshoni) (Moerman, 2002)
Coughs	Common yarrow (*Achillea milleforium L.*)	Infusion of fresh or dried plant (Cheyenne)
		Leaves soaked (Paiute) (Moerman, 2002)
	Common juniper (*Juniperus communis L.*)	Decoction of branch or wood used (Cree)
		Infusion of leaves used (Cheyenne) (Moerman, 2002)
	Catnip (*Nepeta cataria L.*)	Syrup and honey used (Cherokee)
		Infusion of stems used (Iroquois) (Moerman, 2002)

Sources: Anderson, 2000; Chandler, Freeman, & Hopper, 1976; Densmore, 1928, 1974; Hart, 1981; Hamel & Chiltoskey, 1975; Immel, 2001; Leighton, 1985; Moerman, 2002; NLM, 2011; Snow & Stans, 2001; Timbrook, 2007; Train, Hearichs, & Archer, 1941; Vestal, 1952.

(Forster, Rhodes, Poupart, Baker, & Davey, 2007; Nadeau et al., 2012; Paper, 1988; Pego, Hill, Solomon, Chisholm, & Ivey, 1995; Struthers & Hodges, 2004). It is commonly offered by being placed on coals or thrown into a fire so that the smoke will carry prayers to the spirits. It is used as an offering to the Earth (i.e., placed on the ground), thrown into water, placed near sacred objects (i.e., rocks, trees, animals, etc.), or "fanned" around a person.

Sweat Lodge Ceremonies

The sweat lodge is a common and widely recognized purification ceremonial practice among a wide number of American Indian communities. The lodge is often constructed of saplings tied together to form a dome-shaped or inverted bowl structure and covered with tarps, blankets, or quilts. Within the sweat lodge, a pit is formed of heated rocks ("grandfathers") on which is sprinkled sacred water that creates the heated temperature. With the ceremony guided by a spiritual leader, the sweat lodge is used for cleansing and healing through prayer, singing, and drumming (Garrett et al., 2011; Schweigman, Soto, Wright, & Unger, 2011; Wright et al. 2011). For many American Indian communities, the sweat lodge is symbolic of Mother Earth's belly (i.e., womb) and the "rebirthing" of the individual (Lewis, 1990; Portman & Garrett, 2006). "Medicine sweats" are commonly used rituals to maintain traditional balance in mental, physical, and spiritual well-being (Hartman & Gone, 2012).

Chanting

Chanting is a common ceremonial practice that may be used for specific illnesses or life problems. Chanting, or prayers, is used in healing ceremonies. Among the Navajo, chanting ceremonies ("chantway") may be performed for preventive purposes (i.e., to enhance health, social relationships, or financial well-being) or to cure suffering. The chanting ceremony can vary from a short prayer (typically less than one hour) or extend to a nine-night ceremony (Milne & Howard, 2000).

Pipe Ceremonies

As mentioned, tobacco is considered a significant and powerful plant that is commonly used in American Indian healing practices, with the exception of Arctic Native communities. The pipe is considered a sacred vessel that represents the universe ("cosmos") and offers smoke in all directions to sacred beings (Forster et al., 2007; Nadeau et al., 2012; Paper, 1988; Struthers & Hodge, 2004). A medicine man (healer) can incorporate the "sacred pipe"

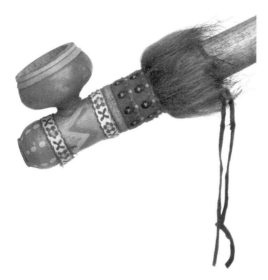

Figure 7.2   Smoke Ceremony Instruments

into a number of ritual ceremonies, including the Sun Dance, sweat lodge, and vision quest preparations (Lewis, 1990). Among the Chumash, sick people may be treated with a ceremony in which smoke is blown onto the sick person's chest and face with a singer who performs curing songs for three to nine days (Walker & Hudson, 1993). Medicine pipe ceremonies are as varied as the ritual ceremonies and styles of individual healers (see Figure 7.2).

Crystals

Crystal stones hold significant healing value for a number of American Indian tribes. Among the Cherokee, the crystal stone possesses powerful healing from the sun that is believed to merge or repel energy (Garrett & Garrett, 1996; Struthers & Eschiti, 2004). The crystal's healing energy comes from its power to restore a person's energy fields and to restore calm. Crystal stones are incorporated into healing ceremonies to realign or repel energy to restore balance. The path of the Crystal Vision results when persons are in harmony and balance with everything around them and with Mother Earth. This sense of balance is essential to physical health.

Vision Quest

The vision quest is a common healing and purification ritual practiced by many American Indian tribal communities. The specific purposes and techniques used during a vision quest vary from tribe to tribe and healer to healer. The ritual may be used for purification, passage into adulthood, to establish self-identity or personal direction, or healing. In terms of a traditional practice, individuals may undergo a vision quest to identify sources of imbalance and disharmony that can lead to illness. The quest is commonly preceded by a purification ceremony, involving a shaman's preparation and the setting up of four poles that represent the four directions, and may incorporate a number of practices, such as fasting, exposure, meditation, use of psychoactive plant substances, and dreams or visions. In general, the vision quest requires individuals to place themselves in isolation and discomfort in order to open their souls to the spirits. Healers are consulted to interpret the meanings of the dreams or visions (Jilek, 1982; Lewis, 1990; Portman & Garrett, 2006).

Healing Ceremonies

Healing ceremonies are an integral part of American Indian traditional practices. There is considerable variation in the types of healing ceremonies, which are as unique and individual as each tribal community and healer. In general, a healing circle ceremony begins and ends with prayer. As the ceremony progresses, sacred plants (i.e., tobacco, sage, sweet grass) are burned and an eagle feather is used to designate speaker turns. Songs, music, and dance are common components of a healing ceremony. Some may involve rituals that call on spirits or ancestors for healing. These ceremonies may last for several hours to several days, depending on the underlying cause of the illness. Healing ceremonies have been used in a wide variety of nontraditional healthcare settings, including mental health, substance abuse treatment, physical illnesses, and traumatic injury (Bassett et al., 2012; Hartman & Gone, 2012; Koithan & Farrell, 2010; Schneider & DeHaven, 2003; Struthers & Eschiti, 2005).

Dance Ceremonies

Dance ceremonies are a part of healing rituals used by many American Indian communities. Most tribal communities have dance ceremonies that incorporate their beliefs on illness and well-being (Koithan & Farrell, 2010). Dance ceremonies require specific preparation of the ceremonial area and ceremonial ritual under the direction of a healer. These ceremonies vary significantly among American Indian communities and traditional healers.

Dance ceremonies can be used for significant life events, life changes, to heal sickness, to give thanks for harvests, to bless hunts, to ensure rain, and other events. For example, the Sun Dance ceremony is used by a number of Plains tribal communities for healing and purification.

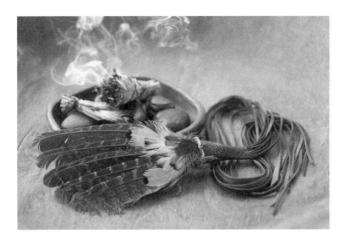

Figure 7.3   Smudge Stick

This ceremony consists of a three- or four-day ritual incorporating fasting, visions, purification, and, in some cases, skin piercing (Lewis, 1990; Portman & Garrett, 2006; Struthers & Eschiti, 2005). Similarly, the potlatch ceremony is used by the Athabascan culture to heal from losing a family and community member and to honor those who have passed to the next spirit world (i.e., died). The community gives their best gifts with love (i.e., hunting game, blankets, beadwork, etc.). The ceremony incorporates food, songs, and speeches from participants. In this way, tribal members can release their grief, and the love, in turn, grows among the community members (Krupa, 1996; Leonard, 2008).

Smudging

Smudging is a common purification practice among many American Indian communities that involves burning sacred medicines to heal or purify the body, mind, and spirit of individuals. Smudging can be used for a variety of purification purposes, including people, homes, and ceremonial grounds. The primary herbs and grasses used for smudging include sage, sweet grass, cedar, and/or tobacco. Most commonly, the smudging ingredients are bundled together with twine creating a smudge stick (see Figure 7.3). This stick is lit, and the flame is blown out to create cleansing smoke used for the ceremony (Portman & Garrett, 2006).

Consumer Issues

Many individuals present themselves as American Indian healers. Consumers should be aware that the credentials of American Indian and Alaska

Native healers are based on treatment outcomes and community validation. As noted, healers may have a gift or be trained in the healing arts. Their practice typically requires many years of training by a recognized healer, which often occurs as a result of their family lineage. Consumers should be wary of individuals who present themselves as healers but do not have the validation of their American Indian/Alaska Native community.

Consumers should be aware that American Indian healers and herbalists guard their medicinal and herbal practices and do not readily disclose "prescriptions" to individuals outside of their communities. Many American Indian and Alaska Native healers typically will not treat persons who are not a member of their community or who do not have Native heritage.

The comprehensive 10-year national objectives for improving the health of all Americans (Healthy People, 2020), focus on the social determinants of health and the disparities across racial/ethnic groups. American Indian and Alaska Native communities often experience high levels of poverty, adverse living conditions, and low education rates (DeNavas-Walt, Proctor, & Smith, 2013; US Census Bureau, 2011). Contrary to many beliefs, not all American Indian and Alaska Native communities have casinos that provide generous incomes to tribal members. Furthermore, American Indians and Alaska Natives have increased rates of death from unintentional injury, suicide, diabetes, certain cancers, chronic liver disease, and alcohol-related mortality (Centers for Disease Control and Prevention, 2014). Because American Indians and Alaska Natives represent a very small segment of the US population, they are not adequately represented in the research literature. They are less than 1% of population, and Healthy People 2020 notes the lack of sufficient data available.

Implications for Health Professionals

For many American Indians, spirituality is an important component of health that cannot be attained through Western medicine. Hsiao et al. (2006) reported that the use of traditional healers and healing rituals was higher among American Indians as compared to other racial/ethnic groups. Marbella and colleagues (1998) reported that 38% of Milwaukee tribal patients (e.g., Ojibwa, Oneida, Chippewa, and Menominee) in an urban Native American health center used a healer, and 86% of those who did not would consider seeing one in the future. However, little current literature on the prevalence of CAIH treatments among American Indians exists.

There also is a lack of contemporary literature on the specific uses of CAM therapies among American Indians. National studies on the use of CAM therapies among racial and ethnic minority adults have not included American Indian practices in their findings (Anderson & Taylor, 2012; Birdee, Phillips, Davis, & Gardiner, 2010; Chao, Wade, Kronenberg, Kalmuss, & Cushman, 2006; Graham et al., 2005). Furthermore, detailed descriptions of healing practices are maintained largely through oral traditions that are passed down to healers. Thus, few written documents detail specific protocols for healing ceremonies or herbal treatments.

Integrative traditional healing with Western medicine has been used for a wide range of illnesses. Numerous researchers (Struthers & Eschiti, 2004; Struthers et al., 2004) reported the incorporation of traditional healers and healing practices (i.e., crystals, healing ceremonies, herbal medicine, and prayers) into Western medical treatments, including for cancer, diabetes, and mental health. Similarly, Marbella, Harris, Diehr, Ignace and Ignace (1998) reported that sweat lodge ceremonies, spiritual healing, and herbal remedies were common practices among urban American Indian patients. Satterfield, Burd, Valde, Hosey, and Shield (2002) used "in-between people" (e.g., respected members of American Indian and Alaska Native communities) to deliver diabetes prevention and management in a healthcare team approach. These lay workers participated in the teams as intermediaries between patients and Western health professionals to ensure culturally appropriate diabetes care. Because of the good results, this approach has been incorporated into education interventions for alcohol and drug prevention, diabetes prevention, and other health-related issues.

Traditional healing practices and ceremonies have been incorporated into mental health and substance abuse treatment programs for American Indians. Garrett et al. (2011) emphasized the need for providers to understand the cultural values that promote wellness among American Indian patients. Novins et al. (2011) described the need to include traditional healing approaches for American Indian substance programs, such as the use of the sweat lodge, tobacco/pipe ceremonies, smudging, herbal medicine, and song/chanting. Portman and Garrett (2006) utilized the sweat lodge ceremony ("Broken Circle") to restore the harmony in an individual in the treatment of alcoholism and substance abuse. BigFoot and Schmidt (2010) proposed the use of a cognitive-behavioral therapy ("Honoring Children, Mend the Circle") to address the mental health needs of American Indian/Alaska Native children and youths.

Traditional American Indian CAM practices continue to be incorporated into Western medical and health practices. The "Circle of Life" cancer education program (Burhansstipanov, Krebs, Grass, Wanliss, & Saslow, 2005; Vogel et al., 2013) was developed to address breast health among American Indian women. The American Cancer Society and Oklahoma American Indian tribal communities incorporated four cultural values into the program: (1) the value of visual communication, (2) the value of interconnected generations, (3) the value of storytelling, and (4) the value of experiential learning. The "Circle of Life" cultural concept also has been used to address HIV/AIDs prevention for American Indian and Alaska Native youth (Kaufman et al., 2012, 2014).

Nonnative health practitioners have a challenge in working with American Indians and the use of traditional medicine for the treatment and healing of physical ailments. It is important that healthcare practitioners and health educators understand the conceptual worldview of American Indians and their interconnectedness with the universe. Furthermore, health professionals must understand that, to American Indians, Western medicine is considered a complementary practice. For American Indians, traditional healing practices represent the first forms of medical care, and those practices are not supplemented with modern treatments for their physical health. The challenge for health educators and other health professionals is to understand and respect the potential blending of traditional healing practices with Western medical treatments. Furthermore, health professionals must differentiate the cultural contexts that define tribal beliefs, values, health, illness, balance, and harmony among the American Indians of their broader community.

Traditional American Indian CAM practices can be considered CAIH modalities since they emphasize health and wellness. As such, it is important that health professionals learn culturally sensitive strategies to integrate those modalities into their healthcare practice.

American Indian and Alaska Natives represent a culturally diverse population. Tribal traditions and beliefs vary greatly among the different communities. Health professionals should recognize that there is no one "tradition" in the American Indian and Alaska Native communities. Thus, American Indian/Alaska Native intermediaries can assist health professionals in acquiring cultural competencies in the healthcare team. Health intermediaries communicate the American Indian and Alaskan perspective in the healing process.

Caveat Emptor

Under the Special General Memorandum 94-8 (Health and Human Services, 1994), the Indian Health Service (IHS) of the US Department of Health and Human Services has implemented policies that protect the religious rights of American Indians as a part of the Traditional Cultural Advocacy Program. The American Indian Religious Freedom Act of 1978 (PL 95-341) ensures the inherent right of all Native Americans and Alaskan Natives to express and exercise their traditional religions. Furthermore, the act recognizes the "value and efficacy to traditional beliefs, ceremonies and practices of the healing of body, mind and spirit." In accordance with this policy, IHS staff must continue to inform patients of their freedom to practice their traditional religion. This includes such efforts as "contacting a native practitioner, providing space or privacy within a hospital room for a ceremony, and/or the authorization of contact health care funds to pay for native healer consultation when necessary." The act requires IHS staff to be sensitive to and respectful of Native Americans' rights to privacy and the practice of their traditional beliefs.

The Affordable Care Act (ACA) has had a significant impact on the health disparities that affect American Indians and Alaska Natives. Under provisions of the act, the Indian Health Care Improvement Act was reauthorized and the current law extended to provide increased affordable coverage and increased investment in prevention and wellness programs for American Indians and Alaska Natives (Warne & Frizzell, 2014). As a part of the ACA, American Indians and Alaska Natives have expanded options, depending on their eligibility and state coverage, which can include (1) continued use of IHS, tribal, and/or urban Indian health programs; (2) enrollment in a qualified health plan through the Health Insurance Marketplace; and/or (3) access to coverage through Medicare, Medicaid, and the Children's Health Insurance Program. As with all Americans, the ACA intends that American Indians and Alaska Natives have access to affordable healthcare at lower costs with improved quality.

Conclusion

The healing practices of American Indians are as varied as the tribal communities and individual healers. American Indians' health beliefs focus on the balance and harmony of the individual and the community and the interconnectedness of everything in the universe. American Indian healing practices include plant-based therapies and spiritual healing rituals. The use of traditional practices is common among American Indians and is often blended with Western healthcare.

Disease is the result of an imbalance, and the goal of traditional healing practices is to restore balance and harmony. Health educators and other health professionals must respect traditional practices as legitimate forms of healthcare that heal the total person, not merely the physical body. Many tribal clinics have retained healers as a part of medical teams to address the total health needs of patients. This integration of Western and traditional healthcare has shown results in the forms of cost-effective treatment and improved American Indian patient care.

Summary

- CAIH therapies are an integral part of health and well-being among American Indians and are often blended with Western healthcare to treat a wide range of ailments.

- Traditional American Indian CAM practices can be considered CAIH modalities since they emphasize health and wellness.

- American Indian healers are specialized practitioners who utilize a wide array of plant-based therapies and/or spiritual healing rituals to treat the total person, not merely the physical body.

- American Indian spiritual beliefs, culture, and practices can vary greatly among the diverse tribal communities. The challenge for health professionals, including health educators, is to understand the context within which American Indians utilize traditional healing practices to restore balance and harmony.

- Understanding the underlying traditional concepts of health and disease (i.e., spiritual beliefs, culture, and practices) is essential in working with American Indian communities. Western practitioners need to be aware of individual and community spiritual beliefs when addressing physical health issues.

Case Study

Description

Daisy is a young American Indian woman who has recently married. She and her husband want to have a child, but have not been able to conceive. Her tribal community places a high value on the role of a wife in producing children. Daisy has recently begun to experience physical symptoms, including bad dreams, insomnia, depression, and headaches. She has seen her doctor for the source of her symptoms and was given a prescription to treat her sleep difficulties and depression. However, she is concerned with her inability to conceive a child.

Questions

1. How are Daisy's physical symptoms related to her spiritual beliefs?

2. How can American Indian CAIH practices be incorporated into the treatment strategies for Daisy's physical symptoms?

3. What other resources should health professionals consider in Daisy's desire to have a child?

KEY TERMS

Herbal medicine. The use of herbs, plants, and roots to maintain wellness and treat diseases and disorders. It includes the use of "herbs, herbal materials, herbal preparations and finished herbal products, that contain as active ingredients parts of plants, or other plant materials, or combinations" (World Health Organization, 2015).

Native American healer or medicine man/woman. A traditional healer who uses information from the spirit world to benefit the community, to provide relief or a cure to illness, or to provide spiritual guidance (NCCAM, 2015).

Spiritual medicine. Used in this chapter to refer to the use of spiritual healing ceremonies to address the spiritual needs of and restore balance to an individual. The Spiritual Science Research Foundation (2012) defines *spiritual healing* as "overcoming the spiritual root causes of problems through spiritual means."

Traditional healer. Used in this chapter to refer to an individual who possesses an extensive knowledge of healing treatments that address the specific needs of the patient. A wide variety of healers are identified for their unique specialities, including herbalists, chanting healers, seers, ceremonial healers, sweat leaders, and others. The World Health Organization (2013) defines a traditional healer as a member of a community who is recognized and accepted by the community as a healer and who has received health-related training within the cultural characteristics of that community.

Traditional medicine. Used in this chapter to refer to the healing beliefs and practices of the indigenous peoples of North America. The World Health Organization (2015) defines *traditional medicine* as "the sum total of the knowledge, skills, and practices based on the theories, beliefs, and experiences indigenous to different cultures, whether explicable or not, used in the maintenance of health as well as in the prevention, diagnosis, improvement or treatment of physical and mental illness."

References

Adams, J. D., Garcia, C., & Lien, E. J. (2010). A comparison of Chinese and American Indian (Chumash) medicine. *Evidence-Based Complementary and Alternative Medicine, 7*(2), 219–225. Retrieved from http://dx.doi.org/10.1093/ecam/nem188

Anderson, M. K. (2000). *Plant guide: Candian wildginger*. Davis, CA: United States Department of Agriculture, Natural Resources Conservation Service, National Plant Data Center, University of Davis.

Anderson, J. G., & Taylor, A. G. (2012). Use of complementary therapies by individuals with or at risk for cardiovascular disease: Results of the 2007 National Health Interview Survey. *Journal of Cardiovascular Nursing, 27*(2), 96–102.

Bailey, C. J., & Day, C. (1989). Traditional plant medicines as treatment for diabetes. *Diabetes Care, 12*(8), 553–564. doi: 10.2337/diacare.12.8.553

Bassett, D., Tsosie, U., & Nannauck, S. (2012). "Our culture is medicine": Perspective of Native healers on posttrauma recovery among American Indian and Alaska Native patients. *Permanente Journal, 16*(1), 19–27.

Bean, L. J., & Saubel, K. S. (1972). *Temalpakh (from the earth): Cahuilla Indian knowledge and usage of plants*. Banning, CA: Malki Museum Press.

BigFoot, D. S., & Schmidt, S. R. (2010). Honoring children, mending the circle: Cultural adaptation of trauma-focused cognitive-behavioral therapy for American Indian and Alaska Native children. *Journal of Clinical Psychology: In Session, 66*(8), 847–856.

Birdee, G. S., Phillips, R. S., Davis, R. B., & Gardiner, P. (2010). Factors associated with the use of complementary and alternative medicine in the United States: Results from the National Health Interview Survey. *Pediatrics, 125*(2), 249–256.

Burhansstipanov, L., Krebs, L. U., Grass, R., Wanliss, E. J., & Saslow, D. (2005). A review of effective strategies for Native women's breast health outreach and education. *Journal of Cancer Education, 20*(1 Suppl.): 71–79.

Carlock, D. (2006). Native American health: Traditional healing and culturally competent health care internet resources. *Medical Reference Services Quarterly, 25*(3), 67–76. doi: 10.1300/J115v25n03_06

Centers for Disease Control and Prevention. (2014). *American Indian and Alaska Native death rates nearly 50 percent greater than those of non-Hispanic Whites*. Retrieved from http://www.cdc.gov/media/releases/2014/p0422-natamerican-deathrate.html

Chandler, R. F., Freeman, L., & Hooper, S. N. (1979). Herbal remedies of the Maritime Indians. *Journal of Ethnopharmacology, 1*, 49–68.

Chao, M. T., Wade, C., Kroenberg, F., Kalmuss, D., & Cushman, L. F. (2006). Women's reasons for complementary and alternative medicine use: Racial/ethnic differences. *Journal of Alternative and Complementary Medicine, 12*(8), 719–720.

Cohen, K. (1998). Native American medicine. *Alternative Therapies in Health and Medicine, 4*(6), 45–57.

Coyhis, D., & Simonelli, R. (2008). The Native American healing experience. *Substance Use and Misuse, 43*, 1927–1949.

Csordas, T. J. (2000). The Navajo Healing Project. *Medical Anthropology Quarterly, 14*(4), 463–475.

Day, D., Silva, D. K., & Monroe, A. O. (2014). The wisdom of indigenous healers. *Creative Nursing*, *20*(1), 37–46.

DeNavas-Walt, C., Proctor, B. D., & Smith, J. C. (2012). Income, poverty, and health insurance coverage in the United States: 2011. *US Census Bureau, Current Population Reports, P60-243*. Washington, DC: US Government Printing Office. Retrieved from http://www.census.gov/prod/2011pubs/p60-239.pdf

DeNavas-Walt, C., Proctor, B. D., & Smith, J.C. (2013). Income, poverty, and health insurance coverage in the United States: 2012. *US Census Bureau, Current Population Reports, P60-245*. Washington, DC: US Government Printing Office.

Densmore, F. (1928). *Uses of plants by the Chippewa Indians*. SI-BAE Annual Report No. 44, pp. 273–379.

Farrer, C. R. (1991). *Living life's circle: Mescalero Apache cosmovision*. Albuquerque, NM: University of New Mexico Press.

Forster, J. L., Rhodes, K. L., Poupart, J., Baker, L. O., & Davey, C. (2007). Patterns of tobacco use in a sample of American Indians in Minneapolis-St. Paul. *Nicotine & Tobacco Research*, *9*(Suppl. 1), S29–S37.

Four Worlds Development Project. (1984–1989). *The sacred tree: Reflections on Native American spirituality*. Wilmot, WI: Lotus Light.

Garrett, M. T. (1999). Understanding the "medicine" of Native American traditional values: An integrative review. *Counseling and Values*, *43*(2), 84–98. doi: 10.1002/j.2161-007X.1999.tb00131.x

Garrett, J. T., & Garrett, M. (1996). *Medicine of the Cherokee: The way of right relationship*. Sante Fe, NM: Bear and Company.

Garrett, M. T., Torres-Rivera, E., Brubaker, M., Portman, T. A. A, Brotherton, D., West-Olatunji, C., . . . Grayshield, L. (2011). Crying for a vision: The Native American sweat lodge ceremony as therapeutic intervention. *Journal of Counseling and Development*, *89*(3), 318–325.

Gilgun, J. F. (2002). Completing the circle. *Journal of Human Behavior in the Social Environment*, *6*(2), 65-84. doi: 10.1300/J137v06n02_05

Graham, R. E., Ahn, A. C., Davis, R. B., O'Connor, B. B., Eisenberg, D. M., & Phillips, R. S. (2005). Use of complementary and alternative medical therapies among racial and ethnic minority adults: Results from the 2002 National Health Interview Survey. *Journal of the National Medical Association*, *97*(4), 535–545.

Greensky, C., Stapleton, M. A., Walsh, K., Gibbs, L., Abrahamson, J., Finnie, D. M., . . . Hooten, W. M. (2014). A qualitative study of traditional healing practices among American Indians with chronic pain. *Pain Medicine*. doi: 10.1111/pme. 12488

Hamel, P. B., & Chiltoskey, M. U. (1975). *Cherokee plants and their uses—a 400-year history*. Sylva, NC: Herald.

Hart, J. A. (1981). The ethnobotany of the Northern Cheyenne Indians of Montana. *Journal of Ethnopharmacology*, *4*, 1–55.

Hartman, W. E., & Gone, J. P. (2012). Incorporating traditional healing into an urban American Indian health organization: A case study of community member perspectives. *Journal of Counseling Psychology, 59*(4), 542–554.

Health and Human Services. (1994). *Special General Memorandum 94-8, Statement of Policy for the Traditional Cultural Advocacy Program. Indian Health Manual.* Rockville, MD: Public Health Service. Retrieved from http://www.ihs.gov/IHM/index.cfm?module=dsp_ihm_sgm_main&sgm=ihm_sgm_9408

Healthy People 2020. (n.d.). *Social determinants.* Retrieved from www.healthypeople.gov/2020/leading-health-indicators/2020-lhi-topics/Social-Determinants

Hill, D. L. (2006). Sense of belonging as connectedness, American Indian worldview, and mental health. *Archives of Psychiatric Nursing, 20*(5), 210–216.

Hodge, F. S., & Nandy, K. (2011). Predictors of wellness and American Indians. *Journal of Health Care for the Poor and Underserved, 22*(3), 791–803. doi: 10.1353/hpu.2011.0093

Hsiao, A. F., Wong, M. D., Goldstein, M. S., Yu, H. J., Andersen, R. M., Brown, E. R., . . . Wenger, N. S. (2006). Variation in complementary and alternative medicine (CAM) use across racial/ethnic groups and the development of ethnic-specific measures of CAM use. *Journal of Alternative and Complementary Medicine, 12*(3), 281–290.

Immel, D. L. (2001). *Plant guide: Sassafras.* Davis, CA: United States Department of Agriculture, Natural Resources Conservation Service, National Plant Data Center, University of Davis.

Jilek, W. G. (1982). *Indian healing: Shamanic ceremonialism of the Pacific Northwest today.* Blaine, WA: Hancock House.

Jimenez, N., Garroutte, E., Kundu, A., Morales, L., & Buchwald, D. (2011). A review of the experience, epidemiology and management of pain among American Indian, Alaska Native, and Aboriginal Canadian peoples. *Journal of Pain, 12*(5), 511–522. doi: 10.1016/j.jpain.2010.12.002

Johnston, S. L. (2002). Native American traditional and alternative medicine. *Annals of the American Academy of Political and Social Science, 583,* 195–213.

Kaufman, C. E., Litchfield, A., Schupman, E., & Mitchell, C. M. (2012). Circle of life HIV/AIDS-prevention intervention for American Indian and Alaska Native youth. *American Indian and Alaska Native Mental Health Research, 19*(1), 140–153. doi: 10.5820/aian.1901.2012.140

Kaufman, C. E., Whitesell, N. R., Keane, E. M., Desserich, J. A., Giago, C., Sam, A., & Mitchell, C. M. (2014). Effectiveness of Circle of Life, an HIV-preventive intervention for American Indian middle school youths: A group randomized trial in a Northern Plains tribe. *American Journal of Public Health, 104*(6), e106–112.

Kim, C., & Kwok, Y. S. (1998). Navajo use of native healers. *Archives of Internal Medicine, 158*(20), 2245–2249.

Kinney, G. (2012). The healers journey: A literature review. *Complementary Therapy and Clinical Practice, 18*(1):31–36. doi: 10.1016/j.ctcp.2011.08.002

Koithan, M., & Farrell, C. (2010). Indigenous Native American traditions. *Journal of Nurse Practitioners, 6*(6), 477–478. doi: 10.1016/j.nurpra.2010.03.016

Krupa, D. J. (1996). *The gospel according to Peter John.* Fairbanks, AK: Alaska Native Knowledge Network.

Lamphere, L. (2000). Comments on the Navajo Healing Project. *Medical Anthropology Quarterly, New Series, 14*(4), 598–602.

Landy, D. (1977). *Culture, disease, and healing: Studies in medical anthropology.* New York, NY: Macmillan.

Leighton, A. L. (1985). *Wild plant use by the Woods Cree (Nihithawak) of East-Central Saskatachewan.* Ottawa, Canada: National Museums of Canada, Mercury Series.

Leonard, B. (2008). Mediating Athabascan oral traditions in postsecondary classrooms. *International Journal of Multicultural Education, 10*(2), 1–16.

Lewis, T. H. (1990). *The medicine men: Oglala Sioux ceremony and healing.* Lincoln, NE: University of Nebraska Press.

Lewton, E. L., & Bedone, V. (2000). Identity and healing in three Navajo religious traditions: Sa'ah Naagháí Bik'eh Hózhǫ. *Medical Anthropology Quarterly, 14,* 476–497. Retrieved from http://www.jstor.org/stable/649717

Locke, R. F. (1990). *Sweet salt: Navajo folklore and mythology.* Santa Monica, CA: Roundtable.

Mackenzie, E. R., Taylor, L., Bloom, B. S., Hufford, D. J., & Johnson, J. C. (2003). Ethnic minority use of complementary and alternative medicine (CAM): A national probability survey of CAM utilizers. *Alternative Therapies, 9*(4), 50–56.

Mails, T. E. (1996). *The Cherokee people: The story of the Cherokees from earliest origins to contemporary times.* New York, NY: Marlowe.

Marbella, A. M., Harris, M. C., Diehr, S., Ignace, G., & Ignace, G. (1998). Use of Native American healers among Native American patients in an urban Native American health center. *Archives of Family Medicine, 7,* 182–185.

McCormick, R. M. (1997). Healing through interdependence: The role of connecting in First Nations healing practices. *Candian Journal of Counselling, 31*(3), 172–184.

McGaa, E. (1989). *Mother Earth spirituality: Native American paths to healing ourselves and our world.* San Francisco, CA: Harper & Row.

Mehl-Madrona, L. E. (1999). Native American medicine in the treatment of chronic illness: Developing an integrative program and evaluating its effectiveness. *Alternative Therapy and Health in Medicine, 5*(1), 36–44.

Miller, M. E. (2004). *Forgotten tribes: Unrecognized Indians and the federal acknowledgment process.* Lincoln, NE: University of Nebraska Press.

Milne, D., & Howard, W. (2000). Rethinking the role of diagnosis in Navajo religious healing. *Medical Anthropology Quarterly, 14*(4), 543–570.

Moerman, D. E. (1996). An analysis of the food plants and drug plants of native North America. *Journal of Ethnopharmacology, 52,* 1–22.

Moerman, D. E. (1998). *Native American ethnobotany.* Portland, OR: Timber Press.

Moerman, D. E. (2002). *Native American ethnobotany database.* Portland, OR: Timber Press. Retrieved from http://herb.umd.umich.edu/

Moerman, D. E., & Estabrook, G. F. (2003). Native Americans' choice of species for medicinal use is dependent on plant family: Confirmation with meta-significance analysis. *Journal of Ethnopharmacology, 89,* 51–59. doi: 10.1016/S0378-8741(03)00105-3

Moodley, R., & West, W. (2005). *Integrating traditional healing practices into counseling and psychotherapy.* Thousand Oaks, CA: Sage.

Nadeau, M., Blake, N., Poupart, J., Rhodes, K., & Forster, J. L. (2012). Circles of tobacco wisdom: Learning about traditional and commercial tobacco with Native elders. *American Journal of Preventive Medicine, 43*(5, Suppl. 3), 222–228. doi: 10.1016/j.amepre.2012.08.003

National Center for Complementary and Integrative Health. (2015). *Terms related to complementary and integrative health.* Retrieved from https://nccih.nih.gov/health/providers/camterms.htm

National Library of Medicine. (2006). *Native voices: Native peoples' concepts of heath and illness.* Bethesda, MD: National Institutes of Health, Health and Human Services. Retrieved from http://www.nlm.nih.gov/nativevoices/exhibition/healing-ways/medicine-ways/healing-plants/images/ob1682.html

National Library of Medicine. (2011). *Native voices: Native peoples' concepts of heath and illness.* Bethesda, MD: National Institutes of Health, Health and Human Services. Retrieved from https://www.nlm.nih.gov/nativevoices/

Norris, T., Vines, P. L., & Hoeffel, E. M. (2012). *The American Indian and Alaska Native population: 2010 Census Briefs.* US Department of Commerce, Economics and Statistics Administration.

Novins, D. K., Aarons, G. A., Conti, S. G., Dhalke, D., Daw, R., Finkenscher, A., . . . Spicer, P. (2011). Use of the evidence base in substance abuse treatment programs for American Indians and Alaska Natives: Pursuing quality in the crucible of practice and policy. *Implementation Science, 6*(63), 1–12.

Paper, J. (1988). *Offering smoke: The sacred pipe and Native American religion.* Moscow, ID: University of Idaho Press.

Pego, C. M., Hill, R. F., Solomon, G. W., Chisholm, R. M., & Ivey, S. E. (1995). Tobacco, culture, and health among American Indians: A historical review. *American Indian Culture and Research Journal, 19*(2), 143–164.

Portman, T. A. A., & Garrett, M. T. (2006). Native American healing traditions. *International Journal of Disability, Development and Education, 53*(4), 453–469.

Satterfield, D., Burd, C., Valdez, L., Hosey, G., & Shield, J. E. (2002). The "In-Between People": Participation of community health representatives in diabetes prevention and care in American Indian and Alaska Native communities. *Health Promotion and Practice, 3*(2), 166–175. doi: 10.1177/152483990200300212

Schneider, G. W., & DeHaven, M. J. (2003). Revisiting the Navajo way: Lessons for contemporary healing. *Perspectives in Biology and Medicine, 46*(3), 413–427.

Schwarz, M. T. (2008). *"I choose life": Contemporary medical and religious practices in the Navajo world.* Norman, OK: University of Oklahoma Press.

Schweigman, K., Soto, C., Wright, S., & Unger, J. (2011). The relevance of cultural activities in ethnic identity among California Native American youth. *Journal of Psychoactive Drugs, 43*(4), 343–348.

Snow, A. M., & Stans, S. E. (2001). *Healing plants: Medicine of the Florida Seminole Indians.* Gainesville, FL: University of Florida Press.

Spiritual Science Research Foundation. (2012). *Principles of spiritual healing.* Retrieved from http://www.spiritualresearchfoundation.org/spiritual-healing/spiritual-healing-principles/

Statistics Canada. (2010). *Aboriginal identity population by age groups, median age and sex, 2006 counts for both sexes, for Canada, provinces and territories.* Retrieved from http://www12.statcan.ca/census-recensement/2006/dp-pd/hlt/97-558/pages/page.cfm?Lang=E&Geo=PR&Code=01&Table=1&Data=Count&Sex=1&Age=1&StartRec=1&Sort=2&Display=Page

Struthers, R. (2003). The artistry and ability of traditional women healers. *Health Care for Women International, 24*(4), 340–354.

Struthers R., & Eschiti, V. S. (2004). The experience of indigenous traditional healing and cancer. *Integrative Cancer Therapies, 3*(1), 13–23.

Struthers, R., & Eschiti, V. S. (2005). Being healed by an indigenous traditional healer: Sacred healing stories of Native Americans: Part II. *Complementary Therapies in Clinical Practice, 11*(2), 78–86.

Struthers, R., Eschiti, V. S., & Patchell, B. (2004). Traditional indigenous healing: Part I. *Complementary Therapies in Nursing and Midwifery, 10*(3), 141–149.

Struthers, R., Eschiti, V. S., & Patchell, B. (2008). The experience of being an Anishinabe man healer: Ancient healing in a modern world. *Journal of Cultural Diversity, 15*(2), 70–75.

Struthers, R., & Hodge, F. S. (2004). Sacred tobacco use in Ojibwe communities. *Journal of Holistic Nursing, 22*(3), 209–225.

Thomason, T. C. (1991). Counseling Native Americans: An introduction for non-Native American counselors. *Journal of Counseling and Development, 69*(4), 321–327.

Timbrook, J. (2007). *Chumash ethnobotany: Plant knowledge among the Chumash people of southern California.* Berkeley, CA: Heyday Books.

Train, P., Henrichs, J. R., & Archer, W. A. (1941). *Medicinal uses of plants by Indian tribes of Nevada*. Washington, DC: US Department of Agriculture.

Unger, J. B., Soto, C., & Baezconde-Garbanati, L. (2006). Perceptions of ceremonial and nonceremonial uses of tobacco by American-Indian adolescents in California. *Journal of Adolescent Health, 38*(4), 443e9–443e16. doi: 10.1016/j.jadohealth.2005.02.002

Uprety, Y., Asselin, H., Dhakal, A. L., & Julien, N. (2012). Traditional use of medicinal plants by Aboriginal people of boreal Canada: Review and perspectives. *Journal of Ethnobiology and Ethnomedicine, 8*, 7. Retrieved from http://ethnobiomed.biomedcentral.com/articles/10.1186/1746-4269-8-7

US Census Bureau. (2011). *Profile America facts for features: American Indian and Alaska Native heritage month: November 2011*. Retrieved from http://www.census.gov/newsroom/releases/archives/facts_for_features_special_editions/cb11-ff22.html

US Department of the Interior, Office of the Secretary, Office of the Assistant Secretary—Indian Affairs. (2014). *2013 American Indian population and labor force report*. Washington, DC: Author.

Vandebroek, I., Calewaert, J., De Jonckheere, S., Sanca, S., Semo, L., van Damme, P., . . . De Kimpe, N. (2004). Use of medicinal plants and pharmaceuticals by indigenous communities in the Bolivian Andes and Amazon. *Bulletin of the World Health Organization, 82*, 243–250.

Vestal, P. A. (1952). The ethnobotany of the Ramah Navaho. *Papers of the Peabody Museum of American Archaeology and Ethnology, 40*(4), 1–94.

Villa-Caballero, L., Morello, C. M., Chynoweth, M. E., Prieto-Rosinol, A., Polonsky, W. H., Palinks, L. A., & Edelman, S. V. (2010). Ethnic differences in complementary and alternative medicine use among patients with diabetes. *Complementary Therapy and Medicine, 18*(6), 241–248. doi: 10.1016/j.ctim.2010.09.007

Vogel, O., Cowens-Alavarado, R., Eschiti, V., Samos, M., Wiener, D., Holander, K., & Royals, D. (2013). Circle of Life cancer education: Giving voice to American and Alaska Native communities. *Journal of Cancer Education, 28*(3), 656–672. doi: 10:1007/s13187-013-0504-y

Walker, P. L., & Hudson, T. (1993). *Chumash healing: Changing health and medical practices in an American Indian society*. Banning, CA: Malki Museum Press.

Warne, D. (2005). Health and healing among American Indians. *Journal of Science and Healing, 1*(2), 122–129.

Warne, D., & Frizzell, L. B. (2014). American Indian health policy: Historical trends and contemporary issues. *American Journal of Public Health, 104*(Suppl. 3), S263–267. doi: 10.2105.AJPH.2013.301682

Weaver, H. N. (2002) Perspectives on wellness: Journeys on the Red Road. *Journal of Sociology and Social Welfare, 29*(1), 5–15.

Wilson, K. (2003). Therapeutic landscapes and First Nations peoples: An exploration of culture, health and place. *Health & Place, 9*, 83–93.

World Health Organization. (2013). *WHO traditional medicine strategy 2014–2023*. Retrieved from http://apps.who.int/iris/bitstream/10665/92455/1/9789241506090_eng.pdf?ua=1&ua=1

World Health Organization. (2015). *Traditional medicine: Definitions*. Retrieved from http://www.who.int/medicines/areas/traditional/definitions/en/

Wright, S., Nebelkopf, E., King, J., Mass, M., Patel, C., & Samuel, S. (2011). Holistic system of care: Evidence of effectiveness. *Substance Use and Misuse, 46*(11), 1420–1430.

Wyman, L. C. (1973). *The red antway of the Navaho*. Sante Fe, NM: Museum of Navaho Ceremonial Art.

Yeh, G. Y., Eisenberg, D. M., Kaptckuk, T. J., & Phillips, R. S. (2012). Systematic review of herbs and dietary supplements for glycemic control of diabetes. *Diabetes Care, 37*(3), 1277–1294. doi: 10.2337/diacare.26.4.1277

Yurkovich, E. E., Hopkins-Lattergrass, I., & Rieke, S. (2012). Health-seeking behaviors of Native American Indians with persistent mental illness: Completing the circle. *Archives of Psychiatric Nursing, 26*(2), e1–e11. doi: 10.1016/j.apnu.2011.11002

COMPLEMENTARY, ALTERNATIVE, AND INTEGRATIVE HEALTH APPROACHES AMONG HISPANICS/LATINOS

Raffy R. Luquis and Joel Arboleda Castillo

Hispanics or Latinos are the largest minority group and one of the fastest-growing populations in the United States. This group includes all those of Cuban, Mexican, Puerto Rican, South or Central American, or other Spanish culture or origin, regardless of race (US Census Bureau, 2011). It is important to note that while some individuals prefer the term *Hispanic*, others prefer the terms *Latino* and/or *Latina*, and yet others prefer to list the name of their country first (e.g., Salvadoran American). In this chapter, terms are used interchangeably to refer to this population group.

In 2012, there were an estimated 52.9 million people of Hispanic/Latino origin living in the United States, which accounted for 16.9% of the total population (US Census Bureau, 2012a). Between 2000 and 2010, the Hispanic population grew at four times the growth in the total population. As a result, it is estimated that by 2060, the Hispanic population will more than double to 128.8 million, accounting for nearly one in three US residents by the end of that period (US Census Bureau, 2012b).

This chapter presents complementary and alternative medicine (CAM) practices and the complementary, alternative, and integrative health (CAIH) approaches most frequently used by the Hispanic/Latino population in the United States. It also discusses their implications for

LEARNING OBJECTIVES

At the completion of this chapter, students will be able to:

- Identify the complementary and alternative medicine practices most frequently used by Hispanics/Latinos as described in the current literature.

- Recognize the similarities and differences in complementary, alternative, and integrative health (CAIH) practices among Hispanic/Latino subgroups.

- Discuss the impact of CAIH practices among Hispanics/Latinos.

- Identify potential challenges and future applications for consumers, health educators, and other health professionals of CAIH approaches used by Hispanic/Latino populations.

consumers and identifies potential challenges for health professionals and health educators when working with this population.

Health professionals and health educators must understand that while the terms *complementary* and *alternative* are often used to describe these practices, the terms *folk* and *traditional* (i.e., customs or rituals followed by Latinos, which may be considered nontraditional by non-Latino individuals in the United States) practices may be more accurate when describing healing modalities among Hispanics (Holliday, 2008). Similarly, several studies have made a distinction between mainstream CAM (i.e., massage therapy, acupuncture) and traditional CAM (i.e., herbal remedies, folk medicine) when discussing these practices among Hispanics (Heathcote, West, Hall, & Trinidad, 2011). In this chapter, the authors focus on traditional CAM practices among Hispanic/Latino individuals residing in the United States, with some historical context from Latin American and other Hispanic countries. It is important to note that while the chapter describes traditional CAM practices among this group, CAIH approaches are also discussed in light of their use, which may be influenced by beliefs, years living in the United States, and acculturation level (i.e., some Latino individuals may no longer subscribe to these traditions).

Theoretical Concepts

Overview

Although Hispanics share many cultural characteristics, there are also distinctions among the Hispanic subgroups. For example, although a majority of Hispanics follow the Roman Catholic faith and speak Spanish, they practice their common religion with many spiritual variations and speak their common language in many different dialects (Pérez & Luquis, 2012, 2014). Similarly, their CAM practices are influenced by their cultural values, religious beliefs, and theories of illness and ailments (Spector, 2009). Examples of CAM practices in this group include visiting shrines; offering prayers; consultation with holistic healers; utilization of *parteras* (midwives); treatment by *sobanderos* (massage healers) and *hueseros* (bonesetters); and use of chamomile, spearmint, orange leaves, and basil teas and infusions (Spector, 2009; Pinzón-Pérez, 2014).

Prevalence of CAM Use among Hispanics in the United States

According to data from the 2012 National Health Interview Survey (NHIS), 22.0% of Hispanic adults reported using CAM, and the use of yoga among this group almost doubled since 2007 to 5% (Clarke, Black, Stussman, Barnes, & Nahin, 2015). Data from the 2007 NHIS provided more detailed information about the use of CAM among Hispanics. The data showed that 23.7% of Hispanic respondents reported using CAM (Barnes, Bloom, & Nahin, 2008). The percentage of CAM use among Hispanics varied by subgroup: Puerto Ricans (29.7%), Dominicans (28.2%), Mexican Americans (27.4%), Central or South Americans (23.4%), Cubans or Cuban Americans (22.9%), and Mexicans (18.2%). The percentage of reported CAM use among Hispanics also differed by modality: biologically based therapies (11.8%), mind-body therapies (10.8%), manipulative and body-based therapies (6.7%), and alternative medical systems (3%) (Barnes et al., 2008). Likewise, there was a difference in CAM modality used by Hispanic subgroups. A higher percentage of Dominicans (18.5%) and Puerto Ricans (16.8%) reported using mind-body therapies than other groups. Within biologically based therapies, Puerto Ricans (14.2%) and Mexicans (14.0%) reported a higher use; and within manipulative and body-based therapies, Cubans (8.5%) and Mexican Americans (7.9%) reported a higher use than other groups (Barnes et al., 2008).

Upchurch and Wexler Rainisch (2012), using data from the 2001–2002 National Longitudinal Study of Adolescent Health, found significant differences in CAM use by subgroups among young Hispanics. For example, Cubans (23.5%) and Central/South Americans (23.6%) reported higher use of biologically based therapies and manipulative and body-based therapies than Puerto Rican (20.0%) and Mexican (18.7%) respondents, respectively. Within mind-body therapies, Puerto Ricans reported the highest use (11.6%) compared to Cubans (10.3%), Central/South Americans (8.0%), and Mexicans (5.0%). Finally, Mexicans reported a higher use of alternative medical systems (7.2%) than Cubans (5.5%), Central/South Americans (5.2%), and Puerto Ricans (3.6%).

Health Beliefs among Latin Americans: Historical Concepts to Current Views

The formation of the concepts and practices of health and healing among Latin Americans is the result of a strong process of syncretism, involving elements of the indigenous world from European conquerors and slaves brought from Africa, Western scientific medicine, and other health models coming from the East and other regions.

Indigenous Health Beliefs

The natural elements that played an important role in the pre-Hispanic indigenous concepts still influence the healing concepts presented today (Gallardo, 2004). In general terms, it can be said that ancient indigenous cultures, which existed and are still present in many Caribbean and in

Central and South American countries, believed that loss of health was associated with an imbalance between human beings and nature. The role of those who cure was, therefore, to reset this balance (Gallardo, 2004). These beliefs can still be found among today's Latino populations (Chifa, 2010). Imbalance that causes disease progression normally was associated with the encounter of humans with supernatural beings or evil gods (Gallardo, 2004; Frisancho, 2012). In this sense, Frisancho (2012) indicated that "the diseases—according to the Aboriginal conception—came from a supernatural world inhabited by gods and spirits, with divine and sacred sense, so the manifestations of any medical condition were attributed to the will of those deities" (p. 122).

The sense of balance between human beings and the surrounding world among indigenous groups is associated with a worldview in which the human being is one part of the world and not its center (Soru, Boris, Carrera, & Duero, 2012). In view of the punitive nature of diseases, prevention and cure meant the development of collective practices to maintain "calm to the gods" (Frisancho, 2012). Moreover, in Latin American indigenous traditional medicine, the visit to the shaman (i.e., healer) is reserved for major issues; everyday health problems are treated at home (Gallardo, 2004; Orzuza, 2013).

Christianity and European Customs and Hispanic Beliefs about Health

European healing approaches that arrived in America were closely related to the Catholic Christian conception of disease, in which illness is not necessarily evil because it can be a divine instrument for the correction of the human being (Maurer, 1979; Rodríguez, 2012). As a result, the saints constituted a fundamental element in Catholic Christian beliefs and ensured conversion into other cultures in the West by virtue of their patronage (Neri, 2001). According to Ros (2002), by popular devotion, people have identified different "miraculous saints" who protect them from adversity. These saints are not always accepted by Rome's religious mainstream. This devotion has dominated the popular tradition to the present day.

Arrival of Slaves and African Beliefs

The African heritage in America is conditioned by the history of slavery (Carvajal, 1999). The country of origin among African slaves determined which religious practices survived. This explains why Bantu rites virtually disappeared while other religions, such as the Yoruba, managed to blend and keep some original rituals (Carvajal & Thoman, 1999; Sampedro, 2006).

Afro-American religions are made up mainly of African and Hispanic heritage and, to a lesser extent, include local pre-Columbian religions (Carvajal & Thoman, 1999). The specific characteristics of each area of the continent are determined by different African religious practices; however, there are some common characteristics, such as the role played by African gods that were intertwined with Christian and pre-Columbian religious figures, the relations of these figures and mystical trances and possessions, and the intervention of priests (Sampedro, 2006). During the last 40 years of the 20th century, African American practices have been strengthened in Latin America and have spread from their main centers (Haiti, Brazil, Cuba, and Jamaica) to Mexico, Peru, Colombia, and Argentina (Carvajal & Thoman, 1999).

Modalities

According to Ortiz, Shields, Clauson, and Clay (2007), the foundations of health beliefs and CAM use among Hispanics can be attributed to a fusion of cultures and historical influences described earlier in this chapter. Hispanics' health beliefs can be traced back from the ancient indigenous people from Central and South America, who believed that the sea, earth, and moon played an important role in a person's health. The beliefs also can be traced back to the arrival of the Spaniards, the Catholic religion, and Hippocrates's humoral theory. In addition, the introduction of spiritual healing (*curanderismo*), magic (*Santería*), and some herbal remedies brought by African slaves in part of South America and the Caribbean, resulted in the development of the hot/cold theory of health and disease that many Hispanics still accept today (Ortiz et al., 2007).

Hot diseases, which are distinguished by vasodilation and high metabolic rate (e.g., pregnancy, diabetes, hypertension), are treated with cold remedies. Similarly, cold diseases, which are believed to be caused by vasoconstriction (e.g., pneumonia, cramps, asthma), are treated with hot remedies (Knoerl, 2007; Ortiz et al., 2007; Tafur, Crowe, & Torres, 2009). For example, diabetes mellitus (a hot illness) is treated with *nopal* (cactus), aloe vera juice, and bitter gourd, all of which are considered cold treatments. Asthma, a cold disease, is treated with hot-quality remedies, such as traditional herbs and massages (Ortiz et al., 2007).

In addition, because of Catholic religious influences, some Hispanics believe that illness is bad luck or punishment from God because of improper behaviors or wrongdoing (Knoerl, 2007; Spector, 2009). Accordingly,

"People are expected to maintain their own equilibrium in the universe by performing the proper way, eating the proper food, and working the appropriate amount of time" (Spector, 2009, p. 288). Likewise, Hispanics can protect their health with prayers; by wearing religious artifacts, such as effigies of their favorite patron saints, and by keeping relics at home (Spector, 2009; Tafur et al., 2009).

Furthermore, Hispanics, especially Mexicans, believe that illnesses can be triggered by other causes (Holliday, 2008; Tafur et al., 2009). Latinos in the United States recognize these common folk illnesses:

- *Caída de mollera* (fallen fontanelle). It refers to the fallen or depressed fontanelle of an infant's head as the result of several events, such as someone touching the child's head, the child falling from a high surface, inefficient suckling, or because the nipple was abruptly removed from the infant's mouth when breastfeeding. Symptoms of *caída de mollera* include colic, crying, diarrhea, vomiting, and fever (Tafur et al., 2009).

- *Susto* (scared-frightened). It is a fearful emotional state that causes the soul to leave the body because of the traumatic event. This condition may result in mental illness; restlessness while sleeping; list-lessness; anorexia; and disinterest in personal hygiene, loss of strength, depression, and introversion (Spector, 2009; Tafur et al., 2009).

- *Mal de Ojo* (evil eye). The evil eye is caused by an adult paying excessive attention to a child or the result of too much admiration from someone else (Tafur et al., 2009). This condition can result in general malaise, sleepiness, fatigue, and severe headaches (Spector, 2009).

- *Envidia* (envy). Envy is an illness caused by intense jealousy. Some Hispanics believe that when "one's success provokes the envy of friends or neighbors, misfortune can befall the person and his or her family" (Spector, 2009, p. 290).

- *Empacho* (upset stomach). Upset stomach is described as "an intestinal blockage and is believed to be caused by eating something that you do not want to eat, eating spoiled food, eating too much, food getting stuck in the stomach" (Tafur et al., 2009, p. 86). Symptoms may include stomach pain and cramps, bloated stomach, and loss of appetite (Spector, 2009; Tafur et al., 2009).

While Puerto Ricans describe these illnesses as part of their folk beliefs, they also define *pasmo* and *ataques* as two other common folk mal-adies. *Pasmo,* a paralysis-like symptom, is caused by the imbalance on the hot/cold humors, while *ataques* are described as hysterical screaming and uncontrollable movement of the arms and legs (Spector, 2009). Sanchez and Shallcross (2012) described *ataques* (also known as *ataques de nervios*) as a condition that often includes episodes of nervousness and crying (i.e., uncontrollable shouting) and can include physical (i.e., sensation of heat, physical aggression), dissociative (i.e., fainting, being out of control), and other emotional symptoms. *Ataques* are often related to family stress, stressful events, or conflict situations, and the individual may return to his or her normal functioning after the *ataque*.

Curanderos and Other Healers

Curanderismo is a "term referring to the Spanish word *curar*, meaning 'to heal,' and is used to describe the practice of traditional healing" (Tafur, Crow, & Torrres, 2009, p. 82) in many Hispanic and Latino cultures. DeBellonia et al. (2008) described *curanderismo* as a form of folk practice associated with spiritual and psychic healing. The *curandero* (folk healer) "is believed to have healing powers and is a common appearing figure in a Mexican community" (p. 228). While some believe that an individual becomes a *curandero* because she or he is born with the innate talent to heal others, there is an emphasis on the education of the healer as an individual becomes a *curandero* after a long traineeship (Tafur et al., 2009). Many members of the Hispanic community consider the *curandero* to be both a religious figure and a medicine healer (DeBellonia et al., 2008; Spector, 2009; Tafur et al., 2009). In addition, many *curanderos* are considered generalists (Spector, 2009), while others have different specializations, including *yerberos* (herbalists), *parteras* (midwives), *sobadores* (massage providers), *espiritistas* (psychics), and tarot card readers. As such, they can use herbal remedies, prayers, rituals, religious ceremonies, and incantations to diagnose, treat, and cure illnesses (DeBellonia et al., 2008; Tafur et al., 2009). Thus, while in some Hispanic communities a *curandero* may perform multiple roles, in others the term describes the name and/or role of the healer.

Although many elements of the figure of the *curandero* come to Latin America as a European heritage, the role *curanderos* play is one of the methods of traditional medicine (Arteaga, 2012). Trotter (2001) pointed out that indigenous tradition highly influences *curanderismo*. This results in the conception of indigenous medicine as a traditional medicine and the identification of shamans, healers, and herbalists (Lámbarri, Flores, & Berenzon, 2012). *Curanderismo* practices are mainly used in Latin American countries with the largest indigenous populations.

Herbs, Natural Remedies, Herbalists, *Yerberos,* and *Sobadores*

Many members of the Hispanic/Latino community commonly use herbs and herbal remedies. According to Tafur et al. (2009), Hispanics use herbs to treat stomach and intestinal problems, sore muscles, burns, for weight loss, cough, acne, and bad breath. They also use them to treat more serious diseases, such as arthritis, cancer, HIV, and diabetes. While some people can find herbs and herbal remedies prepared at local *botánicas* (herbal stores), others prepare the herbal remedies themselves. In some cases healers prefer to prepare the herbal remedies to give to their clients (Tafur et al., 2009; Viladrich, 2006). *Yerberos* are *curanderos* who specialize in the preparation of herbs and herbal remedies for the treatment of illness and diseases (DeBellonia et al., 2008). *Sobadores* are traditional healers who use massage and rub techniques in order to treat patients, prevent disease, and restore health (National Center for Complementary and Integrative Health [NCCIH], 2015c). It is important to note that while many of the herbs are safe, some may have serious side effects or interactions with prescribed medicines. For this reason, it is crucial that healthcare providers be aware of herbal use among Latino patients (Tafur et al., 2009).

Herbal Use

Viladrich's (2006) work has provided a classification of herbs used by Latinos in New York City. Herbs are classified into sweet and bitter, and are mostly used in teas, baths, and rubbing ointments. Sweet herbs, such as *romero* (rosemary), *yerbabuena* (spearmint), and *sabila* (aloe vera), are aromatic, agreeable to the palate, and used in teas to treat physical and organic illnesses. Bitter herbs, such as *aramu* (ginseng of the tropics) and *jengibre* (ginger), are strong in smell and taste and are used in baths to treat stress, relationships, love, bring good luck, and find a job. Viladrich also reported that while most healers prefer to use fresh herbs, consumption of dried herbs and plants is prevalent, as most come from Miami, the Dominican Republic, Puerto Rico, Mexico, Brazil, and Central America. As a result, from time to time, there may be a shortage of the supply of herbs, and some employees of herbal stores and/or healers replace or combine other herbs and plants to get the same effect for their clients.

A study conducted by Howell et al. (2006) found that at least 80% of Hispanic patients reported using herbs; the percentage was higher among Spanish-speaking users and those who had been in the United States for fewer than five years. Moreover, almost 60% reported that they had taken between 6 and 15 different herbs during their lifetime. Most said that they had used herbs to treat cough, stomach pain, sore throat, menstrual cramps, headache , and chest pain. Nonetheless, results of their study showed that the majority of respondents did not inform their doctors about their herbal use. Ortiz and Clauson (2006) found that 75% of Hispanics in South Florida used herbs and herbal remedies for gastrointestinal disturbances and upper respiratory ailments, with most of them citing safety and family traditions as reasons for using them. They also found that a majority of participants (53%) believed that they should tell their healthcare provider about any herb used; yet it was not clear whether participants had done so. Howell et al. (2006) reported that most commonly used herbs by their respondents were cinnamon, cloves, cumin, chamomile, garlic, onion, grass syrup, aloe vera, oregano, and lemon; Ortiz and Clauson (2006) reported chamomile, aloe, linden, star anise, garlic, ginger, ginseng, and valerian as the most commonly used herbs by their participants. As part of their study, Howell et al. (2006) listed some of the most commonly used herbs and their potential drug interactions (see Table 8.1). Given the potential interaction between herbs and medications, healthcare providers and other health professionals (i.e., pharmacists, health educators) must understand and address the use of herbs among the Hispanic population.

It is important to note that the use of herbs for medicinal purposes is widespread among Latin American countries and that such practices are based on knowledge of collective dominance (Chifa, 2010). A special type of use of medicinal herbs is the traditional Dominican *botellas*, or mixtures of root exudates and other parts of plants, spices and other ingredients, prepared in plastic bottles. Their name refers to the bottle or container in which the mixtures are prepared (Vandebroek et al., 2010). They are used for all kinds of problems and illnesses but especially for asthma, female reproductive problems, and male impotence. Dominicans do not consider a *curandero* the person who prepares the bottles but "the man who makes remedies for all ills" (Vanderbroek et al., 2010). Researchers found that the use of *botellas* extends to other parts of the regions. Dominicans living in New York City use a similar mixture of plants as those used by Dominicans in their home country (Vanderbroek et al., 2010). The use of herbs and plants mixtures in *botellas* (aka *galones*) is widespread in the Caribbean, including Cuba, Haiti, Puerto Rico, and Martinique (Benedetti, 1998; Clement et al., 2005; Hernández & Volpato, 2004; Longuesfosse & Nossin, 1996; Volpato, Godínez, & Beyra, 2009).

Botánicas

Botánicas, religious healing stores or herbal markets, have been described as the visible door to the hidden world of Hispanic traditional healing

Table 8.1 Selected Herb Use and Potential Drug Interactions

Herb	Use	Potential Interactions with Prescription Medications
Immortal (Spider milkweed)	Orally, for arthritis, asthma, cough, edema, syphilis, valvular insufficiency, senile heart, to strengthen weak heart muscles following pneumonia, and for diuresis.	Digoxin, diuretics
	Topically, for warts.	
Plumajillo (Pleurisy root)	Orally, for cough, pleurisy, uterine disorders, shortness of breath, pain, spasms, and to promote sweating; for bronchitis, pneumonitis, and influenza.	Digoxin, diuretics, estrogen
Canella (Cinnamon)	Orally, for colds, poor circulation, and as a bitter tonic.	None known
Clavo (Cloves)	Orally, clove for dyspepsia, as an expectorant, for diarrhea, hernia, halitosis, flatulence, nausea, and vomiting.	Antiplatelet and anticoagulant agents
	Topically, for toothache, postextraction alveolitis, pain, a dental anesthetic, mouth and throat inflammation. In combination with other ingredients, topically for premature ejaculation.	
Comino (Cumin)	Orally, as an antiflatulent, stimulant, antispasmodic, diuretic, aphrodisiac, for stimulating menstrual flow, treating diarrhea, colic, and flatulence.	Antidiabetic agents
Manzanilla (Chamomile)	Orally, for flatulence, travel sickness, nasal mucous membrane inflammation, allergic rhinitis, nervous diarrhea, attention deficit-hyperactivity disorder, restlessness, insomnia, gastrointestinal spasms, inflammatory diseases of the gastrointestinal tract, gastrointestinal ulcers associated with NSAIDs [nonsteroidal anti-inflammatories] and alcohol consumption, and as an antispasmodic for menstrual cramps.	Benzodiazepines; CNS [central nervous system] depressants; contraceptive drugs; CYP1A2 substrates (e.g., antipsychotic, calcium channel blocker, beta-blockers); CYP3A4 substrates (e.g., statins, antifungal, antihistamine); estrogens; tamoxifen; warfarin
	Topically, for hemorrhoids, leg ulcers; for skin, anogenital, and mucous membrane inflammation; for bacterial skin diseases; for treating or preventing chemotherapy- or radiation-induced oral mucositis.	
	Via inhalation, for inflammation and irritation of the respiratory tract.	

Ajo (Garlic)	Orally, for hypertension, hyperlipidemia; for prevention of coronary heart disease, age-related vascular changes, and atherosclerosis; for reducing reinfarction and mortality rate post-myocardial infarction, earaches, chronic fatigue syndrome, and menstrual disorders; for HIV-drug-induced lipid disorders and *Helicobacter pylori* infection; for prevention of colorectal, gastric, breast, lung, and prostate cancer; for bladder cancer, benign prostatic hyperplasia, diabetes, arthritis, allergies, traveler's diarrhea, colds and flu; for immune system stimulation, prevention of tick bites, and prevention and treatment of bacterial and fungal infections; for diarrhea, amoebic and bacterial dysentery, tuberculosis, bloody urine, diphtheria, whooping cough, scalp ringworm, hypersensitive teeth, and vaginal trichomoniasis; for fever, cough, headache, stomachache, sinus congestion, athlete's foot, gout, rheumatism, hemorrhoids, asthma, bronchitis, shortness of breath, arteriosclerosis, low blood pressure, hypoglycemia, hyperglycemia, and snakebites; as a diuretic, stimulant, cathartic, aphrodisiac; for enhancing circulation, fighting stress and fatigue.	Anticoagulant and antiplatelet agents; contraceptives; cyclosporine; CYP2E1 substrates (e.g., acetaminophen, ethanol, theophylline); CYP3A4 substrates (e.g., statins, antifungal, antihistamine); nonnucleoside reverse transcriptase inhibitors; saquinavir
Jengibre (Ginger)	Orally, for motion and morning sickness, colic, dyspepsia, flatulence, chemotherapy-induced nausea, rheumatoid arthritis, osteoarthritis, loss of appetite, postoperative nausea and vomiting, migraine headache, anorexia, upper respiratory tract infections, cough, bronchitis, and as a diaphoretic, diuretic, and a stimulant. Fresh ginger: orally, for treating acute bacterial dysentery, baldness, malaria, orchitis, poisonous snake bites, rheumatism, and toothaches. Dried ginger: orally for chest, low back, and stomach pain. Topically, for thermal burns and as an analgesic.	Antiplatelet and anticoagulant agents; antidiabetic agents; calcium channel blockers

(*continued*)

Table 8.1 Selected Herb Use and Potential Drug Interactions (*continued*)

Herb	Use	Potential Interactions with Prescription Medications
Granada (Pomegranate)	Orally, for hypertension, heart failure, myocardial ischemia, atherosclerosis, hyperlipidemia, acidosis, hemorrhage, HIV disease, tapeworm infestations, diarrhea, dysentery, and opportunistic intestinal worms; for preventing prostate cancer, and as an astringent and abortifacient; for chronic obstructive pulmonary disease, influenza, stomatitis, periodontal disease, erectile dysfunction, diabetes, and cancer. Topically, as a gargle for sore throat and to treat hemorrhoids.	Antiplatelet and anticoagulant agents; antidiabetic agents; ACE inhibitors; antihypertensive agents; CYP3A4 substrates (e.g., statins, antifungal, antihistamine); CYP2D6 substrates (e.g., SSRI, tricyclic antidepressants, opiates, antiarrhythmic)
Anis estrella (Star anise)	Orally, for respiratory infections and inflammation, influenza, avian flu, gastrointestinal upset, flatulence, loss of appetite, infant colic, cough, and bronchitis; for increasing milk secretion, promoting menstruation, facilitating childbirth, increasing libido, and treating symptoms of male climacteric. Through inhalation, for respiratory tract congestion.	None known
Estafiate (Wormwood)	Orally, for loss of appetite, indigestion and digestive disorders, biliary dyskinesia, fever, and liver disease; as an anthelmintic, aphrodisiac, tonic, antispasmodic, and to stimulate sweating and the imagination. Topically, for healing wounds and insect bites and as a counterirritant.	Anticonvulsants
Cundeamore (Bitter gourd)	Orally, for diabetes, psoriasis, gastrointestinal upset, ulcers, colitis, constipation, intestinal worms, kidney stones, fever, hepatic disease, and to induce menstruation. Topically, for skin abscesses and wounds, and anorectal herpes lesions.	Antidiabetic agents

Savila (Aloe vera)	Orally, for osteoarthritis, inflammatory bowel disease, fever, itching and inflammation, as a general tonic, for gastroduodenal ulcers, diabetes, asthma, and radiation-related mucositis. Topically, for burns, wound healing, psoriasis, sunburn, frostbite, inflammation, osteoarthritis, and cold sores; and as an antiseptic and a moisturizer.	Oral medications; sevoflurane; diuretics; digoxin; antidiabetic agents
Uña de gato (Cat's claw)	Orally, for diverticulitis, peptic ulcers, colitis, gastritis, hemorrhoids, parasites, Alzheimer's disease, chronic fatigue syndrome, wound healing, arthritis, asthma, allergic rhinitis, cancer (especially of the urinary tract), glioblastoma, gonorrhea, dysentery, birth control, bone pain, "cleansing" the kidneys, and viral infections, including herpes zoster, herpes simplex, and human immunodeficiency virus (HIV).	Antihypertensive agents; immunosuppressants; CYP3A4 substrates (e.g., statins, antifungal, antihistamine)
Pelos de elote (Corn silk)	Orally, for cystitis, urethritis, nocturnal enuresis, prostatitis, inflammation of the urinary tract, diabetes, hypertension, and as a diuretic for congestive heart failure.	Antihypertensive agents; antidiabetic agents; diuretics; corticosteroids; warfarin
Oregano	Orally, for respiratory tract disorders, including cough, asthma, croup, and bronchitis; for gastrointestinal disorders, such as dyspepsia and bloating; for dysmenorrhea, rheumatoid arthritis, urinary tract infections, headaches, heart conditions, intestinal parasites, allergies, sinusitis, arthritis, cold and flu, earaches, and fatigue. Topically, for acne, athlete's foot, dandruff, insect and spider bites, canker sores, gum disease, toothaches, psoriasis, seborrhea, ringworm, rosacea, muscle pain, varicose veins, and warts, and as an insect repellent. In foods and beverages, as a culinary spice and a preservative.	None known

(continued)

Table 8.1 Selected Herb Use and Potential Drug Interactions (*continued*)

Herb	Use	Potential Interactions with Prescription Medications
Limon (Lemon)	Orally, as a source of vitamin C in the treatment of scurvy and colds; as a digestive aid, an anti-inflammatory, diuretic, and to improve vascular permeability.	None known
Valeriana (Valerian)	Orally, as a sedative-hypnotic for insomnia and as an anxiolytic for restlessness; for mood disorders such as depression, mild tremors, epilepsy, attention deficit-hyperactivity disorder, and chronic fatigue syndrome; for muscle and joint pain, asthma, hysterical states, excitability, hypochondria, headaches, migraine, stomach upset, menstrual cramps and symptoms associated with menopause, including hot flashes and anxiety. Topically, as a bath additive for restlessness and sleep disorders.	Alcohol; benzodiazepines; CNS depressants; CYP3A4 substrates (e.g., statins, antifungal, antihistamine)
Tomillo (Thyme)	Orally, for bronchitis, pertussis, sore throat, colic, arthritis, dyspepsia, gastritis, diarrhea, enuresis, dyspraxia, flatulence, skin disorders, as a diuretic, urinary disinfectant, anthelmintic, and as an appetite stimulant. Topically, for laryngitis, tonsillitis, stomatitis, and halitosis; as a counterirritant, an antiseptic in mouthwashes and liniments, and for alopecia areata. Otically, as an antibacterial and antifungal ingredient.	Antiplatelet and anticoagulant agents
Epasote (Wormseed)	Orally, for ascaris and oxyuris infestations.	None known

Source: Reproduced by permission from the American Board of Family Medicine from Howell, Kochhar, Saywell, Zollinger, Koehler, Mandzuk, . . . & Allen (2006), 573–575.

modalities (Tafur et al., 2009; Viladrich, 2006). *Botánicas* play a key role in the Hispanic/Latino communities, as they provide herbs, healthcare products, healing remedies, and informal health advice and refer clients to formal and informal health practitioners. *Botánicas* are usually located in heavily populated Latino neighborhoods or areas undergoing ethnic and racial transformation denoted by growing redevelopment (Viladrich, 2006).

For a health educator or healthcare professional who has never visited a *botánica*, the setting may be similar to a health or natural food store. However, *botánicas* offer medicinal herbs, religious amulets, incense, candles, statues of saints, and other related items (Gomez-Beloz & Chavez, 2001; Viladrich, 2006). According to Gomez-Beloz and Chavez (2001), the Latino owners and employees of the *botánicas* are knowledgeable about the products, provide advice to clients on different herbal remedies and healing practices, and offer these services in a culturally appropriate manner. In addition, *botánicas* are informal settings for healers, herbalists, *curanderos, santeros, espiritistas*, and other community members to network, socialize, and promote their services and healing practices (Viladrich, 2006). While some *botánicas* concentrate on the natural and spiritual aspects of healing and provide primarily herbs, vitamins, and homeopathic and naturopathic remedies, others focus on the magic and religious views of healing and have mainly religious products (Gomez-Beloz & Chavez, 2001). Finally, most *botánicas* have a room in the back of the store or basement for *consultas* (consultations) where the healer provides one-on-one advice to clients.

The *consulta* provides a client with social support, emotional strength, and diagnosis of illness and chronic conditions. Moreover, through the *consulta*, the healer can make a distinction among the spiritual, magical, physical, and mental domains and provide the client with the proper herb, remedy, or treatment (Viladrich, 2006). However, Viladrich (2006) cautioned that the outcome of *consultas* can be inconclusive, ambiguous, and inaccurate, as it depends on the efficacy and competence of the healer. Still, there is no clear method to assess the standards, practices, and impact of the treatments. Nonetheless, healthcare practitioners and health professionals must understand the role of the *botánicas* in the Hispanic community, as they may be the only source of care for this community. In addition, "The *botánica* is a desirable health care option because it overcomes some of the systemic barriers to health care" (Gomez-Beloz & Chavez, 2001, p. 542), such as office hours, health insurance, Spanish-speaking staff, and location.

Finally, Garza and Young (2007), who interviewed herbalists and *botánica* owners in a Texas neighborhood, found that these individuals commonly prescribe herbal remedies for specific medical symptoms.

For example, aloe vera (*savila*) may be prescribed for gastritis/indigestion, senna (*hojasen*) and rhamnus purse (*cascara sagrada*) may be prescribed for constipation, and shave grass (*cola de caballo*) and chamomile (*manzanilla*) may be prescribed for diarrhea. While their results were limited, they concluded that since many of these herbs are not available at mainstream stores, physicians must be aware of *botánicas*, herbalist recommendations, and the use of these products by Latinos.

Espiritismo *and* Santería

Previous sections described natural healing modalities. This section describes two non-Christian spiritual practices, *espiritismo* and *Santería*, which influence the lives of many Puerto Ricans, Dominicans, Cubans, and their descendants living in the United States (Báez & Hernández, 2001). A detailed overview of *espiritismo* and *Santería* is beyond the scope of this chapter. However, the following brief description is presented to help health educators, healthcare practitioners, and other health professionals understand these belief systems.

Espiritismo is a spiritual belief system based on the tenet of spiritual influences and communication with spirits (Báez & Hernández, 2001; Musgrave, Allen, & Allen, 2002). According to Báez and Hernández (2001), *espiritismo* originated in the 1850s with the belief that spirits reincarnated and that each person has an angel or spirit who protects and guides him or her through life's difficulties. In addition, "People also encounter untranquil, unevolved, or evil spirits, sometimes by happenstance, sometimes because of spells (*brujería*), and that spirits of various types can exert a profound influence on human life, causing either good or harm of all types" (Báez & Hernández, p. 411). *Espiritistas*, known as mediums, have the unique ability to perceive and communicate with the spirits and can determine which ritual to use to deal with each situation. *Espiritistas* often use prayers, group healing sessions, house cleansings, and baths with herbs for personal cleansing to resolve the spiritual problem (Báez & Hernández, 2001). *Espiritistas* can also use amulets and medals to protect against evil (Musgrave et al., 2002). Moreover, *espiritistas* believe that the spiritual and material worlds are holistically intertwined; hence, dysfunctions are caused by material, spiritual, or both worlds (Báez & Hernández, 2001). Finally, *espiritismo* also has common roots with *Santería*, as both believe in spiritual causes and share the *orisha*-saint combination presented in the magic-religious beliefs system to be discussed (Pérez y Mena, 1998; Spector, 2009). *Espiritismo* is widely dispersed and practiced in Cuba, Brazil, Argentina, and Colombia (Ludueña, 2013; Prandi, 2012; Ramíres, 2008).

Musgrave et al. (2002) described *Santería* as "an African-Cuban religious tradition combining Catholicism with Nigerian tribal beliefs and practices, includes belief in the magical and medicinal properties of flowers, herbs, weeds, twigs, and leaves" (p. 558). Báez and Hernández (2001) further explained that *Santería* is a religion based on the combination or reconciliation of the religious practices of enslaved Africans (i.e., Yoruba beliefs) in the Caribbean when exposed to Catholicism. As a result, enslaved Africans gave Yoruba's *orishas*, or deities, names of Catholic saints to conceal their devotion (Pérez & Mena, 1998). For example, Obatala, the king of the *orishas*, became the Lady of Mercy and/or Crucified Christ; Chango, the god of fire, became St. Barbara; and Oggun, the god of war, became St. Peter (Báez & Hernández, 2001; Pérez & Mena, 1998; Spector, 2009). The *santero*, skilled practitioner of this religion, possesses magical abilities and receives visions from the *orishas* to determine the causes of the person's illness or magical problem. *Santeros* believe in the use of colorful necklaces, which represent the color of each *orisha* (i.e., Seven African Potencies), and herbs, associated with each *orisha*, to attract good or bad luck toward health, love, and friendship (Viladrich, 2006).

Other Alternative Healing Practices

In addition to the folk and traditional healing practices mentioned in the previous sections, many members of the Hispanic community practice religious rituals such as prayer, devotions, wearing religious medals, and anointing the sick; thus, it is important that health professionals understand and advocate for the inclusion of cultural practices within the patient's plan of healthcare and healing process (Hicks, 2012). Within the cultural framework of the Hispanic culture, prayer is recognized as a folk healing custom as much as a spiritual practice (Easom, 2006). Since folk remedies involve any health practice done at home before seeking healthcare assistance, many Hispanics report that the practice of prayer/spirituality and home remedies are interchangeable (Easom, 2006).

Similarly, Ransford, Carrillo, and Rivera (2010) explained that religion (i.e., prayer and faith) plays an important role in the alternative system of healing of Latinos, as it helps them gain control and boost their health as they face healthcare barriers. As part of a qualitative study, they found that 75% of Latinos residing in the Los Angeles area reported that prayer was important and fundamental to health; as such, they had prayed for their own health and the health of a family member or friend. However, they also found that church attendance was not associated with the importance of prayer, which indicated a distinction between personal and organizational religion (Ransford et al., 2010). In contrast, Heathcote et al. (2011) found that religiosity (i.e., degree of religious behavior, belief, and spirituality) was associated with the use of traditional CAM among a group of foreign-born Hispanics.

Another connection between religious beliefs and healing practices is seen in the use of *juramentos*, or pledges to do or abstain from something, made to the Virgin, a saint, or another religious entity (Cuadrado & Lieberman, 2011). Mexicans and Mexican Americans who often practice *juramento* explain that a *juramento* is done when they want to stop a damaging behavior, hence, making a promise to the "Virgin of Guadalupe provides them with protection from being taunted or ridiculed for not engaging in the behavior they are trying to suppress, usually, drinking, drugging or smoking, even among non-believers of the Church" (p. 924). An exploratory study showed that *juramentos* were used to deal with substance abuse among Hispanic populations in South Florida. These authors concluded that health professionals must understand and accept *juramentos* as a workable form of intervention in conjunction with traditional substance abuse treatment modalities offered in the United States, especially among those who refuse institutional substance abuse treatment.

Consumer Issues

Consumers should be knowledgeable of the benefits and risks associated with Hispanic/Latino CAIH approaches. Several studies have researched the use of *azogue* (mercury) and lead, which are regulated chemicals, as part of many Latino *mágico*-religious rituals (i.e., *Santería*) and folk remedies. Mercury can expose users to toxic mercury vapors (Carter-Pokras, Zambrana, Poppell, Logie, & Guerrero-Preston, 2007; Newby, Riley, & Leal-Almeraz, 2006; Riley, Newby, & Leal-Almeraz, 2006). As part of many of the rituals and traditional remedies, mercury is sold at many *botánicas* or *bodegas* (local stores) to bring "luck, love, or money, as a cleanser, to ward off evil, for cosmetic purposes, to treat intestinal disorders, and in specific acts of divination or religious initiation" (Riley et al., 2006, p. 1206).

Mercury is most commonly sold in gelatin capsules, but it is also sold in other containers and plastic baggies. Moreover, individuals can carry it as an amulet; place it in candles or oil lamps; or add it to perfumes, creams, bathwater, or soap for cleaning floors (Newby et al., 2006; Riley et al., 2006). Carter-Pokras et al. (2007) warned about the mercury exposure in Latino children, as some people sprinkle it around a room or baby's crib as treatment for *empacho* in infants. Acute mercury poisoning or low-level exposure can cause short-term respiratory problems and can lead to "long-term neurological effects, including tremors, insomnia, memory loss, and deteriorated cognitive function" (Riley et al., 2006, p. 1206) and "potentially irreversible neuropsychological deficits and emotional disturbances in children" (Carter-Pokras et al., 2007, p. 310). Thus, it is important that consumers are aware of the potential consequences of exposure to mercury and become educated about it. In addition, CAIH practitioners (i.e., healers, *santeros*) must also become aware and educated about the potential hazards of mercury exposure in its use as part of rituals and healing practices.

Implications for Health Professionals

As previously alluded to, people need to be aware that while many of the herbs and herbal remedies are safe, some may have some serious side effects or potential for interaction with prescribed medications (*Consumer Reports*, 2009; Howell et al., 2006; Ortiz & Clauson, 2006; Tafur et al., 2009). For example, garlic and ginseng may interact with blood thinner and diabetes drugs. Thus, it is important that individuals who take medications consult their physician before using herbs and herbal remedies. Also, as previous survey research showed, many Hispanics do not inform their physicians and other healthcare providers about their use of traditional and folk medicine (Howell et al., 2006; Ortiz & Clauson, 2006). It is important for Hispanic consumers to establish a dialogue with their healthcare providers and other health professionals about the use of herbs, herbal remedies, and other healing practices.

The Food and Drug Administration (2008) warned consumers that while they may continue to use herbs and herbal remedies, they should pay attention to the warnings established by this entity concerning dietary sup-plements, as well as the purity and quality of herbs and herbal remedies sold at many *botanícas*. *Consumer Reports* provided tips to consumers on the safe use of herbal remedies. Similar to general consumers, it is important for healthcare professionals, including health educators, to keep an open mind regarding the use of complementary, alternative, and traditional healing practices among the Latino population. As discussed, many Latinos do not disclose CAM use with their physicians and other healthcare providers. Moreover, the dichotomy between some Latino healing practices (i.e., herbs, spiritual-religious) and health professionals' attitudes about these practices might result in the lack of communication between the individual and the professional as well as a lack of knowledge by the professional. Ortiz et al. (2007) provided recommendations for practitioners when assessing CAM use among Hispanics. Understanding cultural diversity and the different forms of CAM and healing practices among Hispanics is fundamental to providing the best health education and healthcare for this population (DeBellonia et al., 2008). Moreover, when describing the paradigms of health and illness, disease prevention, and healing practices, health professionals must incorporate the "indigenous models of etiology, diagnosis, and treatment," and they "need to be sensitive to their clients' religious, spiritual, and cultural beliefs" (Viladrich, 2006, p. 416). Similarly, health professionals must remember that some Hispanics seek the advice of folk healers and use folk remedies; thus, practitioners need to explore and respect the alternative health modalities that the person may be using, if these are helpful to the individual's health (Knoerl, 2007). Health professionals must understand that some of these healing and religious practices are seen as successful in providing relief from health problems and illnesses and that some Hispanics might use home remedies before seeking the help of healthcare professionals (Easom, 2006).

Health professionals and health educators can play a vital role in providing information on the benefits and risks associated with some of these healing and religious rituals (i.e., herb use and potential interactions) to allow consumers to make informed decisions to improve their health status.

Caveat Emptor

Although there are many laws and regulations regarding healthcare practices, little research and literature examines the regulation of CAIH, traditional, and folk practices among Hispanics. Ortiz and Clauson (2006) stated that although the use of herbs and herbal remedies among Hispanics raised some concerns among healthcare professionals, herbs are classified as dietary supplements; thus, herbal stores such as *botanicas* are not comprehensively regulated. Chapter 3 provides a detailed description of the legal parameters regulating herbal and dietary supplement treatments in the United States.

There is limited information on the education, preparation, or traineeship of *curanderos*, *santeros*, and *espiritistas*, as these individuals are perceived to be born with the innate talent to heal others or as having received their knowledge from prior generations (Ortiz et al., 2007; Tafur et al., 2009). Given the assumed separation of church and state, practices such as prayers and religious rituals do not fall under legal strictures, and their practice is conducted without major regulatory considerations.

The comprehensive National Research Strategy for Complementary and Alternative Medicine from the National Center for

Complementary and Alternative Medicine (NCCAM), now known as the NCCIH, has attempted to provide guidelines in the regulation of traditional healers and other forms of CAM by investing in CAM research, training CAM investigators, expanding outreach, identifying the extent and nature of CAM use among special populations, studying therapeutic interventions to reduce disparities, increasing participation of minority and underserved populations in NCCAM-supported clinical trials, enhancing the ability of minority institutions to support CAM research, and facilitating integration with Western models of care (NCCIH, 2015a). In 2000 the NCCAM developed the first strategic planning document *Expanding Horizons of Health Care*, which was updated in 2005 with the strategic plan for 2005 to 2009, and in 2011 with the document *Exploring the Science of Complementary and Alternative Medicine: Third Strategic Plan 2011–2015* (NCCIH, 2015b). These plans provide guidelines for future development of regulatory actions regarding the practice of traditional healers such as *curanderos, espiritistas, santeros, sobadores*, and *yerberos*, among others.

Conclusion

Hispanic/Latinos are one of the fastest-growing and most diverse population groups in the United States. As discussed in this chapter, Hispanic cultural values, religious beliefs, and theories of illness and disease influence their practices of folk, traditional healing, and CAIH modalities. The literature shows that the Hispanic population continues to use many of the folk and healing modalities employed by their ancestors and prior generations. The roots of the health beliefs, folk medicine, healing, and magico-religious practices came from historical influences and the fusion of cultures of colonist, Latin American, and Caribbean indigenous communities, and African slaves. Today, many Hispanics continue to use herbs and herbal remedies and follow the advice of *curanderos, yerberos, sobadores, espiritistas, and santeros*. As a result, healthcare professionals must understand and respect these practices as they work with this population. In addition, health professionals must educate this population on the use of herbs, herbal remedies, and other healing modalities due to the potential for serious side effects and interactions with prescribed medications.

Summary

- The use of terms such as *folk medicine* and *traditional healing practices* are more appropriate when addressing CAM use among Hispanics.

- There are variations on the frequency and type of CAM use among different Hispanic groups.

- CAM use among Hispanics is rooted in a long history and diverse cultural influences over time.

- Many members of the Hispanic/Latino community commonly use herbs and herbal remedies for ailments and illnesses.

- *Botánicas*, or herbal markets, are the visible entrance to the world of Hispanic/Latino traditional healing practices.

- The practice of *espiritismo* and *Santería* continues to influence the lives of many Puerto Ricans, Dominicans, Cubans, and other Latinos and their descendants living in the United States.

- Many Hispanics use prayer and spiritual rituals to protect their health and cope with illness.

- Consumers need to be aware that some herbs, herbal remedies, and healing practices may have some serious health consequences.

- Traditional healing practices used by Hispanics/Latinos can be classified as complementary, alternative, and integrative health modalities as they are aimed to restore health, promote harmony, and maintain well-being.

- Healthcare professionals, including health educators, must keep an open mind regarding the use of complementary, alternative, and traditional healing practices among the Latino population.

Case Study

Description

As a health professional working in a hospital, you are part of a team who is faced with the following situation. The mother of a six-year-old Mexican believes that he is suffering from *susto* (fright) after he was involved in a car accident. After taking her son to a *curandero*, she bathed him in a preparation of alcohol and herbs and wrapped him in a blanket. A few hours after the child fell asleep, the mother noticed that her son was experiencing seizure-like symptoms, and she could not wake him up. At that point, the mother decided to take him to the hospital.

Questions

1. What is your first reaction to this event?

2. How would you begin to talk about this event with the family?

3. What questions would you ask the family?

4. What education would you offer to the mother concerning Hispanic/Latino folk and traditional healing beliefs?

5. What recommendations would you give to consumers if presented with a similar situation in the future?

KEY TERMS

Botánicas. Religious-healing stores or herbal markets that sell medicinal herbs and other traditional healing modalities. They have been described as the visible door to the hidden world of Hispanic traditional healing modalities (Tafur et al., 2009; Viladrich, 2006).

Consulta. Consultation in which a healer makes a distinction among the spiritual, magical, physical, and mental domains and provides the client with the proper herb, remedy, or treatment (Viladrich, 2006).

Curanderismo. From the Spanish word *curar*, which means "to heal." It is used to describe the practice of traditional healing (Tafur et al., 2009).

Curandero. Type of traditional folk healer from Latin America who specializes in treating illness through the use of supernatural forces, herbal remedies, and other natural medicines (NCCIH, 2015c).

Espiritistas. Individuals with unique abilities to communicate with the spirits. They often use prayers, herbs, group healing sessions, house cleansings, and baths with herbs for personal cleansing to resolve spiritual problems (Báez & Hernández, 2001).

Santería. "An African-Cuban religious tradition combining Catholicism with Nigerian tribal beliefs and practices, including belief in the magical and medicinal properties of flowers, herbs, weeds, twigs, and leaves" (Musgrave et al., 2002, p. 558).

Sobador. A traditional healer who uses massage and rub techniques in order to treat patients, prevent disease, and restore health (NCCIH, 2015c).

Yerberos (or *hierberos*). Individuals who use herbs to treat illness. They specialize in the preparation of herbs and herbal remedies for the treatment of illness and diseases. They are practitioners with knowledge of the medicinal qualities of plants (DeBellonia et al., 2008; NCCIH, 2015c).

References

Arteaga, F. (2012). El proceso de iniciación al curanderismo en La Pampa (Argentina). *Chungará (Arica), 44*(4), 707–715.

Báez, A., & Hernández, D. (2001). Complementary spiritual beliefs in the Latino community: The interface with psychotherapy. *American Journal of Orthopsychiatry, 71*(4), 408–415.

Barnes, P. M., Bloom, B., & Nahin R. (2008). *Complementary and alternative medicine use among adults and children: United States, 2007. National Health Statistics Report, 10*(12), 1–23.

Benedetti, M. (2001). *Hasta los baños te curan! Plantas medicinales, remedios caseros y sanación espiritual en Puerto Rico.* Cayey: Puerto Rico, Verde Luz.

Carter-Pokras, O., Zambrana, R., Poppell, C., Logie, L., & Guerrero-Preston, R. (2007). The environmental health of Latino children. *Journal of Pediatric Health Care, 21,* 307–314.

Carvajal, G., & Thoman, E. (1999). De la religiosidad afroamericana. *Revista Pensamiento Humanista, 5,* 46–57.

Chifa, C. (2010). La perspectiva social de la medicina tradicional. *Boletín Latinoamericano y del Caribe de Plantas Medicinales y Aromáticas, 9*(4), 242–245.

Clarke, T. C., Black, L. I., Stussman, B. J., Barnes, P. M., & Nahim, R. L. (2015). Trends in the use of complementary health approaches among adults: United States 2002–2012. *National Health Statistics Reports, 79 ,* 1–19.

Clement, Y. N., Williams A. F., Aranda D., Chase R., Watson N., Mohammed R., . . . Williamson, D. (2005). Medicinal herb use among asthmatic patients attending a specialty care facility in Trinidad. *BMC Complementary and Alternative Medicine, 5,* 3.

Consumer Reports. (2009). *Dangers of combining herbal medicines with drugs.* Retrieved from http://www.consumerreports.org/cro/2012/05/beware-of-risky-herb-drug-combos/index.htm

Consumer Reports. (2012). *How Latinos use alternative medicine and botanicas for their health: A look at alternative medicine in the Hispanic community.* Retrieved from http://www.consumerreports.org/cro/2012/02/is-it-safe-to-buy-herbs-from-botanicas/index.htm

Cuadrado, M., & Lieberman, L. (2011). The Virgin of Guadalupe as an ancillary modality for treating Hispanic substance abusers: Juramentos in the United States. *Journal of Religion and Health, 50,* 922–930. doi: 10.1007/s10943-009-9304-4

DeBellonia, R. R., Marcus, S., Shih, R., Kashani, J., Rella, J. R., & Ruck, B. (2008). Curaderismo: Consequences of folk medicine. *Pediatric Emergency Care, 24*(4), 228–229.

Easom, L. R. (2006). Prayer: Folk home remedy vs. spiritual practice. *Journal of Cultural Diversity, 13*(3), 146–151.

Frisancho, V. O. (2012). Concepción mágico religiosa de la medicina en la América prehispánica. *Acta Médica Peruana, 29*(2), 121–128.

Food and Drug Administration. (2008). *FDA 101: Dietary supplements.* Retrieved from http://www.fda.gov/ForConsumers/ConsumerUpdates/ucm050803.htm

Gallardo, A. P. (2004). Los especialistas de la curación. Curanderos teenek y nahuas de Aquismón. *Anales de Antropología, 38,* 179–200.

Garza, S., & Young, R. (2007). Herbal and natural medicines in the Latino community. *Family Medicine, 39*(1), 7–8.

Gomez-Beloz, A., & Chavez, N. (2001). The botánica as a culturally appropriate health care option for Latinos. *Journal of Alternative and Complementary Medicine, 7*(5), 537–546.

Heathcote, J. D., West, J., Hall, P.C., & Trinidad, D. (2011). Religiosity and utilization of complementary and alternative medicine among foreign-born Hispanics in the United States. *Hispanic Journal of Behavioral Sciences, 33*(3), 398–408.

Hernández, C. J., & Volpato, G. (2004). Herbal mixtures in the traditional medicine of eastern Cuba. *Journal of Ethnopharmacology, 90*, 293–316.

Hicks, D. (2012). Cultural competence and the Hispanic population. *Medsurg Nursing, 21*(5), 314–315.

Holliday, K. V. (2008). "Folk" or "traditional" versus "complementary" and "alternative" medicine: Constructing Latino/a health and illness through biomedical labeling. *Latino Studies, 6*, 398–417.

Howell, L., Kochhar, K., Saywell, R., Jr., Zollinger, T., Koehler, J., Mandzuk, C., . . . Allen, D. (2006). Use of herbal remedies by Hispanic patients: Do they inform their physician? *Journal of the American Board of Family Medicine, 19*(6), 566–578.

Knoerl, A. M. (2007). Cultural considerations and the Hispanic cardiac client. *Home Healthcare Nurse, 25*(2), 82–86.

Lámbarri, A., Flores, F., & Berenzon, S. (2012). Curanderos, malestar, y daños: Una interpretación social. *Salud Mental, 35*, 123–128.

Longuefosse, J. L., & Nossin, E. (1996). Medical ethnobotany survey in Martinique. *Journal of Ethnopharmacology, 53*, 117–142.

Ludueña, G. (2013). Estudios sociales contemporáneos sobre el espiritismo argentino: Ciencia, religión e institucionalización del espíritu. *Revista Cultura y Religión, 7*(1), 42–59.

Maurer, A. E. (1979). El concepto del mal y poder espiritual en el mundo Maya tzeltal. *Journal de la Societé des Américanistes, 66*, 219–233.

Musgrave, C., Allen, C., & Allen, G. (2002). Spirituality and health for women of color. *American Journal of Public Health, 92*(4), 557–560.

National Center for Complementary and Integrative Health. (2015a). *Development of a comprehensive research strategy for complementary and alternative medicine*. Retrieved from https://nccih.nih.gov/about/offices/od/directortestimony/071100.htm

National Center for Complementary and Integrative Health. (2015b). *Important events in NCCIH history*. Retrieved from http://www.nih.gov/about/almanac/organization/NCCIH.htm

National Center for Complementary and Integrative Health. (2015c). *Terms related to complementary and integrative health*. Retrieved from https://nccih.nih.gov/health/providers/camterms.htm

Neri, V. R. (2001). El papel de los santos en la medicina occidental. *Revista Facultad de Medicina UNAM*, *44*(2), 93–95.

Newby, C. A., Riley, D., & Leal-Almeraz, T. O. (2006). Mercury use and exposure among santería practitioners: Religious versus folk practice in northern New Jersey, USA. *Ethnicity and Health*, *11*(3), 287–306.

Ortiz, B., & Clauson, K. (2006). Use of herbs and herbal products by Hispanics in South Florida. *Journal of the American Pharmacology Association*, *46*, 161–167.

Ortiz, B., Shields, K., Clauson, K., & Clay, P. (2007). Complementary and alternative medicine use among Hispanics in the United States. *Annals of Pharmacotherapy*, *41*, 994–1004.

Orzuza, S. M. (2013). Concepciones y prácticas indígenas sobre la salud y la enfermedad. Conocerlas para respetarlas. *Revista Sujeto, Subjetividad y Cultura*, *5*, 67–78.

Pérez, M. A., & Luquis, R. R. (2012). Getting to know US Latinos: A step toward cultural competence. *Californian Journal of Health Promotion*, 10 (Special Issue: Health Disparities in Latino Communities), 65–69.

Pérez, M., & Luquis, R. (2014). Implications of changing US demographics for health educators. In M. Pérez & R. Luquis (Eds.), *Cultural competence in health education and health promotion* (2nd ed., pp. 87–118). San Francisco, CA: Jossey-Bass.

Pérez y Mena, A. I. (1998). Cuban santería, Haitian vodun, Puerto Rican spiritualism: A multiculturalist inquiry into syncretism. *Journal for the Scientific Study of Religion*, *37*(1), 15–27.

Pinzón-Pérez, H. (2014). Complementary and alternative medicine in culturally competent health education. In M. Pérez & R. Luquis (Eds.), *Cultural competence in health education and health promotion* (2nd ed., pp. 87–118). San Francisco, CA: Jossey-Bass.

Prandi, R. (2012). *Os mortos e os vivos*. São Paulo, Brazil: Três Estrelas.

Ramíres, L. C. C. (2008, January–July). Tecnologías terapéuticas: Sistemas de interpretación en la regla de ocha y el espiritismo bogotano. *Antípoda: Revista de Antropología y Arqueología*, 133–151.

Ransford, H. E., Carrillo, F., & Rivera, Y. (2010). Health care-seeking among Latino immigrants: Blocked access, use of traditional medicine, and the role of religion. *Journal of Health Care for the Poor and Underserved*, *21*(3), 862–878.

Riley, D., Newby, A., & Leal-Almeraz, T. O. (2006). Incorporating ethnographic methods in multidisciplinary approaches to risk assessment and communication: Cultural and religious uses of mercury in Latino and Caribbean communities. *Risk Analysis*, *26*(5), 1205–1221.

Rodríguez, C. Y. M. (2012). Los cultos sincréticos como parte de la cultura popular tradicional en el municipio Jobabo. *Didáctica y Educación*, *3*(5), 107–113.

Ros, C. (2002). *San Pancracio salud y trabajo. Centro de Pastoral Litúrgica, Santos y Santas, 67*. Barcelona.

Sampedro, N. F. (2006). Religiones americanas y afroamericanas. *Veritas*, *1*(14), 11–42.

Sanchez, A., & Shallcross, R. (2012). Integrative psychodynamic treatment of ataque de nervios. *Clinical Case Studies*, *11*(1) 5–23.

Spector, R. (2009). *Cultural diversity in health and illness* (7th ed.). Upper Saddle River, NJ: Pearson Education.

Soru, M. F., Boris, L., Carreras, X., & Duero, D. (2012). Creencias populares sobre la salud, la enfermedad y su tratamiento. *Anuario de Investigaciones de la Facultad de Psicología*, *1*(1), 94–115.

Tafur, M. M., Crowe, T. K., & Torres, E. (2009). A review of curanderismo and healing practices among Mexicans and Mexican Americans. *Occupational Therapy International*, *16*(1), 82–88. doi: 10.1002/oti.265

Trotter, R. T. (2001). Curanderismo: A picture of Mexican-American folk healing. *Journal of Alternative & Complementary Medicine*, *7*(2), 129–131.

Upchurch, D. M., & Wexler Rainisch, B. K. (2012). Racial and ethnic profiles of complementary and alternative medicine use among young adults in the United States: Findings from the National Longitudinal Study of Adolescent Health. *Journal of Evidence-Based Complementary & Alternative Medicine*, *17*(3), 172–179. doi: 10.1177/2156587212450713

US Census Bureau. (2011). *The Hispanic population: 2010*. Retrieved from http://www.census.gov/prod/cen2010/briefs/c2010br-04.pdf

US Census Bureau. (2012a). *ACS demographic and housing estimates: 2012 American Community Survey 1-year estimates*. Retrieved from http://factfinder2.census.gov/faces/tableservices/jsf/pages/productview.xhtml?pid=ACS_12_1YR_DP05&prodType=table

US Census Bureau. (2012b). *2012 National Population Projections*. Retrieved from http://www.census.gov/population/projections/data/national/2012.html

Vandebroek, I., Balick, M. J., Ososki, A., Kronenberg, F., Yukes, J., Wade, C., & Castillo, D. (2010). The importance of "botellas" and other plant mixtures in Dominican traditional medicine. *Journal of Ethnopharmacology*, *128*(1), 20–41.

Viladrich, A. (2006). Botánicas in America's backyard: Uncovering the world of Latino healers' herb-healing practices in New York City. *Human Organization*, *65*(4), 407–419.

Volpato, G., Godínez, D., & Beyra A. (2009). Migration and ethnobotanical practices: The case of Tifey among Haitian Immigrants in Cuba. *Human Ecology*, *37*, 43–53.

COMPLEMENTARY, ALTERNATIVE, AND INTEGRATIVE HEALTH APPROACHES AMONG AFRICAN AMERICANS

Pierre E. Wright and Steven B. Owens

According to the National Center for Complementary and Alternative Medicine (NCCAM, 2012), now known as the National Center for Complementary and Integrative Health (NCCIH), complementary and alternative medicine (CAM) refers to medical and healthcare systems, therapies, and nonconventional products considered as a part of conventional medicine. Although CAM utilization tends to vary among racial and ethnic groups in the United States, research reveals that utilization is increasing among African Americans.

Today African Americans constitute the second largest racial and ethnic minority group. As of April 1, 2010, the total population in the United States was 308.7 million. Among that group, 38.9 million people (13%) identified themselves as Black alone and 3.1 million people (1%) reported being Black in combination with other races. The 2010 Census defined Blacks and African Americans as people having origins in any of the Black racial groups of Africa and the Afro-Caribbean regions, such as Haiti and Jamaica. Most African Americans in the United States are West and Central African descendants. However, some immigrants from African, Caribbean, Central American, and South American nations and their descendants may be identified or self-identify with the term while others may not (US Census Bureau, 2011). According to the Centers for Disease Control and Prevention (2013), in 2012, the African American population in

LEARNING OBJECTIVES

At the completion of this chapter, students will be able to:

- Identify the complementary and alternative medicine practices used most frequently by African Americans as described in the current literature.

- Recognize factors related to African American health and complementary healing practices.

- Discuss the impact of complementary, alternative, and integrative health (CAIH) modalities among African Americans.

- Identify opportunities and challenges related to complementary and alternative medicine and health outcomes of African Americans.

- Discuss the role of health professionals in the use of CAIH among African American populations.

the United States, including those of more than one race, was estimated at 44.5 million, making up 14.2% of the total US population. Those who identified only as African American made up 13.1% of the US population, or over 39 million people (US Census Bureau, 2011).

African American CAM interventions of choice include alternative medical systems, manipulative and body-based therapies, biofeedback, and energy therapies, with prayer being the most widely used. As the US population becomes more diverse, understanding racial/ethnic patterns of CAM use will guide assessment procedures and identify appropriate policies and programs. This knowledge and empathy will help sensitize healthcare providers and health educators to the beliefs and practices of their patients (Kronenberg, Cusham, Wade, Kaimuss, & Chao, 2006).

A Healthy People 2020 (2013) goal is to promote the use of health communication strategies and health information technology to improve population health outcomes and healthcare quality, as well as to achieve health equity in access to health information. The availability of technology has led to increased knowledge of different health practices and treatment modalities, including CAM. Accessibility to health information is essential to patient care; however, information quality is critical to the success of CAM modalities and treatments.

This chapter discusses the impact of complementary healing, alternative medicine, and holistic health among African Americans and identifies CAIH practices used by this group.

Theoretical Concepts

Overview

The diversification of the US population has resulted in noted changes related to health-seeking behaviors and treatments to maintain or restore health. In a 2007 study, nearly 4 out of 10 US adults reported using CAM products and services (Barnes, Bloom, & Nahin, 2008). The research literature suggests that the primary health concerns leading consumers to seek CAM services are to treat illness and to promote health (Davis, West, Weeks, & Sirovich, 2011). Although research on the characteristics of African Americans who use CAM to treat specific conditions is scarce, studies reveal that, like most consumers, African Americans use CAM for a variety of reasons. Among African Americans, women use CAM for treatment and health promotion at greater rates than men (Barner, Bohman, Brown, & Richards, 2010).

CAM healthcare practices in the United States have broadened due to an influx of cultures, values, and beliefs (Cuellar, Aycock, Cahill, & Ford, 2003). Due to these new approaches, there is an increased need for healthcare providers, health educators, and consumers to understand CAM. Understanding scientific knowledge and cultural constructs related to alternative forms of medicine and healing will help consumers and providers make informed decisions about best strategies to promote health.

Findings from the 2002, 2007, and 2012 National Health Interview Surveys (NHIS) indicate that race affects CAM choices. The 2002 and 2007 surveys revealed that 22.9% of African Americans used CAM modalities; the 2012 survey showed that 19.3% did. Regarding medical conditions, African Americans were more likely to use CAM to treat pain (lower back, joint, neck, and recurring), chronic conditions (hypertension, arthritis, high cholesterol, and diabetes), and insomnia and fatigue (Barner et al., 2010). Using data from the 2007 NHIS, Barnes et al. (2008) noted that almost 4 out of 10 adults had used CAM therapy in the past 12 months with the most commonly used therapies being nonvitamin, nonmineral natural products (17.7%), and deep breathing exercises (12.7%). American Indian or Alaska Native adults (50.3%) and White adults (43.1%) were more likely to use CAM therapy than Asian adults (39.9%) or Black adults (25.5%).

The trend analysis between the 2002 and 2007 survey data demonstrated increased use of CAM among adults for acupuncture, deep breathing exercises, massage therapy, meditation, naturopathy, and yoga (Barnes et al., 2008). Arcury et al. (2006) found that ethnicity was the most important characteristic differentiating CAM use among diabetic study participants. African Americans were more likely to use food home remedies and other remedies for diabetes self-management (Arcury et al., 2006). Among the African American study participants, common food and home remedies used for diabetes self-management included honey, lemon, vinegar, garlic, and baking soda. The same study indicated that other treatments included liniments, salves, Epsom salts, and vapor rubs.

Older women in all cultural groups expressed more satisfaction with the use of CAM than younger women did (NHIS, 2007). With respect to racial and ethnic minorities, results indicated that an estimated 34% of Hispanic, non-Hispanic Black, and non-Hispanic White adults in the United States had used at least one CAM therapy (excluding prayer) during the prior 12 months (NHIS, 2002). CAM use was highest for non-Hispanic Whites (36%), followed by Hispanics (27%) and non-Hispanic Blacks (26%). Non-Hispanic Whites were likely to use herbal medicine, relaxation techniques, and chiropractic more frequently than Hispanics and non-Hispanic Blacks. Hispanics had the highest provider nondisclosure rates (68.5%), followed by non-Hispanic Blacks (65.1%) and non-Hispanic Whites (58.1%) (Graham et al., 2005). Results from the CAM Use Self-Rated Health Status report (2007) indicated that 4 out of 10 US adults use CAM therapy (Nguyen, Davis, Kaptchik, & Phillip, 2010). African American CAM use, however,

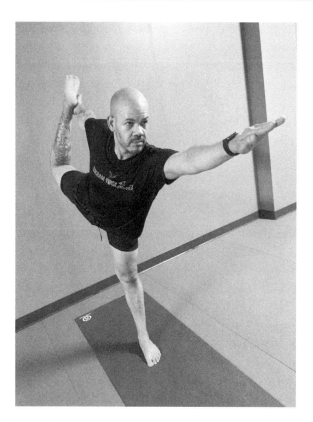

Figure 9.1   Bow Pulling Pose

is not as extensive as other ethnic groups. Barner et al. (2010) reported that approximately one in five African Americans used CAM in the year preceding the study to treat a specific condition. Figure 9.1 shows a modality of CAM used by this ethno-cultural group.

CAM use has been associated with socioeconomic and cultural backgrounds that vary between different racial/ethnic groups (Cui et al., 2012). CAM use tends to be associated with higher education attainment, higher household income, and a history of a chronic disease for African Americans and Whites (Cui et al., 2012). African Americans with higher socioeconomic status tended to use CAM interventions for prevention as well as treatment (Barner et al., 2010). CAM use declines among African Americans as they age or become unemployed (Cui et al., 2012); therefore, employment, insurance, and income play a role in CAM use among this group.

Modalities

The history of African Americans' use of traditional and healing practices has been well documented throughout their history in the United States as well as in their continent of origin. The historical interrelationships of spirituality, culture, health, and illnesses are still prominently observed among African Americans (Savitt, 1978). Traditional healing practices include the use of plants, herbs, seeds, roots, leaves, and Spanish moss for childbearing. According to Anyinam (1997), individuals who deliver care are known as healers, priests, priestesses, or spiritualists. Jolles and Jolles (2000) indicated that when managing forms of illness, the divine provides a diagnosis and the healer chooses a remedy relevant to the specific diagnosis.

According to earlier research as cited by Yoon, Horne, and Adams (2004), older African American women are more likely than White women to use alternative therapies and are less reserved in the use of these products (Cushman, Wade, Factor-Litvak, Kronenberg, & Firester, 1999). Some of the reasons for their preventive and curative self-care practices are rooted in discrimination experienced in the healthcare system (Brandt, 1978; Seto, 2001), the high cost of medications, and more positive results with homeopathic care versus allopathic care. In other studies, excluding prayer, Hispanics and non-Hispanic Blacks used CAM less frequently than Whites and were less likely to disclose their use to healthcare providers (Graham, 2005). Barner et al. (2010) found that African Americans used CAM to treat specific medical conditions and often did not disclose their CAM use with medical providers due to lack of trust.

Since specific results for African Americans' CAM use from the 2012 NHIS are still pending, the results from the 2007 NHIS survey provide a light on CAM use in this race/ethnic group. The 2007 results included four broad categories of CAM: (1) biologically based practices, (2) energy therapy techniques, (3) manipulative and body-based methods, and (4) mind-body medicine. Biologically based practices referred to the use of dietary supplements and include herbal, special dietary, and individual therapies (Tabish, 2008). Energy therapy techniques involved channeling healing energy through the hands of the practitioner into the client's body to restore a normal energy balance and health (Clarke et al., 2015). Manipulative and body-based methods involved manipulation and/or movement of one or more parts of the body (Tabish, 2008). Mind-body medicine focused on the interactions between mind and body and the powerful ways in which emotional, mental, social, and spiritual factors can directly affect health (NCCAM, 2012).

The most prevalent CAM modalities used by African Americans are prayer, herbals, and relaxation. These modalities fall into three use categories: primarily treatment (prayer), both treatment and prevention (herbals), and prevention (relaxation) (Barner et al., 2010). African American women who tend to use religion/spirituality (prayer) to treat serious conditions, such as cancer, heart disease, osteoporosis, and depression, were more likely to see a physician for their health problems. These uses imply complementary behaviors with CAM use among African American women (Barner et al., 2010). Additionally, common examples of CAM used by rural elderly African Americans are prayer, vitamins, exercise, meditation, herbs, chiropractic medicine, glucosamine, and music therapy (Cuellar et al., 2003). Health professionals must be aware that elders are using CAM and are satisfied with their use. Patterns of CAM use and ethnic-specific CAM utilization vary across racial/ethnic groups. Evaluation of CAM use in ethnically diverse populations should identify ethnic-specific modalities and variations across ethnicity.

Prayer

For decades, the influence of religion and prayer among African Americans has been well documented, although less is known about prayer for health concerns (Graham et al., 2005). According to Freeman (2009), prayer is difficult to conceptualize and research. African American women were more likely to use prayer/spirituality for health reasons. The high use of prayer may be attributed to the central theme of religious and spiritual beliefs as an integral part of many traditional health systems (Graham et al., 2005). Theologians and researchers conceptualize prayer into distinct types: prophetic and verbal prayer that can be used either to request a desired outcome or to improve one's relationship with God (Barnes, 2005).

The exact role of prayer is difficult to determine. Prayers can be employed by an individual or by someone on behalf of another person. Researchers have attempted to measure the impact of prayer via interviews. Questions included: Did you pray specifically for the purpose of your *own* health? Did you ask others to pray for your *own* health? Did you participate in a prayer chain or prayer group for your *own* health? And did you have a healing ritual or sacrament performed for your *own* health or treatment? (Graham et al., 2005). African Americans have used prayer for treatment, as prevention, and in conjunction with other CAM modalities.

Vitamins and Herbal Supplements

CAM therapies from Africa include plants, herbs, seeds roots, leaves, minerals, thorns, incantations, needles, and powder of bones (Revell, 2012). According to Barner (2010), almost half of African Americans who used CAM in the past 12 months used herbals for treatment and other forms of CAM. African Americans have used herbal CAM therapies to treat diabetes, HIV/AIDS, and prostate and breast cancer (Butler et al., 2011; Kaufman & Gregory, 2007; Villa-Caballero et al., 2010). According to

Villa-Caballero et al. (2010), diabetic African Americans used pharmacological CAM (herbs and vitamins) and nonpharmacological CAM (prayer, yoga, and acupuncture) for treatments. Prayer and Vitamin E were the most-used CAM therapies among African American patients with diabetes. Additionally, multivitamins, glucosamine, gingko biloba, and green tea were other supplements used commonly among African American patients with diabetes.

Yoon et al. (2004) documented patterns of herbal product use for health promotion and self-care management among older African American women. Subjects included 57 African American women aged 65 and older in a select north-central Florida county area recruited for the study. Participants completed questionnaires related to their overall health status, use of herbal products, reasons for use, and demographic information. Users of herbal products in the last 12 months were assigned to Group 1 and nonusers assigned to Group 2. Of the 57 women interviewed, 19 (33.3%) reported using at least one herbal product within the past 12 months. Glucosamine products (5 participants, 26.3%), garlic products (5 participants, 26.3%), aloe products (3 participants, 15.8%), and gingko biloba (3 participants, 15.8%) were the most commonly taken herbal products out of 33 products. Of the herbal products used, 23 products (69.7%) were used for maintaining health or preventing possible health problems. Seven products (21.2%) were taken to treat actual health problems. Three products (9.1%) were used to both treat and prevent health problems.

Herbal users did perceive their total health (physical and emotional) to be better than nonusers did, although there was no significant difference with perceived control over health outcomes or management of self-care. The majority of participants in both groups (57.9%) rated their overall health as good or excellent. Yoon et al. (2004) noted, based on the medical history data, that herbal customers used more over-the-counter (OTC) drugs but fewer prescription drugs than nonusers did. Table 9.1 lists disease states with commonly used treatments by African Americans.

African Americans commonly use echinacea, lemongrass, green tea, wheatgrass juice, and goldenseal for illness prevention, wellness, and overall health (Ryder et al., 2008). African Americans also engage in alternative medical modalities, such as acupuncture, ayurveda, homeopathy, and naturopathy. Additionally, African Americans use manipulative and body-based therapies (chiropractic and massage) for treatment. Biologically based therapies, such as folk medicine and herbals, were used more for prevention among African Americans (Barner et al., 2010). Twenty percent of African Americans who used CAM in the past year were treating a specific condition. Alternative medical systems, manipulative and body-based

Table 9.1   Selected Conditions and CAM Treatments Commonly Used by African Americans

Disease State/Conditions	Commonly Used Treatments
Pain/aching joints	WD-40
Hypertension	Garlic or vinegar and herbal tea
Arthritis	Apple cider vinegar, witch's broom, cranberry juice/honey, chondroitin sulfate, fish oils, and Omega-3 fatty acids
Recurring, lower back and neck pain	Lemon juice topical treatment—liniment and solvents
Insomnia	Herbal tea
High cholesterol	Oatmeal
Diabetes	Nutritional advice and lifestyle diets, spiritual healing, herbal remedies, massage therapy and meditation (Egede, Ye, Zheng, & Silverstein, 2002); cayenne pepper and garlic, orange juice; diabeticine and cinnamon green tea, multivitamins and vitamin E

Source: Arcury et al., 2006; Bannett et al., 2003; Egede, Ye, Zheng, & Silverstein, 2002; Ryder et al., 2008; Silverman, Nutini, Muse, King, & Albert, 2008; Tamhene, et al., 2014; Villa-Caballero et al., 2010.

therapies, folk medicine, prayer, biofeedback, and energy/reiki are common CAM therapies used by African Americans (Barner et al., 2010). Figure 9.2 shows another modality of CAM used by this ethno-cultural group.

According to Bright-Gbebry et al. (2011), CAM use is the highest among breast cancer survivors, but limited data are available for CAM usage specific to African Americans. Bright-Gbebry et al. (2011) studied the prevalence of multivitamin, folic acid, and herbal supplement use among 998 African American women who were breast cancer survivors and who completed the 1999 Black Women's Health Study questionnaire, the CAM use questionnaire, and self-reported diagnoses of breast cancer between 1995 and 1999. Participants identified which of these herbal products they used: echinacea, garlic, ginger, St. John's wort, gingko, chamomile, feverfew, hawthorn, milk thistle, goldenseal, ginseng, aloe, ephedra products, and cat's claw. Separate questions asked about multivitamin and/or folic acid. Breast cancer survivors were classified as users if they used any herbals, multivitamins, or folic acid at least three days per week during the previous two-year period. Among the 998 breast cancer survivors, 681 (68.2%) had used either herbal or vitamin supplements or both; 53.6% of the women had used vitamin supplements; and 39% had used one or more herbal supplements. The three most frequently used herbals were garlic (21.2%), gingko (12.0%), and echinacea (9.4%).

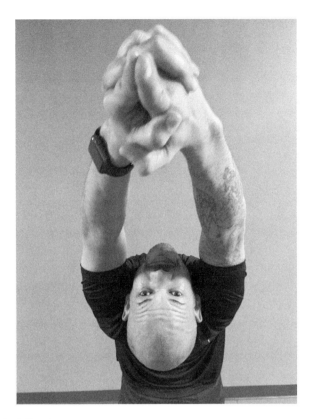

Figure 9.2   Fascia Stretch

According to the data, CAM use was significantly higher among survivors who were well educated, postmenopausal, and nonsmokers. Obesity and smoking were significantly associated with lower use of herbs and multivitamins among African American breast cancer survivors in this study. Although this study contributes to the understanding of CAM usage among a specific cohort of African Americans, it does not include feedback on these participants' reasons for using these resources for disease treatment or disease prevention (Bright-Gbebry et al., 2011). The study also did not clarify whether the women who used herbs and multivitamins/supplements also used other CAM modalities, such as prayer or home remedies.

Consumer Issues

Many scholars have written about the historical underpinnings and likely consequences of African Americans' distrust of the American healthcare system (Jacobs, Rolle, Ferrans, Whitaker, & Warnecke, 2006). A major barrier to African Americans seeking healthcare services is widespread cultural mistrust of the healthcare system and healthcare providers (Moore et al., 2013). Interpersonal trust between a physician and patient has been a predictor of perceived quality of care (Jacobs et al., 2006). Jacobs et al. (2006) conducted a qualitative study with a focus group of 32 African American women and 34 African American men discussing their trust and distrust of healthcare professionals, as well as their perceptions of providers whom they do not trust. Some participants cited racism (favoring White patients over Black patients) or greed, such as refusal of care because of a possible lack of insurance to pay for services, as sources of distrust.

Moore et al. (2013) underscored this notion of racism and lack of trust as a source of stress and an obstacle in receiving adequate healthcare among African American men. Respondents indicated that distrust of a healthcare provider led them to forgo care by refusing surgeries or other methods of treatment, withdrawing from care altogether, or not seeking care in the first place (Jacobs et al., 2006). This finding is consistent with those of earlier research. O'Malley et al. (2004) found that in their African American sample, higher trust was associated with a greater use of health services (Benkert, Peters, Clark, & Keves-Foster, 2006). The majority of participants in the Jacobs et al. (2006) study indicated that the physician's race did not influence their trust. However, what did matter was the physician's ability to communicate across language and cultural barriers. A limitation of this study was the small sample size ($n = 66$); therefore, these findings may not be generalizable to all African Americans. It is worth conducting a further examination of the connection between past exploitation and expected discrimination with regard to African Americans and their CAM health behaviors (Jacobs et al., 2006).

Brown et al. conducted a study in 2007, utilizing national data ($N = 23,828,268$) sets from the 2002 NHIS survey, to determine (1) characteristics of CAM use among the African American population, (2) the prevalence of CAM use, and (3) CAM for treatment and prevention of disease. According to the authors, a substantial number of African Americans used CAM (67%), with use varying across sociodemographic characteristics. Prayer was the most commonly used therapy (60%), when prayer for health was included. Overall, CAM is often used for the treatment of specific conditions as opposed to prevention, and its use was common among African Americans with disease states of pain/aching joints, recurring pain, and migraine.

Complementary therapies are used together with allopathic or con- ventional medicine, whereas alternative therapies are used in place of conventional treatment (Cui et al., 2012). It has been reported that one reason why some patients seek CAM therapies is because they are

BOX 9.1   ENGAGING AFRICAN AMERICANS ABOUT CAM USE

- African Americans are not likely to use CAM to treat chronic diseases, such as hypertension, high cholesterol, and diabetes.

- African Americans who suffer from anxiety and depression are likely to use prayer, herbals, and relaxation to treat their condition.

- When encountering patients who suffer from chronic pain, health professionals should ask the patient if any type of CAM is being used to treat their condition.

- African Americans with poorer health status are likely to use CAM because of failures of mainstream medicine or to complement mainstream medicine.

- Health professionals should engage patients in a dialogue regarding the role of prayer to treat specific conditions.

Source: Adapted from Barner et al. (2010); revised from National Center for Complementary and Alternative Medicine (2012).

disappointed in allopathic medicine, which implies that CAM therapies can be used as a substitute for conventional treatment in a subset of users. Excluding prayer, Hispanics and non-Hispanic Blacks used CAM less frequently than Whites used it and were less likely to disclose their use to healthcare providers (Graham, 2005). Barner et al. (2010) found that African Americans used CAM to treat specific medical conditions and did not often disclose their CAM use to medical providers due to lack of trust. When encountering any patient, health professionals should consider cultural beliefs and health-seeking behaviors. Some strategies that Barner et al. suggested to consider when encountering African American patients using CAM are presented in Box 9.1.

The NCCIH provides general recommendations for consumers when selecting CAM practitioners. These recommendations are presented in Box 9.2.

Implications for Health Professionals

Health educators and health professionals must be aware of health beliefs held by their patients in relationship to health outcomes. George (2012) conducted a literature review on health beliefs, treatment preferences, and CAM use for lung diseases—asthma, smoking, and lung cancer self-management—in Black communities. The review highlighted the importance of providers discussing unconventional beliefs and preferences.

BOX 9.2   NCCIH RECOMMENDATIONS FOR SELECTING A COMPLEMENTARY HEALTH PRACTITIONER

1. Check with your doctor or other healthcare provider if you need advice on CAM.

2. Seek information that you consider helpful about a practitioner such as education, training, licensing, and certifications.

3. Determine if the practitioner is willing to work with your conventional healthcare provider.

4. Explain all of your health conditions to the practitioner and find out about the practitioner's training and experience in working with people who have your condition(s).

5. Don't assume that your health insurance will cover the practitioner's services.

6. Tell your healthcare provider about all complementary approaches you use and about all practitioners who are treating you.

Source: National Center for Complementary and Integrative Health (2015).

When patients' unconventional beliefs and preferences are not discussed with providers, Black patients were at greater risk of not benefiting from self-management treatments for lung disease and were at increased risk for employing potentially dangerous CAM practices.

Data from the 2002 and 2007 NHIS highlighted several CAM therapies used in the African American community, including provider-based CAM, chiropractic care, massage, homeopathy, and acupuncture. African Americans used other provider-based therapies to a lesser extent, such as energy healing therapy/reiki, hypnosis, naturopathy, biofeedback, ayurveda, and folk medicine (Su & Li, 2011). Most African Americans reported using at least one CAM therapy with prayer (Su & Li, 2011).

It is important for healthcare providers to be knowledgeable regarding herbal product use and to be open to communicating with patients, particularly older people who may use more herbal products. Many persons taking herbal products do not discuss these products with their providers (Yoon et al., 2004). According to Yoon et al. (2004), patients who use herbal products do not consider herbs as part of their medication regimen. The authors identified the lack of specific inquiry into such use and suggested that someone must take responsibility for monitoring the use of Over the Counter (OTC) medications and herbal products when combined with prescription medications. They also stated that older African American women prefer some sense of control and empowerment for their own healthcare. Thus, it is important for healthcare professionals, including health educators, to ask consumers what they use to manage their health. Consumers should clearly inform their health provider of self-prescribed treatments, and providers must help consumers to understand that they should rely on professional healthcare sources for their health information.

Due to the array of products and modalities of CAM use, the Food and Drug Administration (FDA) does not regulate most CAM therapies. According to FDA (2006) guidelines, if a CAM product meets the statutory definition of a drug, device, biological product, or food, it is subject to regulations under the Federal Food, Drug, and Cosmetic (FDC) Act and the Public Health Service (PHS) Act. However, for CAM products and services, the FDA may become involved only after problems have been reported.

CAM therapies frequently used by African Americans that fall under the category titled biologically based practices (which include botanicals, animal-derived extracts, vitamins, minerals, fatty acids, amino acids, proteins, prebiotics and probiotics, whole diets, and functional foods) are subject to statutory and regulatory requirements (FDA, 2006). Biologically based practices other than food that claim to diagnose, cure, mitigate, treat, or prevent disease in human beings are considered drugs and are regulated by FDA. For example, biologically based practices using herbal products to treat diabetes are considered drugs and are subject to FDA regulations.

Manipulative and body-based methods, such as chiropractic manipulation and massage therapy, involve a practitioner manipulating a person's body. Generally, if a device is not involved in these practices, these body-based therapies are not subject to FDA regulations. Manipulative and body-based therapies that use equipment or involve the application of products, ointments, creams, and lotions to the skin are subject to FDA regulations through the FDC or PHS acts (FDA, 2006). For example, the FDA regulates needles used in acupuncture; however, this body-based practice does not fall under the FDA's regulations. Most manipulative and body-based methods require the provider to undergo some type of training, formal or informal, to deliver the therapy. According to the NCCIH, local and state governments and professional organizations establish the credentials for complementary health practitioners who treat patients.

Healthcare professionals must inquire about CAM use and any adverse reaction their clients may have experienced using CAM therapies. Serving as a resource for health education, health educators can provide their clients with the FDA's website form for reporting adverse reactions to dietary and herbal supplements. The FDA's Safety Reporting Portal (SRP), http://www .fda.gov/NewsEvents/PublicHealthFocus/ucm212845.htm#, is a safe and a convenient way for health educators to assist their patients and clients when reporting adverse reactions to dietary supplements.

CAM use continues to increase in the United States. According to Nahin, Barnes, Stussman, and Bloom (2009), in 2007 over $34 billion was spent on out-of-pocket CAM services and products. As CAM use continues to grow and influence health-seeking behaviors, health professionals must be informed of the CAM practices and modalities used by their clients.

Among health professionals, health educators play a key role in providing accurate information to promote individual and community health. The Master Certified Health Education Specialist and Certified Health Education Specialist are trained and credentialed professionals who passed a competency-based examination demonstrating skill and knowledge of the Seven Areas of Responsibility of Health Education Specialists (National Commission for Health Education Credentialing, 2008). Health educators possess sound theoretical knowledge that could assist them with assessment, serving as a health resource and advocating for health education, but many lack information specific to the use of CAM, as this topic is not covered in most health education programs in the United States.

Expansion of CAM use in the United States requires health educators and health professionals to be knowledgeable of CAM practices among ethnic/racial groups. Competencies in health education are important in understanding the interplay between health-seeking behaviors related to CAM use, especially among African Americans. Although CAM use is prevalent in the United States, broad examinations of CAM practices among African Americans often exclude the socioeconomic and physical context of their use (Ryder et al., 2008).

Seven Areas of Responsibility are the competencies that define the role of a health education specialist. Areas of Responsibility VI and VII from the National Commission for Health Education Credentialing (NCHEC) provide the foundation for health educators who are charged with understanding, developing, and delivering health promotion services to African Americans who use CAM. Area of Responsibility VI, which involves serving as a health education resource person, requires health educators to possess competencies to assess information needs, analyze resources, and convey health information (NCHEC, 2008). Health educators must be knowledgeable and understand CAM use and practices among ethnic and racial groups. Serving as a health education resource, health educators should stay abreast of and knowledgeable about CAM practices among African Americans. Manipulative and body-based therapies, folk medicine, herbal supplements, and prayer are CAM modalities that African Americans employ to treat conditions (Barner et al., 2010). Through culturally competent approaches, health educators can serve as resource persons who provide comprehensive information about the risks and benefits of CAM and conventional therapies.

As CAM use continues to gain popularity in the United States, health educators are reminded of Responsibility VII: communicate and advocate for health and health education. This area offers many opportunities for health educators to demonstrate their competencies. Competencies related to assessing and prioritizing health information, developing communication strategies, and delivering health messages related to CAIH will empower individuals and communities. Moore et al. (2013) highlighted how African American mistrust in the conventional healthcare system may cause them to delay treatment for health conditions. Because of this mistrust, African Americans may use CAM therapies to treat different conditions. Health educators and other health professionals must understand the emerging use of CAIH therapies and how they influence behavior among African American groups. Tailoring messages about CAIH benefits and risks will empower African American communities to make informed choices about CAIH approaches and to understand their limitations.

Since the use of CAM is significant in the African American population, health professionals working with this racial/ethnic group should emphasize wellness and health. The healing power of CAIH modalities is of particular importance for African Americans. Health professionals must advocate for laws and regulations on CAIH use and licensure of providers in order to protect consumers.

Caveat Emptor

There is no standardized national system for credentialing CAM practitioners. The extent and type of credentialing varies from state to state and from one CAM modality to another (NCCAM, 2013). Some African Americans use nonregulated CAM therapies. The benefits and limitations of CAM therapies require ongoing investigation and exploration by healthcare professionals and consumers to increase the understanding of their impact on health.

The most commonly used modalities of CAM among African Americans are prayer, vitamins, exercise, meditation, music therapy, chiropractic medicine, and herbs (Barner et al., 2010; Cuellar et al., 2003). Their potential impact on treatment and health promotion practices must be acknowledged and explored. Often health professionals in clinical settings ignore or do not discuss the use of folk remedies (Cuellar et al., 2003; Ryder et al., 2008). Users seek CAM providers for specific health issues (Hawk, Ndetan, & Evans, 2012). Inquiring about the use of folk remedies must also be part of a health promotion strategy. Likewise, Hawk, Ndetan, and Evans (2012) identified the need to train CAM providers on the inclusion of evidence-based health promotion and counseling. CAM providers also need to acknowledge the importance of working closely with the patients' primary care providers.

The use of CAM continues to increase each year; however, few federal or state regulations guide consumer choices among CAM therapies. Many consumers use CAM to promote health or in addition to treatments and plans prescribed by a healthcare provider. A common hidden problem encountered in clinical practice is the interaction of natural products and drugs. The interactions between natural products and drugs share pharmacokinetic and pharmacodynamic principles of any other regular drug-drug interaction (Bushra, Aslam, & Yar Khan, 2011). Biologically based products such as herbal remedies can interact with prescription drugs. For example, some CAM therapies may adversely affect the efficacy of conventional HIV medications (Owen-Smith, McCarthy, Hankerson-Dyson, & Diclimente, 2012). Other CAM therapies have been shown to interact with blood pressure medicine and prevent the anticoagulation properties of some drugs. As the human body ages, changes in physiology and metabolism occur. The use of herbs in African American elders generates specific concerns related to their metabolism, specifically in absorption, distribution, and excretion (Cuellar et al., 2003). Healthcare providers must be knowledgeable regarding potential effects of CAM with standard medication treatments (Cuellar et al., 2003). CAM and herbal supplement use are not right for everyone. Consumers must be vigilant when considering CAM therapy or a CAM practitioner.

CAM and other integrative healing practices present many opportunities to promote health and overall wellness among African Americans, specifically African American women. CAM use has many benefits. Mind-body and other contemplative forms of exercise, such as yoga, tai chi, meditation, and prayer, support the individual's wellness. These types of practices help to increase body awareness and mindfulness, which may aid in the therapeutic relationship between patient and provider. In addition, CAM use among African Americans focuses on the prevention of disease and illness.

Although CAM use has increased in popularity over the years, there are limitations of CAM use and a need for consumer education on CAM products' use and benefits. Knowledge and education regarding the side effects of herbs and supplements are key to patient success. Because supplements and some CAM treatments may interfere with prescription drug regimens administered by a medical practitioner, communication and awareness are necessary to gain the maximum benefits of CAM use. For example, consumers should maintain an appropriate regimen and avoid overmedicating to prevent negative drug reactions or interactions of CAM. Consumers must recognize the importance of talking to qualified health professionals prior to taking any supplements not prescribed by a medical practitioner and of researching potential reactions or side effects of drug use. Legislation and regulation of CAM practices is an important step toward improving the practice of CAIH.

Conclusion

The NHIS surveys of 2002, 2007, and 2012 collected a significant amount of data on CAM use. These data present the national scope of CAM usage among cultural and racial groups, including factors such as socioeconomic status and disease prevention strategies. More data are needed with respect to African Americans' use of CAIH therapies. Additional research is also required to determine motivations for CAM use as well as geographic factors affecting accessibility to CAM services.

Collecting a national data set of CAM use specific to persons who consider themselves African American or Black would be very beneficial. This data set would further expand existing theoretical and empirical knowledge regarding CAM use specific to this population. Moreover, health professionals are instrumental in researching the outcomes that will speak directly to generalizations about African American use of CAIH therapies. Small sample sizes and the lack of diversity in many studies have limited the understanding of CAIH use among African Americans. Through research, we know that 19.3% of US adults using CAM are African American or Black. We also know that African American CAM interventions of choice include alternative medical systems, manipulative and body-based therapies, biofeedback, and energy therapies, with prayer being the most widely used. We also know that African American patients may be more likely to disclose CAM use and follow up on recommended treatments if they trust their healthcare providers. Future research should expand the understanding of the impact of socioeconomic status on CAM use among African American groups.

Although health information about CAM is easily accessible via the Internet, it does not substitute for discussing health concerns with a qualified health professional. Some information in the Internet is not reliable. Factors such as health literacy play a major role in the understanding of the benefits and risks of CAIH practices used by African Americans. African Americans disproportionately live in poverty and have limited educational opportunities. Health professionals should work to equip this population with the health literacy tools necessary to use CAIH practices effectively and safely.

Summary

- Understanding the value of integrating CAIH practices with traditional medical treatments is very important in the healthcare management of African American individuals.

- Consideration of cultural views and values on both CAM and traditional medicine helps to maximize the effectiveness of treatment among African Americans.

- Prayer and religion influence health-seeking behaviors of African Americans.

- It is important that health practitioners inquire about the use of all therapeutic interventions and their efficacy from the patient's perspective.

- Health professionals should be aware of CAIH use in African American elders, specifically those who live in rural areas and who may be familiar with folk medicine and alternative interventions.

- Patients in poverty may not have the benefits of expensive interventions and may rely on CAIH practices as a first line of treatment for illnesses and diseases.

- Healthcare providers must recognize that CAM use varies among racial groups. Among African Americans, the use of CAM modalities is significant, and it may be related to historical mistrust in the conventional healthcare system.

- Underserved populations use CAM therapies largely in part because they cannot afford access to conventional healthcare (Graham et al., 2005). Even without the language barriers, English-speaking, non-White patients may not inform their doctors of nonconventional treatments because they may think their use is irrelevant, are embarrassed to discuss them, or feel that the healthcare provider will object to their use.

- Health professionals must be proactive in asking African American patients about CAM use (Graham et al., 2005).

Case Study

Description

An African American faith-based organization invites you to speak at a health fair on the benefits of decreasing healthcare costs by taking herbal supplements to promote health and prevent disease. After you polled the audience to identify the health conditions and topics, you realize that many of the participants have diabetes, hypertension, and high cholesterol.

Questions

1. What strategies would you use to assess the needs of this audience?
2. What strategies would you use to identify and analyze factors that influence the health behaviors of this audience?
3. How would you prioritize the health education needs of this group?
4. What information and resources would you provide to this audience about CAIH and chronic diseases?

KEY TERMS

African Americans. Persons having origins in any of the Black racial groups from Africa and the Afro-Caribbean regions, such as Haiti and Jamaica (US Census Bureau, 2011).

Complementary and alternative medicine. Therapies not usually taught in US medical schools or generally available in US hospitals. Group of diverse medical and healthcare systems, practices, and products that are not generally considered to be part of conventional medicine.

Herbal supplement. A type of biologically based therapy that includes plants and other botanicals (Tabish, 2008).

Prayer. A type of mind-body practice that involves the active process of communicating with and appealing to a higher spiritual power (Graham et al., 2005).

Provider-based therapy. A type of therapy in which practitioners are required to provide care or advice on a specific CAM modality (Su & Li, 2011).

References

Anyinam, C. A. (1997). The role of female spiritualists in Africa: Persistence with change. *Canadian Women Studies: Les Cashiers De La Femme, 17*(1), 103–106.

Arcury, T. A., Bell, R. A., Snively, B. M., Smith, S. L., Skelley, A. H., Wetmore, L. K., & Quandt, S. A. (2006). Complementary and alternative medicine (CAM) use as health self-management: Rural older adults with diabetes. *Journals of Gerontology, 61B*(2), S62–S70.

Barner, J. C., Bohman, T. M., Brown, C. M., & Richards, K. M. (2010). Use of complementary and alternative medicine (CAM) for treatment among African-Americans: A multivariate analysis. *Research in Social and Administrative Pharmacy, 6*(3), 196–208.

Barnes, P. M., Bloom, B., & Nahin, R. L. (2008). Complementary and alternative medicine (CAM) use among adults and children: United States, 2007. *National Health Statistics Reports, 12*, 1–23.

Barnes, P. M., Powell-Griner, E., McFann, K., & Nahin, R. (2004, May 27). Complementary and alternative medicine use among adults: United States, 2002. *Advance Data*, no. 343, 1–19.

Barnes, S. L. (2005). Black church culture and community. *Special Forces, 84*(2), 967–994.

Barnett, M. C., Cotroneo, M., Purnell, J., Martin, D., Mackenzie, E., & Fishman, A. (2003). Use of CAM in local African American communities: Community-partnered research. *Journal of the National Medical Association, 95*(10), 943–950.

Benkert, R., Peters, R. M., Clark, R., & Keves-Foster, K. (2006). Effects of perceived racism, cultural mistrust and trust in providers on satisfaction with care. *Journal of the National Medical Association, 98*(9), 1532.

Bushra, R., Aslam, N., & Yar Khan, A. (2011). Food–drug interactions. *Oman Medical Association, 26*(2), 77–83.

Butler, S., Owen-Smith, A., DiIorio, C., Goodman, M., Liff, J., & Steenland, K. (2011). Use of complementary and alternative medicine among men with prostate cancer in a rural setting. *Journal of Community Health, 36*, 1004–1010. doi: 10.1007/s10900-011-9402-6

Bright-Gbebry, M., Makambi, K. H., Rohan, J. P., Llanos, A. A., Rosenberg, L., Palmer, J. R., & Adams-Campbell, L. L. (2011). Use of multivitamins, folic acid and herbal supplements among breast cancer survivors: The black women's health study. *BioMed Central Complementary and Alternative Medicine, 11*(1), 30.

Brown, C., Barner, J., Bohman, T., & Richards, K. (2009). A multivariate test of expanded health care utilization model for complementary and alternative medicine (CAM) use in African Americans. *Journal of Alternative and Complementary Medicine, 15*(8), 911–919.

Centers for Disease Control and Prevention. (2013). *Health of Black or African-American non-Hispanic Population.* (2016, April 27). Retrieved from http://www.cdc.gov/nchs/fastats/black-health.htm

Cuellar, N., Aycock, T., Cahill, B., & Ford, J. (2003). Complementary and alternative medicine (CAM) use by African American and Caucasian American older adults in a rural setting: A descriptive, comparative study. *BioMed Central Complementary and Alternative Medicine, 3*(8), 1–7. doi: 10.1186/1472-6882-3-8

Cui, Y., Hargreaves, M. K., Xiao-Ou, S., Liu, J., Kenerson, D., Signorello, L., & Blot, W. J. (2012). Prevalence and correlates of complementary and alternative medicine (CAM) services use in low-income African American and Whites: A report from the Southern Community Cohort Study. *Journal of Alternative and Complementary Medicine, 18*(9), 844–849.

Cushman, L. F., Wade C., Factor-Litvak, P., Kronenberg, F., & Firester, L. (1999). Use of complementary and alternative medicine among African-American and Hispanic women in New York City: A pilot study. *Journal of the American Medical Women's Association, 54*(4), 193–195.

Davis, M. A., West, A. N., Weeks, W. B., & Sirovich, B. E. (2011). Health behaviors and utilization among users of complementary and alternative medicine (CAM) for treatment versus health promotion. *Health Services Research, 46*(5), 1402–1416.

Egede, L. E., Ye, X., Zheng, D., & Silverstein, M. D. (2002). The prevalence and pattern of complementary and alternative medicine use in individuals with diabetes. *Diabetes Care, 25*(2), 324–329.

Food and Drug Administration. (2006). *Complementary and alternative medicine (CAM) products and their regulation by the Food and Drug Administration.*

Freeman, L. W. (2009). *Mosby's complementary and alternative medicine: A research-based approach* (3rd ed.). St. Louis, MO: Mosby Elsevier.

George, M. (2012). Health beliefs, treatment preferences and complementary and alternative medicine for asthma, smoking and lung cancer self-management in diverse Black communities. *Patient Education and Counseling, 89*(3), 489–500.

Graham, R. E., Ahn, A. C., Davis, R. B., O'Connor, R. B., Eisenberg, D. M., & Phillips, R. S. (2005). Use of complementary and alternative therapies among racial and ethnic minority adults: Results from the 2002 National Health Interview Survey. *Journal of the National Medical Association, 97*(4), 535–545.

Hawk, C., Ndetan, H., & Evans, M. (2012). Potential role of complementary and alternative health care providers in chronic disease prevention and health promotion: An analysis of National Health Interview Survey data. *Preventive Medicine, 54*(1), 18–22.

Healthy People 2020. (2013). *Health communication and health information technology.* Retrieved from https://www.healthypeople.gov/2020/topics-objectives/topic/health-communication-and-health-information-technology

Hsiao, A., Wong, M., Goldstein, M., Yu, H., Andersen, R., Brown, E., . . . Wenger, N. (2006). Variation in complementary and alternative medicine (CAM) use across racial/ethnic groups and the development of ethnic-specific measures of CAM use. *Journal of Alternative and Complementary Medicine, 12*(3), 281–90.

Jacobs, E. A., Rolle, I., Ferrans, C. E., Whitaker, E. E., & Warnecke, R. B. (2006). Understanding African Americans' views of the trustworthiness of physicians. *Journal of General Internal Medicine, 21*(6), 642–647.

Jolles, F., & Jolles, S. (2000). Zulu ritual immunization in perspective. *Journal of the International African Institute, 70*(2), 229–248.

Kaufman, K., & Gregory, W. (2007). Discriminators of complementary and alternative medicine (CAM) providers use among men with HIV/AIDS. *American Journal of Health Behavior, 31*(6), 591–601.

Kronenberg, F., Cusham, L., Wade, C., Kaimuss, D., & Chao, M. (2006). Race/Ethnicity and women's use of complementary and alternative medicine in the United States: Results of a national survey. *American Journal of Public Health, 96*(7), 1236–1242

Moore, A., Hamilton, J., Knafl, G., Godley, P., Carpenter, W., Bensen, J., . . . Mishel, M. (2013). The influence of mistrust, racism, religious participation, and access to care on patient satisfaction for African American men: The North Carolina-Louisiana Prostate Cancer Project. *Journal of the National Medical Association, 105*(1), 59–68.

Nahin, R. L., Barnes, P. M., Stussman, B. J., & Bloom, B. (2009). Costs of complementary and alternative medicine (CAM) and frequency of visits to CAM practitioners: United States, 2007. *National Health Statistics Reports, 18*, 1–16.

National Center for Complementary and Alternative Medicine. (2012). *What is complementary and alternative medicine?* Retrieved from https://www.nlm.nih.gov/medlineplus/complementaryandintegrativemedicine.html

National Center for Complementary and Alternative Medicine. (2013). *Credentialing: Understanding the education, training, regulation, and licensing of complementary health practitioners.* Retrieved from https://nccih.nih.gov/health/decisions/credentialing.htm

National Center for Complementary and Integrative Health. (2015). *6 things to know when selecting a complementary practitioner.* Retrieved from https://nccih.nih.gov/health/tips/selecting

National Commission for Health Education Credentialing. (2015). *Areas of responsibilities, competencies and sub-competencies for the Health Education Specialist 2015.* Retrieved from http://www.nchec.org/responsibilitiesand-competencies

National Institute of Health & National Library of Medicine. (2013). *Herbs and supplements.* MedlinePlus. Retrieved from http://www.nlm.nih.gov/medlineplus/druginfo/herb_All.html

Nguyen, L., Davis, R., Kaptchuk, & Phillip, R. (2010). Use of complementary and alternative medicine (CAM) and self-rated health status: Results from a national survey. *Journal of General Internal Medicine, 26*(4), 399–404.

O'Malley, P., Trimble, N., & Browning, M. (2004). Are herbal therapies worth the risks? *Nurse Practitioner, 29*(10), 71–75.

Owen-Smith, A., McCarthy, F., Hankerson-Dyson, D., & Diclemente, R. (2012). Prevalence and predictors of complementary and alternative medicine (CAM)

use in African-Americans with acquired immune deficiency syndrome. *Focus on Alternative Complementary Therapies*, *17*(1), 33–42.

Revell, M. (2012). Use of complementary and alternative medicine in the African American culture. *International Journal of Childbirth Education*, *27*(3), 55–59.

Ryder, P. T., Wolpert, B., Orwig, D., Carter-Pokras, O., & Black, S. (2008). Complementary and alternative medicine use among older urban African Americans: Individual and neighborhood associations. *Journal of the National Medical Association*, *100*(10), 1186–1192.

Savitt, T. L. (1978). *Medicine and slavery: The disease and health care of blacks in antebellum Virginia*. Urbana, IL: University of Illinois Press.

Silverman, M., Nutini, J., Musa, D., King, J., & Albert, S. (2008). Daily temporal self-care responses to osteoarthritis symptoms by older African Americans and whites. *Journal of Cross Cultural Gerontology*, *23*(4), 319–337.

Su, D., & Li, L. (2011). Trends in the use of complementary and alternative medicine in the United States: 2002–2007. *Journal of Health Care for the Poor and Underserved*, *22*, 296–310.

Sullivan, G. (2010). Plantation medicine and health care in the Old South. *Legacy*, *10*(1). Retrieved from http://opensiuc.lib.siu.edu/legacy/vol10/iss1/3

Tabish, S. A. (2008). Complementary and alternative healthcare: Is it evidence-based? *International Journal of Health Sciences*, *2*(1), v–ix.

Tamhane, A., McGwin, G., Redden, D., Hughes, L., Brown, E., Westfall, A., . . . Callahan, L. (2014). Complementary and alternative medicine use in African Americans with arthritis. *Arthritis Care and Research*, *66*(2), 180–189.

Villa-Cabalelero, L., Morello, C., Chynoweth, M., Prieto-Rosinol, A., Polonsky, W., Palinkas, L., & Edelman, S. (2010). Ethnic differences in complementary and alternative medicine use among patients with diabetes. *Complementary Therapies in Medicine*, *18*, 241–248.

Yoon, S. L., Horne, C. H., & Adams, C. (2004). Herbal product use by African American older women. *Clinical Nursing Research*, *13*(4), 271–288.

US Census Bureau. (2011). *The Black population: 2010 Census Briefs*. Retrieved from http://www.census.gov/prod/cen2010/briefs/c2010br-06.pdf

COMPLEMENTARY, ALTERNATIVE, AND INTEGRATIVE HEALTH APPROACHES AMONG ASIAN AMERICANS, NATIVE HAWAIIANS, AND PACIFIC ISLANDERS

Liliana Rojas-Guyler and Mariamma K. Mathai

Diversity within a group is an asset to the culture and richness of any ethnic constituency. The Asian American group is a very diverse one, and it includes people with origins from a number of countries and regions. According to the Centers for Disease Control and Prevention (CDC, 2013a), people in this group trace their origins to approximately 25 countries in Southeast Asia, the Far East, and the Indian subcontinent. Examples of countries in these regions include Malaysia, Pakistan, Thailand, and Cambodia, as well as the Philippines, China, Korea, Japan, and Vietnam (Hoeffel, Rastogi, Kim, & Shahid, 2012). It is evident from the plethora of countries and regions from which Asians originate that they are a very heterogeneous group. In fact, the 2003 President's Advisory Commission on Asian Americans and Pacific Islanders (PACAAPI) indicated that the ethno-cultural group called "Asians" consists of people from 52 different countries. The vast number of countries exemplifies the variety and heterogeneity of the Asian cultures. Each country in itself likely represents a multitude of traditions, religions, belief systems, and languages, which consequently produces a wide range of points of view and health beliefs.

LEARNING OBJECTIVES

At the completion of this chapter, students will be able to:

- Identify the complementary, alternative, and integrative health (CAIH) practices most frequently used by Asian Americans, Native Hawaiians, and Pacific Islanders as described in the current literature.

- Analyze current health needs of Asian American, Native Hawaiian, and other Pacific Islander communities.

- Discuss complementary, alternative, and integrative health (CAIH) modalities utilized in Asian American, Native Hawaiian, and Pacific Islander communities.

- Discuss possible limitations and necessary precautions to

(continued)

LEARNING OBJECTIVES
(*continued*)

   be considered with the use of
   CAIH modalities.

 • Describe the role of health
   professionals in supporting
   Asian American, Native
   Hawaiian, and Pacific Islander
   communities in their use of
   CAIH modalities.

The Native Hawaiian or Other Pacific Islander group includes people with Native Hawaiian, Samoan, Guamanian or Chamorro, Fijian, Tongan, or Marshallese origins. It also includes Melanesia (Fijian, Guinean, and Solomon Islander), Micronesia (Marshallese, Palauan, and Chuukese), and Polynesia (Tahitian, Tongan, and Tokelauan) (Hixson, Hepler, & Kim, 2012).

This chapter provides an overview of the demographic characteristics of Asian American, Native Hawaiian, and Other Pacific Islander American communities and presents complementary, alternative, and integrative health (CAIH) practices being used by this ethno-cultural group, modalities that promote wellness and restore health in this group.

Theoretical Concepts

Overview

Asian Americans, Native Hawaiians, and Pacific Islanders display a number of similar cultural traits, such as placing high importance in preserving traditions, fomenting strong family values, valuing academic achievement, and upholding the value of personal relationships (PACAAPI, 2003). The diversity within the Asian cultures can be observed in the heterogeneity of socioeconomic, educational, and cultural traditions. A wide variety in religious practices, selections of food, cooking methods, clothing customs, and forms of entertainment is a testament to the multiple influences and traditions within this group (PACAAPI, 2003). Additionally, differences are found in the multitude of languages. In the United States, the Census Bureau recognizes 33 Asian, Native Hawaiian, and Pacific Islander spoken languages with approximately three out of four Asians speaking a language other than English at home (Ryan, 2013).

The 2011 report on Asian Americans by the Asian American Center for Advancing Justice synthesized national data from the US Census Bureau, the CDC, and the US Departments of Education, Homeland Security, and State (Asian Pacific American Legal Center [APALC] & Asian American Justice Center [AAJC], 2012). There are over 17.3 million Asian Americans and 1.2 million Asian and Native Hawaiian and Other Pacific Islanders living in the United States, making up 6% and 0.4% of the US population, respectively.

Asian Americans, Native Hawaiian, and Other Pacific Islanders are both among the fastest-growing racial groups, with a population growth of over 40% in the last decade alone (Hixson et al., 2012; Hoeffel et al., 2012). The value of Asian Americans, Native Hawaiians, and Pacific Islanders is widely recognized. They have had "substantial contributions to the economy through entrepreneurial activity, job creation, and consumer spending" (APALC & AAJC, 2012, p. 3). For example, there has been a significant growth in the buying power of Asian American communities, and Asian American–owned businesses make major contributions to the US economy (APALC & AAJC, 2012). Asian Americans, Native Hawaiian, and Pacific Islanders are becoming citizens, registering to vote, and casting ballots. However, there are several barriers to the health status of Asian Americans, Native Hawaiian and Pacific Islanders, such as language barriers, that continue to reduce opportunities and generate health disparities for millions of people in this group.

The educational attainment of this ethno-cultural group varies. Many Asian American communities enjoy economic stability, but others experience severe poverty. For example, Hmong Americans rank as having the lowest per-capita income of any racial or ethnic group nationwide; while Bangladeshi and Cambodian Americans have poverty rates close to those of African Americans and Latinos (APALC & AAJC, 2012).

Healthcare access and quality have been deficient for the Asian Americans, Native Hawaiian, and Pacific Islanders group. Asian Americans, Native Hawaiians, and Pacific Islanders were two times as likely to report not having seen a healthcare provider in the prior five years than both non-Hispanic Whites and African Americans. An important fact is that they are more likely than non-Hispanic Whites to develop hepatitis, stomach, and liver cancer (APALC & AAJC, 2012).

An important consideration in interpreting data available about health and other characteristics of Asian Americans, Native Hawaiians, and Pacific Islanders is the inconsistency in the terminology historically utilized to denominate this group. In the past, the US Census Bureau had only one Asian category. "Asian" and "Pacific Islander" categories other than "Chinese" and "Japanese" were introduced with the 1910 census. In 1950, the categories for race included White, Black, American Indian, Asian, and Other race. In 1980, the Asian and Pacific Islander category as well as Hawaiian were used for the first time in census tabulations at the state and national level (Gibson & Young, 2005). It was not until the 2010 census that the two separate categories of Asian American and Native Hawaiian and Other Pacific Islander were utilized (Hixson et al., 2012; Hoeffel et al., 2012).

There are a variety of ethnicities under the racial categories of Asian, Native Hawaiians, and Pacific Islanders. These distinctions are key in comparing differences among people with different cultural backgrounds. Moreover, it is important to understand differences in how they receive medical treatment and what home remedies they use to treat illnesses. This chapter provides an overview of the health status of Asian Americans, Native Hawaiians, and Pacific Islanders as well as their medicinal beliefs and CAIH practices with a close look at the social determinants of health for this group.

Health Status of Asian Americans

The health indicators for Asian Americans show extremes in their health outcomes. According to the CDC (2013a), Asian American women have the longest life expectancy in the United States (85.8 years). Among Asian Americans, the leading causes of death in 2010 included cancer, heart disease, stroke, unintentional injuries due to accidents, and diabetes. The death rates for the leading causes of death are lower than for other populations. Asian Americans are at risk for chronic obstructive pulmonary disease, hepatitis B, HIV/AIDS, and tuberculosis. Asian Americans are more likely to smoke and to live in counties with air quality not meeting US standards for particulate matter and ozone. Liver disease has a lower prevalence in the overall Asian American population, but there is a higher incidence of hepatitis B among young adults (ages 19–24). There are similar rates of diabetes when compared to the White population (CDC, 2013a).

Socioeconomic characteristics of Asian Americans help shape their life experience. According to the CDC (2013a), "They are less likely to live in poverty (12.8%), more likely to be college graduates or hold graduate degrees (50%), and more likely to be employed in management, business, science, and arts occupations (48.5%) compared with the total US population (15.9%, 28.5%, 36.0%, respectively)" (p. 1). However, at times Asian Americans confront many factors that could affect their health. These can include infrequency in visiting healthcare providers due to the fear of deportation, limited English language skills, varied cultural barriers, and lack of health insurance (CDC, 2013a). All of these factors can contribute to delayed diagnoses and treatments. Additionally, lower healthcare access rates impede delivery of prevention services, which are two determinants of negative health outcomes.

Health Status of Native Hawaiians and Other Pacific Islanders

There is a dearth of information on the health status and health behaviors of Native Hawaiians and Other Pacific Islanders in the research literature.

Much of what is available is based on data that combines them with Asian Americans into one Asian and Pacific Islander race/ethnicity category. In this chapter, we utilize specific data for each group when available. Where the data refers to a combined sample, we use the term *Asian American and Pacific Islander*.

Park, Gardner, and Nordyke (2009) report that life expectancy for Native Hawaiians (71.5 years for men and 77.1 years for women) is lower than for the overall population of the state of Hawaii (77.5 years for men and 83.6 years for women). Similarly, their life expectancy is lower than that of the overall US population (Park et al., 2009). Further, the infant mortality rate for Native Hawaiians was 9.6 per 1,000 live births in 2002, and the rate for all Asian and Pacific Islanders combined was 4.8, whereas the rate for all US populations was 7.0 (CDC, 2013b).

According to the CDC (2013b), the top five causes of death for Native Hawaiians and Other Pacific Islanders include: cancer, heart disease, stroke, unintentional injuries, and diabetes. Among this group there exists a disproportionately high prevalence of alcohol use and abuse, hepatitis B, HIV/AIDS, overweight and obesity, smoking and tobacco use, and tuberculosis. Native Hawaiians and Other Pacific Islanders have a higher cancer death rate and a lower five-year relative survival rate for all cancers as compared to other racial and ethnic populations.

Disparities also exist in the prevalence of chronic conditions such as diabetes. In 2010, the age-adjusted prevalence of diabetes was three times greater among Native Hawaiians and Other Pacific Islanders. In 2008, this group had the third-largest incidence of HIV infection among racial and ethnic groups behind African American and Hispanic populations. Native Hawaiians and Other Pacific Islanders are also more likely to live in environments with poor air quality (CDC, 2013b). Determinants of these disparities are similar to those for Asian Americans and other minority or vulnerable populations. Native Hawaiians and Other Pacific Islanders are "more likely to live in poverty (21.5%), less likely to be college graduates or hold graduate degrees (14.5%), and less likely to be employed in management, business, science, and arts occupations (24.0%) compared with the total US population (15.9%, 28.5%, 36.0%, respectively)" (CDC, 2013b, p. 2).

Modalities

According to Su and Li (2011), the use of complementary and alternative medicine (CAM) grew significantly in the United States between 2002 and 2007. In particular, there was growth in the rate of utilization of provider-based CAM therapies, including acupuncture, massage, and chiropractic care.

Using information from the 2007 National Health Interview Survey (NHIS), Su and Li (2011) found that 31.8% of Asian Americans reported utilizing at least one CAIH modality. Unfortunately, the data are reported only for one general Asian race/ethnic category. The use of medicinal and healing systems and modalities that we call CAIH are not alternative or complementary in many Asian countries. In many Asian countries, these modalities are traditional and conventional, not merely alternatives to a Western norm. For example, in China and Japan, "the use of very advanced modern Western medicine coexists with traditional Eastern medicine" (Bomar, 2013, p. 2). Many of these traditions transcend immigration status and generations. Thus, understanding and studying these practices may prove integral to better serving a changing and more diverse society.

As America grows in diversity, so does our spectrum of health beliefs, behaviors, and attitudes about CAIH. There are already established patterns of traditional medicine and healing among Asian American, Native Hawaian, and Pacific Islander cultures. Traditional medicine and healing practices among people of Asian origin are in many instances similar for all subgroups. Some ancient health beliefs are shared in the use of customary medical systems among subgroups, such as traditional Chinese medicine (TCM). These beliefs include that: (1) the human body is a part of the larger surrounding universe; (2) harmony between opposite energies (i.e., yin which is the female principle and yang which is the male principle) supports health; and (3) an imbalance in energy can result in disease (National Center for Complementary and Integrative Health [NCCIH], 2013a). Additionally, traditional ancient Asian medicines are based on the principle that five elements (fire, earth, wood, metal, and water) are symbolic representations of everything, including stages in human life. These elements can explain the functioning of the human body and the presence of disease. Another principle is that *qi* is a vital energy that flows throughout the human body, where it performs a variety of functions to maintain health (NCCIH, 2013a).

Although there is some knowledge within Western medical practice of the more readily recognized CAIH modalities such as acupuncture, in which specific body points are stimulated by putting needles in the skin (NCCIH, 2014), and TCM, there is much more to consider. It is known that there is variability in the modalities used and the fidelity to CAIH practices among Asian American and Pacific Islander communities. As immigrants spend more time in the United States, their CAIH preferences may change. According to Lee, Goldstein, Brown, and Ballard-Barbash

(2010), Asian immigrants of Japanese, Chinese, and Korean descent in California who had lived in the United States longer were less likely to have used provider-based CAIH modalities, such as seeing an acupuncturist or massage therapist. Acculturation was found to be a predictor of CAIH provider preferences; those more acculturated to America were more likely to also use mainstream provider-based CAIH, such as massage and chiropractic (Lee et al., 2010). Tanaka, Gryzlak, Zimmerman, Nisly, and Wallace (2008) found a higher likelihood of using herbs among Asian Americans, Native Hawaiians, and Pacific Islanders than other ethnicities. The use of herbs was evident primarily among those 60 years or older and among women and younger generations with higher education and income levels.

Chinese Practices and Traditions

TCM incorporates a multitude of practices. According to the National Center for Complementary and Alternative Medicine, now known as the NCCIH. These practices include "acupuncture, moxibustion (burning an herb above the skin to apply heat to acupuncture points), Chinese herbal medicine, tui na (Chinese therapeutic massage), dietary therapy, and tai chi and qi gong (practices that combine specific movements or postures, coordinated breathing, and mental focus)" (NCCIH, 2013a, p. 2).

TCM centers upon the principle of energy balance in the body and universe. It is based on ancient beliefs, including the need for balance of *qi* (energy) in maintaining health and wellness and that the five elements mentioned earlier represent the stages of life and disease (NCCIH, 2013a). Rooted in Taoism, an ancient philosophy dating back more than 2,500 years, TCM is a long-accepted and effective practice (Institute of Medicine [IOM], 2005). The rule of Tao ("the way" or "the law") is to live in complete harmony with our natural world. TCM has specific diagnostic methods and systematic approaches to healing and preventing disease that utilize a unique combination of medicinal pharmacology, acupuncture, massage, herbal medicine, and qi gong (IOM, 2005).

In TCM, herbal medicine includes the use of plant seeds, berries, roots, leaves, bark, or flowers for medicinal purposes. Qi gong, which can be translated literally as "energy cultivation," includes exercises designed to bring about harmony in addition to promoting health and longevity. This harmony is achieved by using breathing, movement, the power of the mind, and vision. In moxibustion, also known as cupping, burning mugwort is placed on the body's acupuncture points to stimulate *qi* and healing. Mugwort is a plant that holds essential oils, such as camphor (IOM, 2005).

Some traditional Chinese practices are rare but still found in the United States. For example, tui na is a 2,000-year-old Chinese massage practice similar to acupuncture but without utilizing needles. In tui na, the *qi* energy of patients is manipulated to bring about balance (IOM, 2005). Other Chinese traditional practices that have become more common in the United States include reiki and tai chi.

Reiki, originally from Tibet, is an ancient tradition that includes the use of hand symbols and breathing. Movement of air and manipulation of energy forces bring balance to the body and the spirit. The source of energy from the healer travels to the client through the practitioner's body. In tai chi, people use balanced and very gentle movements that incorporate a combination of breathing and meditation. The movements are planned to dissolve physical and karmic layers (deposits of past actions) that can cause tension by opening the spiritual space inside and creating a positive effect on the physical and energy bodies (IOM, 2005).

Japanese Practices and Traditions

TCM systems also exist in other East and South Asian countries, including Japan and Korea. In Japan, the traditional herbal medicine practice is termed *kampo*. According to Watanabe et al. (2011), kampo itself refers to the practices of the Han period of China, dating from around 206 BC to AD 220. Kampo emphasizes diagnostic methods that directly link symptoms and therapy. Formulations of crude herbal drugs in Japan were administered as early as 1,500 years ago. Recently there has been a revival of kampo in contemporary medical practice. This resurgence is accompanied by a "scientific reevaluation and critical examination of its relevance in modern health care" (p. 1).

Other Japanese traditions include Jin Shin Jyutsu and shiatsu. In Jin Shin Jyutsu, gentle manipulation is placed using the fingertips on 26 specific "safety energy locks" found on the body in order to harmonize and restore balance. In shiatsu, body energy is manipulated through the acupuncture meridians by applying finger pressure in order to activate and balance the *qi* (or *chi*). A more recent practice derived from Japanese shiatsu is Watsu, which is an innovative combination of Zen shiatsu, meridian stretches, *chakra* (Indian energy points) work, yoga movements, and acupressure performed in warm water (IOM, 2005).

Korean Practices and Traditions

One traditional healing and medicinal method popular with Native Koreans and Korean immigrants is *Han bang* (or *hanbang*). A combination of herbal medicine and acupuncture, the practice includes four major modalities. The first is *ch'im*, which is a type of acupuncture. The second is *hanyak*, which is a traditional set of Korean herbal formulations. Third is *d'um*, which is the practice of moxibustion (direct or indirect burning with a stick made of the mugwort plant). The fourth, *buhwang*, is the practice of cupping (formation of a vacuum by applying heated glass cups directly to the skin). Han bang treatment aims to restore balance of life energy, *um*, and also includes assessment of the voice, medical history, and observation of the patient (Sohn, 2010).

Southeast Asian Practices and Traditions

Southeast Asia is defined by the Association of Southeast Asian Nations (ASEAN) as having 10 distinct nations: Brunei Darussalam, Burma, Cambodia, Indonesia, Laos, Malaysia, the Philippines, Singapore, Thailand, and Vietnam (Office of the US Trade Representative, 2013). It is important to consider historical transitions in order to understand any cultural tradition and health beliefs of a group of people. The Southeast Asia region is no exception. For example, there is much common in belief and practice between Chinese living on the mainland and the Hmong people, who have origins in China and who migrated in large numbers during the 19th century, following conflicts with the Han dynasty, to Vietnam, Laos, and Thailand (Gerdner, 2010).

Vietnam, Laos, Cambodia, and Thailand Practices and Traditions

Among the Hmong people, traditional healing modalities similar to TCM continue to thrive among immigrants. Home remedies for physical symptoms are common. Ailments such as headaches, muscle aches, swelling, tingling, back pains, chest pains, abdominal pains, and others are believed to result from an increase in pressure from everyday life that must be released (Gerdner, 2010). The four healing techniques include: (1) *txhuav* or *nqus* (cupping); (2) *kav* (coining/spooning/rubbing); (3) *zuaj ib ce* (massage); and (4) *hno* (pricking the skin with a needle). These techniques are used to *dim pa* (to release the pressure that is causing the ailment). *Dim pa* results in residual marks on the skin surface where the procedure was applied. These are usually the back, neck, temple, bridge of the nose, and the chest area. The marks usually dissipate within a couple of days. Although *txhuav or Nqus*, *kav*, and *zuaj ib ce* are common in TCM, *hno* is not as widely utilized in TCM among Chinese in the United States (Gerdner, 2010).

Hno, which involves the pricking of skin with a needle,

can be done alone, after massage, or in conjunction with cupping and coining. Pricking often occurs at the bruised skin site after cupping or coining or at the fingertips after massage. Pricking is conducted both to release pressure and toxins causing the illness, as well as to determine the severity of the illness by examining the released drop of blood. The color and consistency of the blood are visually analyzed; the darker and thicker the blood, the more severe the illness. (Gerdner, 2010, p. 15)

The Khmer people of Cambodia also believe that balance of all elements is integral to good health. For example, excess air or wind can cause illness. One such illness is *kyol goeu*, also known as wind overload or fainting syndrome. One traditional healing method utilized by the Khmer for *kyol goeu* is *cạo gió*, or coining (Hinton, Um, & Ba, 2001).

In Vietnam, traditional Eastern medicine (*Thuốc Đong Y*) reflects the effects of environmental factors, such as wind and spirits. These factors can offset the internal balance of a person, which in turn can lead to illness. For example, a Vietnamese person may refer to a cold or flu as having been exposed to "poisonous wind" (*gió độc*) or "catching the wind" (*trung gió*) instead of the common American term of "catching a cold." And like Cambodians, Laotians, and Filipinos, Vietnamese also use coining (*cạo gió*) and or cupping (*giác hơi*) to heal the resulting imbalance from such exposure (Tran & Hinton, 2010).

Filipino Practices and Traditions

Pranic healing is a comprehensive system of subtle energy healing, and it utilizes *prana* (life force) in balancing, harmonizing, and transforming the body's energy process (IOM, 2005). According to De la Cruz and Periyakoil (2010), a central concept in Filipino health beliefs and behaviors is that of *timbang*, or balance. As in other Asian ancient medical practices, harmony and balance are integral. Among Filipino immigrants in the United States, specific aspects of *timbang* appear to be more prevalent among older and rural immigrants. A range of humoral balances can influence Filipino health perceptions. As adapted from Becker (2003) and presented by De la Cruz and Periyakoil (2010), these beliefs include:

- Rapid shifts from "hot" to "cold" lead to illness
- "Warm" environment is essential for maintaining optimal health
- Cold drinks or cooling foods should be avoided in the morning

- An overheated body is vulnerable to disease; a heated body can get "shocked"
- When cooled quickly, it can cause illness
- A layer of fat maintains warmth, protecting the body's vital energy
- Imbalance from worry and overwork create stress and illness
- Emotional restraint is a key element in restoring balance
- A sense of balance imparts increased body awareness (2010, p. 12)

De la Cruz and Periyakoil (2010) go on to explain that Filipino health beliefs and practices adapt to protecting the body. For example, behaviors conducive to protection and rebalance include: flushing (e.g., sweating, vomiting, or expelling gas), heating (e.g., balancing hot and cold to prevent illness), and protection (e.g., safeguarding against external effects of supernatural or natural powers).

Native Hawaiian Practices and Traditions

Historical context often aids in understanding health status, beliefs, and needs. Today's Native Hawaiians are the descendants of ancestors who endured years of sociopolitical conflict and underserved community environments. These have helped shape Native Hawaiian health beliefs, practices, and behaviors. Many cultural values are important to Native Hawaiians, and some of these are particularly relevant to health and health-care systems. The most relevant include *lokahi* (balance), *'ohana* (family), *aloha* (love, compassion), and *malama* (to care for) (Mau, 2010).

Lokahi is relevant as a health concept in that without it, the physical body cannot be healed. Lack of balance can cause immediate problems within the mental or spiritual realms. Native Hawaiians see health as a holistic entity, and physical, mental, and spiritual harmony are required to attain health. These three entities are the "points of the triangle" and encompass not only the physical health of the body but also the environment in which one lives. This environment includes relationships with others, including family, ancestors, and gods. It also includes mental and emotional states (Mau, 2010). Any existing problems with any of these environmental factors can prevent healing in the body. It is believed that healers (and healthcare providers) ought to take time to understand all of these factors and how the patient might go about remedying or making amends for any past wrongdoing (Mau, 2010).

'*Ohana*, the family, includes the extended family, as it is a primary social structure of Native Hawaiians. It is usual for Hawaiians to live in homes composed of several generations, where grandparents often play an integral role in child rearing; thus, illness affects the entire family. Typically, all family members are involved in health decision making and the necessary treatments. Native Hawaiians are a cooperative, helping, and collectively responsible people (Mau, 2010).

One specific and integral aspect of the health professional relationship with Native Hawaiians is their need to feel respected and valued in order to be "willing partners in the patient-physician relationship" (Mau, 2010, p. 20). The concepts of *aloha* and *malama* reflect this tradition. The primary meaning of *aloha* centers around love, caring, and compassion. Thus, establishing trust is important when addressing health and healing. Inclusion of the family in health issues reinforces their collective responsibility to care for one another (Mau, 2010).

As Mau (2010) explained, Native Hawaiians often seek the traditional healing practices of their ancestors. These practices may include massage (*lomilomi*), herbal or plant-based healing (*la'au lapa'au*), prayer (*la'au Kahea*), and conflict resolution (*ho'oponopono*). Health practitioners utilize one or all of these practices in traditional healing. These strategies often involve prayer, a reflection of the belief that healing comes from a god or higher power. It is also important that the patient be willing in the attempt to bring back health, harmony, and balance (Mau, 2010). One specific traditional healing practice is *huna (t*he original arts and sciences of healing and spiritual development), which utilizes a combination of ancient Hawaiian healing and investigation of body, mind, and spirit through shamanism. It is believed that *huna* practice increases both the spirituality and the healing powers of the patient (IOM, 2005).

Traditions and Practices of Other Pacific Islanders

Pacific Islanders and Hawaiians, like other Asian groups, share similarities in their traditional healing values, beliefs, and practices. For instance, the Micronesian model follows the Native Hawaiian model of family very closely. To Micronesians, family includes extended family and adopted siblings plus a multitude of cousins (Mau, 2010). Among Samoans, customary cultural beliefs continue to dominate health behaviors. At the core of Samoan communities is *aiga*, which is an extended family system. The head of the *aiga* is a *matai* chief. In Samoan culture, kinship ties play a very important role in social and economic life. All kindred (by birth or adoption) are accepted as belonging to one *aiga*, containing more than a hundred people (Mau, 2010).

Table 10.1   Selected CAM Modalities of Asian Americans and Pacific Islanders

Modality	Description
Acupuncture	The stimulation of specific body points, most often by putting needles in the skin (NCCIH, 2014)
Buhwang	Korean method of cupping (Sohn, 2010)
Cao gio	Cambodian method of coining (Hinton et al., 2001)
Chakra	Indian practice, manipulation of energy points (IOM, 2005)
Ch'im	A type of Korean acupuncture (Sohn, 2010)
D'um	Korean practice of moxibustion (Sohn, 2010)
Dim pa	Hmong method used to release pressure that is causing an ailment (Gerdner, 2010)
Hanyak	A set of traditional Korean herbal combinations (Sohn, 2010)
Hno	Chinese tradition of pricking of the skin with a needle (Gerdner, 2010)
Huna	A combination of ancient Hawaiian healing and investigation of body, mind, and spirit through shamanism (IOM,2005; Mau, 2010)
Jin Shin Jyutsu	Japanese method of gentle manipulation placed with fingertips on 26 specific "safety energy locks" of the body in order to harmonize and restore balance (IOM, 2005)
Kampo	Traditional Japanese herbal medicine practice that emphasizes diagnostic methods that directly link symptoms and therapy and bypass the more speculative concepts of the Chinese tradition from which *kampo* is derived (Watanabe et al., 2011)
La'au lapa'au	Hawaiian herbal or plant-based healing (Mau, 2010)
Lomilomi	Hawaiian massage (Mau, 2010)
Shiatsu	Japanese method where body energy is manipulated through acupuncture meridians by applying finger pressure in order to activate and balance the *chi* (IOM, 2005)
Moxibustion	Burning a herb above the skin to apply heat to acupuncture points (NCCIH, 2013)
Reiki	An ancient Tibetan tradition that includes the use of hand symbols and breathing; movement of air and manipulation of energy forces brings about balance (IOM, 2005)
Watsu	A water-based innovative combination of Shiatsu, meridian stretches, chakra work, yoga movements, and acupressure performed in warm water (IOM, 2005)
Tai chi	The use of balanced and very gentle movements that incorporate a combination of breathing and meditation (IOM, 2005)
Tui na	Chinese therapeutic massage, similar to acupuncture but without needles, also called acupressure (IOM, 2005)

Pacific Islanders share many of the traditional healing practices of Hawaiian Natives, such as the belief in balance. It is evidenced in the prevalence of massage and herbal remedies, in addition to social involvement and maintenance of harmony in families. As with Native Hawaiian ancient traditions, often Samoans and Micronesians observe the hierarchical structure within families. In health-related situations, precedent and preference are given to elders and male family members. This may be especially relevant when the elderly are involved. Additionally, among Samoan women issues related to modesty are still very sensitive and may limit the types of discussions or health topics that can be addressed with more traditional community members (Mau, 2010). Table 10.1 presents selected CAM Modalities of Asian Americans and Pacific Islanders.

Consumer Issues

Asian American and Pacific Islanders are savvy consumers who participate actively in the selection of CAIH practitioners who ensure safety and client protection. The NCCIH (2013) recommended six strategies for selecting such healthcare providers:

1. Seeking referrals from primary care providers

2. Thoroughly reviewing providers prior to being seen

3. Seeking providers who will work with CAIH and conventional medicine practitioners

4. Establishing open communication about health history and the practitioner's experience with particular ailments

5. Awareness of insurance and coverage limitations or exclusions for CAIH

6. Complete disclosure of all CAIH modalities utilized

When engaging in traditional healing methods, such as moxibustion, Watsu, *Hno*, and other forms of CAIH therapies, Asian Americans, Native Hawaiians, and Pacific Islanders need to be cognizant of the benefits and risks associated with such practices. To increase understanding of Asian American, Native Hawaiian, and Pacific Islander healing traditions, consumers should advocate for research on these modalities.

Health professionals can play an important role in the use of CAIH by Asian Americans, Native Hawaiians, and Pacific Islanders. They ought to be knowledgeable about the modalities used by the communities they serve. Although it is difficult, in most instances, to learn specific modalities in sufficient depth to educate about precise risks, health professionals can play a critical role as resources—for example, helping communities increase their knowledge of conventional US healthcare systems and how to interact successfully with healthcare providers. Research shows that health educators have an overall positive attitude toward CAIH (Johnson, Priestley, Porter, & Petrillo, 2010) and that CAIH needs to be included as a content area in their professional preparation.

Implications for Health Professionals

Health professionals are encouraged to promote positive patient-healthcare provider interactions. Further, they can design health-promotion programs that take into consideration CAIH modalities utilized and appreciated by their priority communities. For example, Chang et al. (2013) combined acupuncture and nicotine replacement therapy with a traditional smoking cessation curriculum. The results of their retrospective evaluation study of a three-year program showed that the "real-world community program offering acupuncture as a cultural adjunct to a tobacco cessation" was effective with engaging Chinese American male participants in their tobacco cessation program (p. 80S).

Pinzón-Pérez (2014) addressed the role and responsibilities of health educators in incorporating CAIH practices into their profession. Specific recommendations included acknowledging the relevance of CAIH as a part of health education, facing the challenge to increase the body of knowledge about CAM among health education professionals, and further developing the body of knowledge regarding CAIH in health education professional development and research.

According to Frampton et al. (2008), there are key aspects of successful interactions between health professionals and patients or clients. Although not limited to these key strategies, addressing them can increase the richness of health-related interactions and health outcomes. Communicating in an effective way with patients and their families is the cornerstone of quality healthcare interactions with Asian Americans, Native Hawaiians, and Pacific Islanders. Also it is important to personalize care and interactions with individual patients and their sociocultural group.

Ensuring continuity of care throughout the entire system (from information gathering to healing treatment) can also help guarantee positive outcomes and client satisfaction. Similarly, providing ample access to information and patient education can result in a more engaged and satisfied patient. Maintaining positive family involvement can also increase beneficial interactions and limit disengagement. Other issues that Frampton et al. (2008) considered key to positive and effective health-system interactions include the environment of care, acknowledgment of the role of spirituality and faith, and the inclusion of integrative medicine principles.

Communication and Personalization Considerations for Health Interactions

Given the collective and family-centered values of many Asian American, Native Hawaiian, and Pacific Islander cultures, it is important to consider that successful interactions between health professionals (healthcare providers, health promoters, and health education specialists) depend on cultural paradigms affecting adoption of positive health behaviors. "Patients who understand their providers are more likely to accept their health problems, understand their treatment options, modify their behavior and adhere to follow-up instructions. If the single most important criterion by which patients judge us is by the way we interact with them, it stands to reason that effective communication is at the core of providing patient-centered care" (Frampton et al., 2008, p. 78). Further, customizing the patient's or client's experience is a key strategy for minimizing possible anxiety, fear, or stress that often is associated with formal Western healthcare settings (Frampton et al., 2008). Hospitals, for example, are places where one can quickly lose autonomy and, more important in the eyes of Asian American, Native Hawaiian, and Pacific Islander community members, lose family interaction and involvement.

CAIH modalities can be good management approaches in that they can allow the combination of traditional healing beliefs and practices with Western standards of care. As indicated by Frampton et al. (2008), patient-centered care can empower clients with the knowledge, support, and resources needed to arrive at informed decisions in their management of health and wellness. Acknowledging and expecting that many Asian American, Native Hawaiian, and Pacific Islander clients and patients are familiar with CAIH modalities traditional to their culture could lead to more openness and forthrightness on the part of patients. Further, familiarity and acceptance could prevent discontinuation of care or increased reluctance in seeking preventive or early treatment of illnesses.

As the World Health Organization (WHO, 2013) explained in a strategic report, traditional or complementary medicine practices are "an important and often underestimated part of health services" with an extensive "history of use in health maintenance and in disease prevention and treatment, particularly for chronic disease" (p. 11). Further, the WHO director explained relevant reasons for continued global support of

CAIH modalities, including the contribution toward the access by all to "traditional medicines, of proven quality, safety, and efficacy," given that this type of care often for many is "the main source of health care, and sometimes the only source of care. This is care that is close to homes, accessible and affordable. It is also culturally acceptable and trusted by large numbers of people. The affordability of most traditional medicines makes them all the more attractive at a time of soaring health-care costs and nearly universal austerity" (p. 16).

In the United States, CAIH utilization is common in immigrants and Asian communities. Among Asian communities, a few characteristics have been found to be correlated with higher likelihood of CAIH use. These characteristics include higher acculturation to their native culture, older age, lower socioeconomic status, and lower educational attainment (Lee et al., 2010). No cohesive pattern can be found in the literature to describe the diverse set of characteristics among CAIH users, especially in light of the recent increased utilization of alternative modalities alongside mainstream medicinal practices. It is important to remember the diversity of all communities and thus the uniqueness of each potential client.

As previously stated, there are commonalities among the CAIH modalities, health beliefs, and practices of Asian American and Pacific Islander community members. As a whole, they share a strong emphasis on family and extended family, group harmony, and interdependence within members of a group; veneration of natural influences on health; and varying degrees of spirituality (Palmer, 2015). These principles emphasize body and mind connectedness and the ideal of wellness in all areas of life, not simply physical health. As Asian American, Native Hawaiian, and Pacific Islander communities continue their fast growth in the United States, so will the use of CAIH modalities. Therefore, the need for knowledge, awareness, and promotion of diversity in professional preparation and practice in the health professions is increasing.

Caveat Emptor

Health professionals often confront diverse situations and health beliefs. Likely, they are continuously learning and growing to address the diverse needs of their patients and clients. As evidenced by the dearth of professional literature on CAIH modalities specific to Asian American, Native Hawaiian, and Pacific Islander communities, there is much more to be explored and studied.

Bomar (2013) described the convergence of Western and Eastern health systems and CAM modalities into a global healthcare system that merges pharmacological, biotechnical, and surgical specialties with mind, body, and spirit. Further, Bomar made specific recommendations for health professionals, including: (1) respecting clients' CAM requests; (2) knowing common CAM modalities; (3) networking with CAM healthcare provider referral networks; (4) appraising professional CAM literature and research; and (5) engaging in rigorous CAM research (p. 4). Bomar also encouraged health professionals to merge evidence-based CAM with standard Western conventional care in a way that is empowering to culturally diverse communities.

It is also important to keep in mind that currently the United States lacks a standard for national credentialing of CAIH providers and that it is up to each state and local government to delineate standards of practice and credentialing. Further, there is a large degree of variation between states and disciplines on the specific credentials or certifications required to practice CAIH modalities (NCCIH, 2013b). It is also important to consider that "regulations, licenses, or certificates do not guarantee safe, effective treatment from any provider—conventional or complementary" (NCCIH, 2013b, p. 1).

As with conventional US medical modalities, CAIH includes a certain level of risk and possible side effects; however, regulatory standards help alleviate and prevent them. Some TCM herbal remedies have been found to be contaminated with metals (e.g., mercury), and others can accumulate in the liver (e.g., kava, germander, and valerian root), potentially causing toxicity.

Conclusion

A rich institution of traditional healing practices is evident in the use of CAIH modalities by Asian Americans, Native Hawaiians, and Pacific Islanders. Many of these modalities are based in the ancient principles of balance and harmony. Energy forces—when out of balance—can result in illness. CAIH modalities used by Asian Americans, Native Hawaiians, and Pacific Islanders aim to restore balance in a variety of ways. These modalities include the use of alternative medical systems (e.g., *buhwang* by Korean Americans), biologically based therapies (e.g., *kampo* by Japanese Americans), manipulative and body-based therapies (e.g., *tui na* by Chinese Americans), mind-body medicine (e.g., pranic healing by Filipino Americans), and energy therapies with prayer (e.g., *Thuốc Đong Y* by Vietnamese Americans).

Current understanding of the meaning and uses of these modalities is limited due to the lack of empirical literature. Multiple efforts are under way across the nation and the world to improve health professionals' knowledge and understanding of CAIH methods in general and their use among Asian American, Native Hawaiians, and Pacific Islander communities. The NCCIH supports research studies based on evidence-based empirical methods to measure the effectiveness of various complementary and integrative health modalities for specific health concerns, symptoms, and diagnoses (NCCIH, 2015).

Summary

- Asian Americans, Native Hawaiians, and other Pacific Islander communities are very diverse and represent a multitude of countries, origins, and traditions.

- There are several health disparities among Asian Americans, Native Hawaiians, and Pacific Islanders that may affect their interaction with the conventional US healthcare system. Integrating CAIH use and conventional healthcare systems is a relevant consideration for this population.

- The underlying commonality among traditional healing modalities of Asian Americans, Native Hawaiians, and Pacific Islanders is that they are based on the value of harmony and balance among humans and nature.

- Younger Asian Americans, Native Hawaiians, and Pacific Islanders may not follow traditional native customs in the same way their elders do. However, the cultural values and beliefs are still present and can influence their decision making.

- In their interactions, health professionals should consider the diversity within the Asian American, Native Hawaiian, and Pacific Islander groups and develop strategies to evaluate CAIH.

Case Study

Description

Mrs. Gao, a 69-year-old mother of two and wife of 41 years, immigrated from Thailand to New York in 1988 with her immediate family. She has limited English proficiency despite years of formal English ESL classes. She studied through the 11th grade before entering the workforce as a young woman and then marrying in her '20s. She has worked cleaning restaurants and commercial buildings since she immigrated to the United States. She has experienced persistent stomachache, bloating, pain after meals, and indigestion with heavy, condiment-rich foods. This has lasted all of her life, and she has dealt with it by taking digestive pills and watching what she eats.

Mrs. Gao has been having more issues with her digestion, primarily upset stomach and nausea after meals. She tried a "cleansing" traditional medicine and some supplements. The cleansing appeared at first to be working, but after a week she started having pain again. Two weeks passed and the pain intensified and became constant. Mrs. Gao continued to self-treat with herbal remedies, meditation, and acupuncture. Approximately four weeks later, Mrs. Gao had lost nearly 20 pounds and was very weak and in severe pain. Despite her discomfort, she continued to resist the Western medicine recommendations given by her healthcare provider.

Her family was finally able to convince her to go to the hospital, where she was admitted for rehydration and treatment. At the hospital, Mrs. Gao cautiously accepted pharmacological treatment for the pain. She underwent a couple of diagnostic procedures, after which results were consistent with Crohn's disease. Mrs. Gao was given the diagnosis, and after six days in the hospital was able to go home on a soft diet. While at the hospital, her major complaints were the coldness of people, being handled by strangers, the large amount of medications, and the bad energy in a place of illness and death.

Mrs. Gao completed the prescribed two weeks of steroids while she investigated her condition on the Internet and through her circle of family and friends. She found limited information in her native language and none that incorporated her traditional beliefs. She longed to be able to have someone knowledgeable of both traditions with whom to talk and ask for advice. Afterward, she consulted her traditional healer. The healer explained that, in his opinion, it was not Crohn's but a parasitic infection that resulted from an imbalance in her gut. Mrs. Gao started a course of probiotics and changed her diet to help prevent future inflammation and ulcers in her colon. She saw improvement in her signs and symptoms.

Currently, Mrs. Gao does not comply with her prescribed Western medication, nor does she continue to visit the specialist to whom she was referred. Instead, she relies on family and friends and her traditional beliefs. She continues to meet with her social circle of friends at her neighborhood community center where she volunteers.

Questions

1. What CAIH approaches were used by Mrs. Gao in this case study?

2. What role did Mrs. Gao's traditional health beliefs and practices play in her situation?

3. What could the healthcare provider do to ensure that Mrs. Gao understands the diagnosis given for her ailment?

4. Can you identify potential professional collaborations in this story? What are they? How can health professionals include such collaborations in community settings?

KEY TERMS

Herbal medicine. The use of plant seeds, berries, roots, leaves, bark, or flowers for medicinal purposes (IOM, 2005).

Prana. The life force (IOM, 2005).

Qi (chi). Energy, necessary in maintaining health and wellness (NCCIH, 2013a).

Qi gong. Energy cultivation, including exercises designed to bring about harmony in addition to promoting health and longevity (IOM, 2005).

Tao. "The way" or "the law." The rule of Tao is to live in complete harmony with our natural world (IOM, 2005).

Traditional Chinese medicine. An ancient philosophy dating back more than 2,500 years. It is a long-accepted and effective practice (IOM, 2005).

Yin and yang. Harmony between opposite energies (NCCIH, 2013a).

References

Asian Pacific American Legal Center & Asian American Justice Center. (2012). *Asian American Center for Advancing Justice: A community of contrasts: Asian Americans in the United States, 2011.* Retrieved from http://napca.org/wp-content/uploads/2012/11/AAJC-Community-of-Contrast.pdf

Becker, G. (2003). Cultural expressions of bodily awareness among chronically ill Filipino Americans. *Annals of Family Medicine, 1*(2), 113–118.

Bomar, P. J. (2013). Comments on complementary and alternative healing modalities. (Editorial). *International Journal of Nursing Practice, 19*(2), 1–6.

Centers for Disease Control and Prevention. (2013a). *Asian American populations.* Retrieved from http://www.cdc.gov/minorityhealth/populations/REMP/asian.html#CHDIR

Centers for Disease Control and Prevention. (2013b). *Native Hawaiian and Other Pacific Islander populations.* Retrieved from http://www.cdc.gov/minorityhealth/populations/REMP/nhopi.html

Chang, E., Fung, L., Li, C., Lin, T., Tam, L., Tang, C., & Tong, E. K. (2013). Offering acupuncture as an adjunct for tobacco cessation: A community clinic experience. *Health Promotion Practice, 14*(1S), 80–87.

De la Cruz, M. T., & Periyakoil, V. J. (2010). *Health and health care of Filipino American older adults.* In V. S. Periyakoil (Ed.), *eCampus—Geriatrics.* Stanford, CA. Retrieved from http://geriatrics.stanford.edu/wp-content/uploads/downloads/ethnomed/filipino/downloads/filipino_american.pdf

Frampton, S., Guastello, S., Brady, C., Hale, M., Horowitz, S., Bennett Smith, S., & Stone, S. (2008). *Patient-centered care: Improvement guide.* Derby, CT: Planetree, and Picker Institute. Retrieved from http://planetree.org/wp-content/uploads/2015/03/Patient-Centered-Care-Improvement-Guide-10.10.08.pdf

Gerdner, L. (2010). *Health and health care of Hmong American older adults.* In V. S. Periyakoil (Ed.), *eCampus—Geriatrics.* Stanford, CA. Retrieved from http://geriatrics.stanford.edu/ethnomed/hmong.html

Gibson, C., & Young, K. (2005*). Historical census statistics on population totals by race, 1790 to 1990, and by Hispanic origin, 1970 to 1990, for the United States, regions, divisions, and states.* Washington, DC: Population Division of the US Census Bureau. Retrieved from http://www.census.gov/population/www/documentation/twps0076/twps0076.html

Grzywacz, J., Lang, W., Suerken, C., Quandt, S. A., Bell, R. A., & Arcury, T. A. (2005). Age, race, and ethnicity in the use of complementary and alternative medicine for health self-management: Evidence from the 2002 National Health Interview Survey. *Journal of Aging and Health, 17*, 547–572.

Hinton, D., Um, K., & Ba, P. (2001). *Kyol goeu* ("wind overload"), Part I: A cultural syndrome of orthostatic panic among Khmer refugees. *Transcultural Psychiatry, 38*(4), 403–432. doi: 10.1177/136346150103800401

Hixson, L., Hepler, B. B., & Kim, M. O. (2012). *Native Hawaiian and Other Pacific Islander population: 2010.* Retrieved from http://www.census.gov/prod/cen2010/briefs/c2010br-12.pdf

Hoeffel, E. M., Rastogi, S., Kim, M. O., & Shahid, H. (2012). *The Asian population: 2010.* Retrieved from https://www.census.gov/prod/cen2010/briefs/c2010br-11.pdf

Institute of Medicine. (2005). *Complementary and alternative medicine in the United States.* Washington, DC: National Academies Press. Retrieved from http://www.nap.edu/catalog/11182/complementary-and-alternative-medicine-in-the-united-states

Johnson, P., Priestley, K., Porter, K. J., & Petrillo, J. (2010). Complementary and alternative medicine: Attitudes and use among health educators in the United States. *American Journal of Health Education, (41)*3, 167–177. doi: 10.1080/19325037.2010.10598858

Lee, J. H., Goldstein, M. S., Brown, E. R., & Ballard-Barbash, R. (2010). How does acculturation affect the use of complementary and alternative medicine providers among Mexican- and Asian-Americans? *Journal of Immigrant and Minority Health, 12*, 302–309. doi: 10.1007/s10903-008-9171-1

Mau, M. (2010). *Health and health care of Native Hawaiian and Other Pacific Islander older adults.* In V. S. Periyakoil (Ed.), *eCampus—Geriatrics.* Stanford, CA. Retrieved from http://geriatrics.stanford.edu/ethnomed/hawaiian_pacific_islander.html

National Center for Complementary and Integrative Health. (2013a). *Traditional Chinese medicine: An introduction.* Retrieved from http://NCCIH.nih.gov/health/whatiscam/chinesemed.htm

National Center for Complementary and Integrative Health. (2013b). *Credentialing: Understanding the education, training, regulation, and licensing of complementary health practitioners.* Retrieved from https://nccih.nih.gov/sites/nccam.nih.gov/files/CAM_Basics_Credentialing_09-13-2013.pdf

National Center for Complementary and Integrative Health. (2014). *Acupuncture: What you need to know.* Retrieved from https://nccih.nih.gov/sites/nccam.nih.gov/files/Get_The_Facts_Acupuncture__10-28-2014.pdf

National Center for Complementary and Integrative Health. (2015). *Complementary, alternative, or integrative health: What's in a name?* Retrieved from https://nccih.nih.gov/sites/nccam.nih.gov/files/Whats_In_A_Name_08-11-2015.pdf

Neiberg, R. H., Aickin, M., Grzywacz, J. G., Lang, W., Quandt, S. A., Bell, R. A., & Arcury, T. A. (2011). Occurrence and co-occurrence of types of complementary and alternative medicine use by age, gender, ethnicity, and education among adults in the United States: The 2002 National Health Interview Survey (NHIS). *Journal of Alternative and Complementary Medicine, 17*(4), 363–370.

Office of the Press Secretary. (2013, May 29). *Remarks by the President at AAPI heritage month celebration.* Retrieved from http://www.whitehouse.gov/the-press-office/2013/05/28/remarks-president-aapi-heritage-month-celebration

Office of the US Trade Representative. (2013). *South East Asia and Pacific.* Retrieved from https://ustr.gov/countries-regions/southeast-asia-pacific/association-southeast-asian-nations-asean

Palmer, P. H. (2015). Pacific Islander health and disease. In R. M. Huff, M. V. Kline, & D. V. Peterson (Eds.), *Health promotion in multicultural populations* (3rd ed.). Los Angeles, CA: Sage.

Park, C. B., Gardner, R. W., & Nordyke, E. C. (2009). Longevity disparities in multiethnic Hawaii: An analysis of 2000 life tables. *Public Health Reports, 124,* 579–584.

Pinzón-Pérez, H. (2014). Complementary and alternative medicine in culturally competent health education. In M. A. Pérez & R. R. Luquis (Eds.), *Cultural competence in health education and health promotion* (2nd ed.). San Francisco, CA: Jossey-Bass, 87–118.

President's Advisory Commission on Asian Americans and Pacific Islanders. (2003). *Asian Americans and Pacific Islanders addressing health disparities: Opportunities for building a healthier America.* Washington, DC: Government Printing Office.

Ryan, C. (2013). Language use in the United States: 2011. *American Community Survey Reports.* Retrieved from http://www.census.gov/prod/2013pubs/acs-22.pdf

Sohn, L. (2010). *Health and health care of Korean American older adults.* In V. S. Periyakoil (Ed.), *eCampus-Geriatrics.* Stanford, CA. Retrieved from http://geriatrics.stanford.edu/ethnomed/korean.html

Su, D., & Li, L. (2011). Trends in the use of complementary and alternative medicine in the United States: 2002–2007. *Journal of Health Care for the Poor and Underserved, 22*(1), 296-310.

Tanaka, M. J., Gryzlak, B. M., Zimmerman, M. B., Nisly, N. L., & Wallace, R. B. (2008). Patterns of natural herb use by Asian and Pacific Islanders. *Ethnicity and Health, 13*(2), 93–108.

Tran, C., & Hinton, L. (2010). *Health and healthcare of Vietnamese American older adults.* In V. S. Periyakoil (Ed.), *eCampus—Geriatrics.* Stanford, CA. Retrieved from http://geriatrics.stanford.edu/ethnomed/vietnamese.html

Watanabe, K., Matsuura, K., Gao, P., Hottenbacher, L., Tokunaga, H., Nishimura, K., & Witt, C. M. (2011). Traditional Japanese Kampo medicine: Clinical research between modernity and traditional medicine—the state of research and methodological suggestions for the future. *Evidence-Based Complementary and Alternative Medicine.* Article ID 513842. Retrieved from http://www.ncbi.nlm.nih.gov/pmc/articles/PMC3114407/pdf/ECAM2011-513842.pdf

World Health Organization. (2013). *WHO Traditional Medicine Strategy 2014–2023.* Geneva, Switzerland: WHO. Retrieved from http://www.who.int/medicines/publications/traditional/trm_strategy14_23/en/

COMPLEMENTARY, ALTERNATIVE, AND INTEGRATIVE HEALTH APPROACHES AMONG CAUCASIAN/EUROPEAN AMERICANS

Kara N. Zografos

The term *Caucasian* is often used interchangeably with *White*; however, the two terms are not synonymous (Lee, Mountain, & Koenig, 2001). *Caucasian* refers to individuals with origins in Europe, the Middle East, or North Africa, and who indicate their race as being White, Irish, German, Italian, Lebanese, Arab, or Moroccan (US Census Bureau, 2012a). According to the US Census Bureau (2012b), in 2012, Whites constituted the majority (77.9%) of the US population. Although the non-Hispanic White population is expected to peak in 2024 at 199.6 million, it is projected to decrease by approximately 20.6 million from 2024 to 2060.

This chapter examines the use of healthcare practices outside of mainstream Western medicine for specific health conditions and for the overall well-being of Caucasian/European Americans. It also discusses complementary and alternative medicine (CAM) therapies used by Caucasians/Europeans in the United States and their relation to complementary, alternative, and integrative health (CAIH) approaches.

Theoretical Concepts

Overview

The terms *alternative* and *complementary* are often used to describe nonmainstream approaches to health care such

LEARNING OBJECTIVES

At the completion of this chapter, students will be able to:

- Identify the complementary and alternative medicine (CAM) practices most frequently used by Caucasian/European Americans as described in the current literature.

- Identify CAM therapies used by Caucasians/Europeans in the United States that could be considered complementary, alternative, and integrative health (CAIH) approaches.

- Describe some of the regulatory and practical realities associated with complementary and alternative practices.

- Explain some of the recommendations offered to consumers of CAIH modalities.

(continued)

LEARNING OBJECTIVES
(continued)

• Provide some practical advice for health professionals working with Caucasian/European consumers who use CAIH approaches.

as chiropractic care, acupuncture, and massage therapy; and although these terms are often used interchangeably, they refer to different concepts. *Complementary* generally refers to using a nonmainstream approach together with conventional medicine, while *alternative* generally refers to using a nonmainstream approach in place of conventional medicine (National Center for Complementary and Integrative Health [NCCIH], 2013b). Box 11.1 presents definitions of selected traditional and alternative healing practices.

The National Center for Health Statistics released findings on trends for 2002, 2007, and 2012 in the use of CAIH approaches among 88,962 US adults 18 and older using the National Health Interview Survey (NHIS). According to this survey, 34% reported using a CAIH therapy in the past 12 months. Nonvitamin, nonmineral dietary supplements were the most frequently practiced CAIH therapy for each of the time periods studied, while deep breathing exercises were the second most frequently practiced CAIH therapy for each time period. Yoga, tai chi, and qi gong use increased over the study period (5.8% in 2002; 6.7% in 2007; and 10.1% in 2012), with yoga being the most frequently practiced therapy when compared to tai chi and qi gong. Ayurveda, biofeedback, guided imagery hypnosis, and energy healing were the least frequently practiced CAM therapies for each of the time periods studied.

The use of CAM therapy was also examined against selected sociodemographic variables, including sex, age, Hispanic or Latino origin and race, educational attainment, poverty status, and health insurance coverage. Overall, the most significant differences were for age and Hispanic or Latino origin and race. With regard to yoga and age, adults 18 to 44 had the highest prevalence of use across each of the time periods studied (1.6% increase from 2002 to 2007; 3.3% increase from 2007 to 2012). With regard to Hispanic or Latino origin and race, Hispanic and non-Hispanic black adults reported less CAM use compared to non-Hispanic White adults (Clark, Black, Stussman, Barnes, & Nahin, 2015). These factors are important for health professionals to consider as they integrate CAIH therapies within their practice and into their prevention strategies.

BOX 11.1   SELECTED TRADITIONAL AND ALTERNATIVE HEALING PRACTICES

Acupuncture. A technique involving stimulation of specific points on the body by penetrating the skin with thin, solid, metallic needles (NCCIH, 2013b).

Ayurveda. A system of medicine that originated in India several thousand years ago. The aim of ayurveda is to cleanse the body of substances that can cause disease, which helps to reestablish harmony and balance (Barnes, Powell-Griner, McFann, & Nahin, 2004).

Biofeedback machine. An electronic device that teaches clients how to consciously regulate bodily functions, such as breathing, heart rate, and blood pressure, in order to improve overall health (Barnes et al., 2004).

Chelation therapy. Therapy in which a substance is used to chemically bind molecules, such as metals or minerals, in order to remove them from the body (Barnes et al., 2004).

Chiropractic care. Treatment that involves adjustment of the spine and joints to influence the body's nervous system and natural defense mechanisms to alleviate pain and improve health (NCCIH, 2012a).

Deep breathing. A conscious and slow style of breathing. A focus on taking regular and deep breaths (NCCIH, 2013f).

Energy healing therapy. Therapy that involves channeling healing energy through the hands of a practitioner into a client's body to restore a normal energy balance (Barnes et al., 2004).

Guided imagery. A process in which one focuses on pleasant images to replace negative or stressful feelings (NCCIH, 2013f).

Homeopathy. A system of medical practices based on the theory that any substance that can produce symptoms of disease or illness in a healthy person can be used to cure those symptoms in a sick person (NCCIH, 2013c).

Hypnosis. An altered state of consciousness characterized by increased responsiveness to suggestion (NCCIH, 2013f).

Massage therapy. A number of different techniques in which practitioners manually manipulate soft tissues in the body (NCCIH, 2013b).

Meditation. A group of techniques, mostly originating from Eastern religious or spiritual traditions, where a person focuses attention and suspends thoughts that normally occupy the mind (Barnes et al., 2004).

Naturopathy. An alternative medical system that suggests there is a healing power in the body that establishes, maintains, and restores health. It is based on the theory that diseases can be treated or prevented without the use of drugs (NCCIH, 2012b).

Natural products. A large and diverse group of substances from a variety of sources. They are produced by marine organisms, bacteria, fungi, and plants. This term also includes vitamins, minerals, and probiotics (NCCIH, 2014).

Qi gong. An ancient Chinese discipline combining gentle physical movements, mental focus, and deep breathing toward specific parts of the body (NCCIH, 2013d).

Reiki. An energy medicine practice that originated in Japan. It involves the practitioner placing his or her hands on or near the client, with the intent to transmit *qi* (or *chi*), which is believed to be life force energy (NCCIH, 2013e).

Tai chi. A mind-body practice that originated in China as a martial art. It involves specific movements, coordinated breathing, and mental focus (NCCIH, 2013b).

Yoga. A combination of physical postures or movement, breathing techniques, and meditation (NCCIH, 2013e).

Source: National Center for Complementary and Integrative Health (NCCIH). (2013a). Complementary, alternative, or integrative health: What's in a name? Retrieved from http://www.nccih.nih.gov/health/whatiscam

This chapter provides an overview of CAIH modalities and describes traditional and alternative healing practices among Caucasians/Europeans in the United States. Additionally, it provides information on the regulatory and practical realities associated with CAIH, along with applications for consumers and health professionals. This chapter concludes with a case study designed to provide hands-on opportunities for learners to practice critical thinking skills related to CAIH.

Modalities

Traditional medicine is defined as "the sum total of the knowledge, skills, and practices based on the theories, beliefs, and experiences indigenous to different cultures, whether explicable or not, used in the maintenance of health as well as in the prevention, diagnosis, improvement, or treatment of physical and mental illness" (World Health Organization, 2014, para. 2). Traditional medicine covers a wide range of therapies and practices, which vary from country to country and from region to region.

The history of CAIH in the United States has been shaped by scientific, economic, and social factors (White House Commission on Complementary and Alternative Medicine Policy, 2002). Until the middle of the 19th century, most primary medical care was provided by botanical healers, midwives, chiropractors, homeopaths, and a wide variety of other lay healers (Whorton, 1999). In the latter part of the 19th century, however, the situation began to change with the development of the germ theory and significant advances in antiseptic techniques, anesthesia, and surgery. In the 20th century, infectious diseases were less of a threat, people began living longer, and there was an increase in the prevalence of chronic conditions, all of which led to an increased reliance on Western medicine (White House Commission on Complementary and Alternative Medicine Policy, 2002).

The relative popularity of traditional and alternative healing practices among Caucasians in the United States is strong and growing. Kronenberg, Cushman, Wade, Kalmuss, and Chao (2006) examined the patterns of CAM use among 3,068 women in four racial/ethnic groups: non-Hispanic Whites, African Americans, Mexican Americans, and Chinese Americans. Between one-half and one-third of the women from all of the groups indicated using at least one CAM modality in the year preceding the survey.

Overall, CAIH use among Caucasians surpassed that of all other racial/ethnic groups. Similarly, Bausell, Lee, and Berman (2001) conducted a secondary analysis to examine the extent to which demographic and health-related variables were related to visits to a CAM practitioner. Gender, education, age, geographic location, and race were all found to be statistically significant predictors of visits to CAIH practitioners. In general, however, Caucasians were more likely to visit a CAIH practitioner than Hispanics and African Americans. Upchurch and Chyu (2005) used data from a 1999 survey to assess sociodemographic and other characteristics associated with CAM use. An estimated 35% of American women reported using CAIH in the past 12 months, with spiritual healing/prayer and herbal medicine among the most commonly reported. Additionally, individuals in poorer health and those suffering from mental, musculoskeletal, and metabolic disorders were more likely to visit a CAIH practitioner. Multivariate analyses revealed that Caucasians were more likely to use CAM than were African Americans, Hispanics, and Asians.

A limited number of studies exist on the use of traditional and alternative healing practices among Europeans who reside in the United States. Molassiotis et al. (2005) conducted a study aimed at exploring the use of CAM among 956 cancer patients across a number of European countries. The data suggested that CAM was popular among cancer patients with 35.9% using some form of CAM. The most common therapies used were herbal medicines and remedies together with homeopathy, vitamins/minerals, medical teas, spiritual therapies, and relaxation techniques. Multivariate analyses revealed that younger individuals, females, and those with higher educational levels were more likely to use CAM, which is consistent with some of the previous findings for CAM users in the United States.

As mentioned, this chapter examines the use of healthcare practices outside of mainstream Western medicine for specific health conditions and for overall well-being among the Caucasian/European American population. The next sections contain information pertaining to the German, Greek, Irish, and Italian heritages. For each heritage, a discussion on spirituality, healthcare practices, and a cultural alert is provided.

German Heritage

Spirituality

The major religions among those of German heritage in the United States include Roman Catholicism, Methodism, and Lutheranism. Other religions, such as Judaism, Islam, and Buddhism, also have substantial membership in this group (Thernstrom, 1980). Prayer is used to ask for healing, for effectiveness of treatments, for strength to deal with the symptoms of an illness, and for acceptance of the outcome of the course of an illness. Prayers are often recited at the patient's bedside, with all who are present joining hands, bowing heads, and receiving a blessing from clergy (Purnell & Paulanka, 2005).

Healthcare Practices

In traditional families, the mother usually ensures that children receive checkups, get immunizations, and take vitamins. Women in the family often administer folk/home remedies and treatments. Common, natural folk medicinal agents include roots, herbs, soups, poultices, and medicinal agents such as camphor, peppermint, and spirits of ammonia. Folk medicine includes "powwowing," use of special words, and wearing charms (Purnell & Paulanka, 2005).

Cultural Alert

To assess potential contraindications with prescription medication, it is important for healthcare professionals to ascertain if over-the-counter and folk remedies are being used. Healthcare professionals may not be able to identify verbal or nonverbal clues about pain among Germans. Careful interviewing and observation is necessary to accurately assess the level of pain experienced (Purnell & Paulanka, 2005).

Greek Heritage

Spirituality

When the Greeks first arrived in this country, it was common for them to attend Eastern-rite services in already established Eastern Orthodox churches. The pressure to build parish churches in which both the priest and the service would be Greek Orthodox, however, increased as the number of Greek immigrants grew (Thernstrom, 1980). The central religious experience is the Sunday morning liturgy, which is a church service with icons, incense, and singing or chanting by the choir. When a person is ill, the icon of the family saint or the Virgin Mary may be placed above the bed (Purnell & Paulanka, 2005). Many Greeks also sprinkle their home and places of work with holy water from Epiphany Day church services to protect from evil (Father J. Pappas, personal communication, January 16, 2014).

Healthcare Practices

Matiasma refers to "bad eye" or "evil eye." While the eye is able to harm a wide variety of things, including inanimate objects, children are particularly susceptible to attack (S. Booras, personal communication, July 28, 2008). Common symptoms include headache, chills, irritability, restlessness, and lethargy (Purnell & Paulanka, 2005). The Greeks employ a variety of preventive mechanisms to thwart the effects of the evil eye, including protective charms, amulets consisting of blessed wood or incense, or blue "eye" beads (see Figure 11.1), which "reflect" the eye (S. Booras, personal communication, July 28, 2008).

Practika are herbal and humoral treatments used for initial self-treatment. Chamomile, the most popular herb, is generally used in teas for gastric distress or abdominal pain, including infant colic and menstrual cramps. It is also used as an expectorant to treat colds. Liquors, including anisette, ouzo, and mastika, are used primarily for colds, sore throats, and coughs. These liquors are consumed by themselves or in combination with tea, lemon, honey, or sugar (Purnell & Paulanka, 2005). *Vendousas* is a

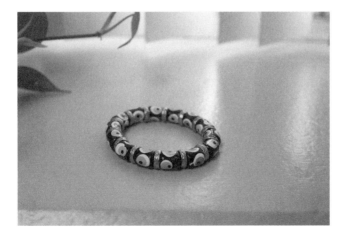

Figure 11.1 Greek Eye

healing practice that is used as a treatment for colds, high blood pressure, and backache. It consists of lighting a swab of cotton held on a fork, then placing the swab in an inverted glass while creating a vacuum in the glass, which is then placed on the back of the ill person. The skin on the back is drawn into the glass. This practice is similar to cupping methods used among other ethnic groups. *Kofte* is considered "cut *vendousa*." The same procedure is followed, except that a cut in the shape of a cross is made on the skin. Blood is drawn in when the glass is placed over the cut (P. Kourafas, personal communication, April 2, 2014). The therapeutic rationale for cut *vendousa* surrounds its counterirritant effect: The technique increases and revitalizes circulation, draws out poisons and "cold," and prevents blood coagulation (Purnell & Palanka, 2005).

Cultural Alert

The family generally assumes responsibility and care for a sick family member. Healthcare professionals should encourage empowerment and help the family care for the ill person. Healthcare professionals should not remove protective charms against the bad or evil eye from the patient or from the bedside (Purnell & Palanka, 2005).

Irish Heritage

Spirituality

The predominant religion of most people of Irish heritage in the United States is Catholicism, and the church is a source of strength and solace (Thernstrom, 1980). In times of illness, Irish Catholics receive the Sacrament of the Sick, which includes anointing, communion, and a blessing by the priest. The Eucharist, a small wafer made from flour and water, is given to the sick as the food of healing and health (Purnell & Palanka, 2005).

Healthcare Practices

Illness or injury may be linked to guilt and considered to be the result of having done something morally wrong. Restraint is a modus operandi in the Irish culture, and temptation must be guarded against. Irish folk practices include eating a balanced diet, getting a good night's sleep, exercising, dressing warmly, and not going out in the cold air with wet hair. Other folk practices include wearing religious medals to prevent illness, using cough syrup made from honey and whisky, taking honey and lemon for a sore throat, drinking hot tea for nausea, drinking tea and eating toast for a cold, and putting a damp cloth on the forehead for a headache. Some common folk practices might be harmful; these include the use of senna to cleanse the bowels every eight days, eating a lot of oily foods, and avoiding seeing a physician (Purnell & Palanka, 2005).

Cultural Alert

Many Irish people ignore symptoms and delay seeking medical attention. Irish Americans tend to limit and understate problems. Health professionals should encourage early intervention and explain its importance (Purnell & Palanka, 2005).

Italian Heritage

Spirituality

The predominant religion among those of Italian heritage in the United States is traditional Roman Catholicism. Sacraments include the celebration of Mass and the Eucharist, baptism, confirmation, confession, matrimony, ordination, and anointing of the sick (Thernstrom, 1980). When a loved one becomes ill, prayers are said at home and in church for the person's health. Most of those of Italian heritage pray to the Virgin Mary (see Figure 11.2) or the Madonna, and a number of saints. Prayer and

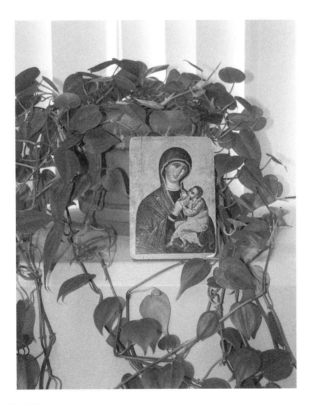

Figure 11.2   Virgin Mary

having faith in God and the saints help Italian Americans through illnesses (Purnell & Palanka, 2005).

Healthcare Practices

Nervousness, hysteria, and many other mental illnesses are attributed to an evil spirit entering the body and remaining there until it is cast out by making the place where it abides so unpleasant that it is forced to leave. *Il mal occhio* (the evil eye), which is also called *occhio cattivo* (bad eye), *occhio morto* (eye of death), and *occhio tristo* (wicked eye), has its roots in ancient Greece. Individuals can protect themselves from the evil eye by using magical symbols and by learning the rituals of the *maghi* (witch). Amulets, miniature representations of natural or manmade weapons that fight off the evil eye, include teeth, claws, and replicas of animal horns that are worn on necklaces or bracelets, held in a pocket, or sewn into clothing.

Common plant derivatives used in folk healing are olive oil, lemon juice, wine, vinegar, garlic, onion, lettuce, and tobacco. A crown of lemon leaves is believed to cure a headache. The leaves and flowers of the wild mallow herb, malva, are used to make tea, providing cool energy and positive effects on the lungs and stomach. A person is given hot rather than cold drinks when suffering from a fever. For indigestion, a mixture of coffee grounds and sugar is taken (Purnell & Palanka, 2005).

Cultural Alert

Women are more likely to report pain experiences, and they expect immediate attention. Health professionals should be careful to avoid an overdose of pain medication. Assigning health professionals from the same culture, when possible, can be advantageous (Purnell & Palanka, 2005).

Consumer Issues

CAM/CAIH therapies have become more popular in recent years (Mayo Clinic, 2014a), and their increased use may be influenced by a number of factors, including the rise of the Internet, the self-care movement, and various changes in the eating patterns of Americans. The Internet provides an opportunity for consumers to access a variety of health information quickly, with more than 70,000 health-related websites available (Grandinetti, 2000). The Internet can pose a problem, however, for users with limited literacy skills and/or limited experience. To assist in addressing this concern, health communication and health information technology is a topic area in the Healthy People 2020 document. This topic area contains a number of objectives, including improving the health literacy of the population, increasing individuals' access to the Internet, and increasing the proportion of quality health-related websites (US Department of Health and Human Services, 2015).

The self-care movement might also be responsible for the increase in CAIH therapy use since self-care is essential to the prevention and management of chronic conditions, which are now the leading cause of death and disability worldwide (Dickson, Clark, Rabelo-Silva, & Buck, 2013). Finally, various changes in eating patterns, including "green movements" that emphasize organic and nonchemical solutions to health problems, might also contribute to the increase in CAIH therapy use (Coulter & Willis, 2004). CAIH diets typically are low in fat, high in fiber, high in fruit, and high in vegetable intake. These diets also include detoxification and various supplements. According to findings from observational studies, predominantly plant-based diets reduce the risk for some cancers, including breast and prostate. These findings must be interpreted with caution, however, as evidence does not exist in support of these claims (Weitzman, 2008).

The increased popularity of CAIH therapy makes it essential for consumers to understand a therapy's potential benefits and risks. Scientific research is limited, and information may not be available for every CAIH therapy (Mayo Clinic, 2014a). Box 11.2 lists some general recommendations, based on the professional literature, for consumers to consider before using various CAIH modalities.

Implications for Health Professionals

Cultural diversity permeates most societies throughout the world. Multicultural holistic healthcare encompasses diverse populations of consumers who need culturally sensitive and culturally competent care from healthcare providers. Although it is impossible for health professionals, including health educators, to understand differences between and among all groups of individuals, it is important to be aware and culturally sensitive to these differences. The goal should always be to promote cultural sensitivity and culturally competent care that respects each person's right to be understood and treated as a unique individual (Purnell & Paulanka, 2005).

Box 11.3 lists general recommendations, based on the professional literature, for professionals as they work with consumers who practice various CAIH therapies.

BOX 11.2 RECOMMENDATIONS FOR CONSUMERS TO CONSIDER BEFORE USING CAM/CAIH MODALITIES

- *Take charge of your health.* It is important to be an informed consumer who reads scientific studies on the safety and efficacy of CAM/CAIH modalities. As you conduct this research, keep in mind the strengths and limitations associated with various study designs. As we have seen throughout this chapter, there is limited scientific evidence that supports the safety and efficacy of the various CAIH modalities. Be sure to also discuss your findings with your healthcare provider.

- *Research your complementary medicine practitioner.* Generally speaking, most practitioners have home pages that list specialties, certifications, education, and other information. Try to avoid randomly picking a practitioner from a health provider list or from a phone book. Talk to people you trust: a friend, a family member, or your general health practitioner. It is also important to determine the type of insurance your provider accepts and whether the services you are considering are covered under that insurance policy. As a result of Section 2706 (Nondiscrimination in Health Care) of the Patient Protection and Affordable Care Act, CAIH services may become more accessible to consumers. This section requires that insurers include and reimburse licensed healthcare providers. These providers may include: chiropractors, medical doctors, naturopathic providers, acupuncturists, massage therapists, osteopaths, optometrists, nurse practitioners, and licensed or direct-entry midwives and podiatrists. The intent of this regulation is to provide consumers with greater choice regarding the type of healthcare provider they wish to visit.

- *Talk to your doctor or primary care provider before taking a dietary supplement.* You and your practitioner need to discuss any potential side effects associated with the selected supplement. Additionally, it is possible that the new supplement might interact with other medications you are currently taking.

- *Refrain from replacing a conventional medical treatment for a CAM/CAIH therapy without appropriate evidence regarding its safety and efficacy.* Be aware that some CAIH practitioners make exaggerated claims about curing diseases and may suggest that you forgo your conventional treatment. For these reasons, some practitioners may be conservative about recommending CAIH modalities. Use the NCCIH, which was established to foster CAM/CAIH research, as a reputable and credible resource.

- *Tell your healthcare provider about any CAIH therapy you use.* It is important to share with your practitioner all the CAIH modalities you use to manage your health. This will help to ensure safe and coordinated care.

Sources: Integrative Health Policy Consortium, n.d.; Mayo Clinic, 2014b; NCCIH, 2013a; Responsible Reform for the Middle Class, n.d.

BOX 11.3   RECOMMENDATIONS FOR HEALTH PROFESSIONALS REGARDING CAM/CAIH USE

- *Refrain from removing religious art or icons from the patient's bedside.* As a healthcare practitioner or health educator, it is important to respect the patient's religious beliefs and practices. This recommendation draws on professional competence in recognizing the role that culture plays in health, specifically the importance of religion and spirituality.

- *Ask whether sick individuals wish to see a member of the clergy.* As we have seen throughout this chapter, religion is important to various populations. Consider asking if the patient would like to speak to a member of the clergy. If patients wish to involve a clergy member, respect their beliefs and incorporate the clergy members into the patient's care.

- *Inquire about home treatments in a nonjudgmental manner, as some individuals from European cultures lack trust in healthcare professionals.* This recommendation draws on professional competence in assessment and communication. Health professionals must be capable of talking with patients to assess home treatment use without being offensive or rude.

- *Encourage patients to reveal all traditional and home remedies being used to treat symptoms.* As we have seen, research on many of the CAIH modalities is limited, and the safety and efficacy of some traditional and/or home remedies is uncertain. Therefore, it is important for health professionals to have cultural competence in communication and to be culturally humble, as they will need skills in asking questions in a culturally sensitive manner.

- *Provide factual information about potentially harmful folk and traditional practices.* It is important to provide accurate and reliable information to patients. This recommendation draws upon professional competence in the public health sciences, specifically in the ability to retrieve scientific evidence from a variety of sources, including text and electronic media.

Sources: Council on Linkages between Academic and Public Health Practice, 2010; Purnell & Paulanka, 2005.

Caveat Emptor

An important responsibility of health professionals related to CAIH practices is to ensure adequate consumer protection. One of the challenges, however, is to discover ways in which to protect consumers without restricting their right to choose. Consumer education has been cited by many in the field as a key component of consumer protection. If consumers are to rely on the advice of physicians and other healthcare professionals, it is imperative that these individuals are knowledgeable and appropriately trained (Trachtenberg, 2002).

The number of medical schools in the United States that offer courses in CAIH has risen dramatically in recent years. Brokaw, Tunnicliff, Raess, and Saxon (2002) collected data from 123 CAM/CAIH course directors at 74 US medical schools in an effort to gather information about the specific topics being taught and the objectives behind the instruction. The main topics covered were acupuncture (76.7%), herbs and botanicals (69.9%), meditation and relaxation (65.8%), spirituality/faith/prayer (64.4%), chiropractic (60.3%), homeopathy (57.5%), and nutrition and diet (50.7%). Although the instruction appeared to be founded on the assumption that CAIH was effective, little scientific evidence exists to support this conclusion.

Similarly, the National Center for Complementary and Integrative Health (NCCIH) from the National Institutes of Health provided funding for a program called the CAM Education Project, which aimed to integrate CAM into health profession curricula. The grants were awarded in cohorts of five per year in 2000, 2001, and 2002–2003. The rationale for this program was to enable future health professionals to provide informed advice to patients who use CAM. Overall, several benefits of the program were noted, including increased faculty development activities, the creation of new programs, and the development of new collaborations among universities (Lee et al., 2007).

Selected Regulatory CAIH Practices

The 1994 passage of the Dietary Supplement Health and Education Act in the United States classified dietary supplements as foods, which prevented the Food and Drug Administration (FDA) from regulating them as strictly as drugs with respect to their efficacy, safety, or marketing claims (Ventola, 2010). Although consumers often consider these supplements to be "natural" and "safe," there is still the potential for them to be harmful as a result of drug interactions, toxicities, contamination, and other dangers (Gardiner et al., 2008; Kantor, 2009; Kroll, 2004). Manufacturers are not required to submit clinical efficacy and safety data for their products to the FDA before obtaining marketing approval, which results in a lack of information about significant health risks to the public (Cohen, Cerone, & Ruggiero, 2002).

To address this lack of information, the NCCIH was established to sponsor research and disseminate scientific data on CAIH therapies and dietary supplements (Kantor, 2009; Micozzi, 2003). Proposals also exist for governmental policy changes that will enhance the FDA's regulatory authority over dietary supplements, ensure that NCCIH-sponsored research meets quality standards comparable to research on conventional medicines, and integrate the therapies determined to be safe and effective into mainstream medicine as "standards of care" (Cohen et al., 2002; Kantor, 2009). Although some CAIH therapies and dietary supplements are scientifically evaluated, important safety and efficacy questions still remain for many others that have not yet been evaluated by NCCIH or by other investigators (Ventola, 2010).

Safety and Efficacy of CAIH Practices

There is some evidence to support the efficacy of massage therapy for cancer patients. Post-White et al. (2003) placed 230 cancer outpatients randomly in three groups (therapeutic massage, healing touch, and standard care) to assess relaxation and symptom reduction. Physiologic effects, such as decreased heart rate and respiration, were noted in all three groups. Therapeutic massage lowered pain and anxiety, and healing touch also lowered anxiety. Additionally, Cassileth and Vickers (2004) conducted a large, retrospective, observational study on pre- and postmassage symptom scores for 1,290 in- and outpatients seen over a three-year period at Memorial Sloan Kettering Cancer Center. Patients rated symptoms such as pain, fatigue, anxiety, nausea, and depression on a scale from 1 to 10. On average, a 50% reduction in symptoms was seen following massage. Although this was not a randomized design, the authors felt the results were clinically significant and in support of the use of massage in symptom control for patients with cancer.

There is also some evidence on the safety and efficacy of CAIH therapies for menopausal symptoms. The majority of the studies focused on hot flashes, as they are the primary symptom for which menopausal women seek "natural" treatments. A control trial conducted by Jacobson et al. (2001) examined the use of black cohosh for menopausal symptoms among 85 women and found no significant differences in the frequency and intensity of hot flashes. The benefits of black cohosh, however, are noted in studies outside of the United States; but these results need to be interpreted with caution as there is insufficient data on the safety of long-term use of this herb (Lehmann-Willenbrock & Riedel, 1988 as cited in Jacobson, 2001). Irvin, Domar, Clark, Zuttemzeister, and Friedman (1996) examined the efficacy of elicitation of the relaxation response for the treatment of menopausal hot flashes and concurrent psychological symptoms among 33 women between the ages of 44 and 66. The participants were randomly assigned to one of three groups: relaxation response, reading, or control. Daily elicitation of the relaxation response led to significant reductions in hot flash intensity and the concurrent psychological symptoms of tension-anxiety and depression.

Despite the existing evidence, healthcare professionals and consumers need to be aware that research on many of the CAIH therapies is limited. The popularity of CAIH therapies and their therapeutic potential, however, necessitates more definitive safety and efficacy studies (Kronenberg & Fugh-Berman, 2002). Experts argue that CAIH and dietary supplements should be subject to the same level of critical assessment as conventional therapies (Cohen et al., 2002). Without this scrutiny, there could be a risk for creating a healthcare system that is less efficient, less cost effective, and less safe.

Conclusion

Many Americans use healthcare approaches outside of mainstream Western medicine. A variety of CAIH approaches are used among the Caucasian and European cultures, including those related to spirituality. Some of these therapies, however, have not been scientifically tested for safety and efficacy. Consumers must be smart when considering CAIH therapies by being informed and asking the right questions. Health professionals need to work toward promoting cultural sensitivity and culturally competent care that is respectful of the differences between and among all groups of individuals.

Summary

- CAIH therapies have become more popular in recent years.

- More research is needed on the safety and efficacy of CAIH approaches.

- Common CAIH modalities for the Caucasian/European American population include those that rely on spirituality, natural folk medicinal agents, and the use of magical/religious medals and charms.

- As a consumer of CAIH therapies, it is important to be informed and to ask questions.

- As a health professional, it is important to be aware of the CAIH practices of various cultural groups.

Case Study

Description

Anastasia has a common cold and is choosing to practice *vendousas*, a healthcare practice specific to the Greek culture. As a health professional from a different cultural background, this practice is unfamiliar and concerning to you. You are meeting with Anastasia today to discuss various methods to prevent and treat the common cold.

Questions

1. What CAIH approaches are being used by Anastasia?
2. List at least five questions you would ask Anastasia about *vendousas*.
3. List at least three sources you could use to gather more information about *vendousas*.
4. What topics would you cover regarding the prevention of the common cold?
5. What topics would you cover regarding the treatment of the common cold?
6. What elements would you take into account when designing a culturally sensitive health plan for Anastasia?

KEY TERMS

Alternative medicine. Using a nonmainstream approach in place of conventional medicine (NCCIH, 2013b).

Caucasian/European. Individuals with origins in Europe, the Middle East, or North Africa and who indicate their race as being White, Irish, German, Italian, Lebanese, Arab, or Moroccan (US Census Bureau, 2012a).

Complementary medicine. Use of a nonmainstream approach together with conventional medicine (NCCIH, 2013b).

Multicultural holistic healthcare. Encompasses diverse populations of consumers who need culturally sensitive and culturally competent care from health providers (Purnell & Paulanka, 2005).

Section 2706 (Nondiscrimination in Health Care) of the Patient Protection and Affordable Care Act. Requires that insurers include and reimburse licensed healthcare providers, including chiropractors, medical doctors, naturopathic providers, acupuncturists, massage therapists, osteopaths, optometrists, nurse practitioners, and licensed or direct-entry midwives and podiatrists (Integrative Health Policy Consortium, n.d.).

References

Barnes, P., Powell-Griner, E., McFann, K., & Nahin, R. (2004). Complementary and integrative health use among adults: United States, 2002. *Seminars in Integrative Medicine*, 2(2), 54–71.

Bausell, R. B., Lee, W. L., & Berman, B. M. (2001). Demographic and health-related correlates to visits to complementary and alternative medical providers. *Medical Care*, *39*(2), 190–196.

Brokaw, J. J., Tunnicliff, G., Raess, B. U., & Saxon, D. W. (2002). The teaching of complementary and alternative medicine in US medical schools: A survey of course directors. *Academic Medicine*, *77*(9), 876–881.

Cassileth, B. R., & Vickers, A. J. (2004). Massage therapy for symptom control: Outcome study at a major cancer center. *Journal of Pain and Symptom Management*, *28*(3), 244–249.

Clark, T. C., Black, L. I., Stussman, B. J., Barnes, P. M., & Nahin, R. L. (2015). Trends in the use of complementary health approaches among adults: United States, 2002–2012. *National Health Statistics Reports*, *79*, 1–15.

Cohen, K. R., Cerone, P., & Ruggiero, R. (2002). Complementary/Alternative medicine use: Responsibilities and implications for pharmacy services. *Pharmacy and Therapeutics*, *27*(9), 440–446.

Coulter, I. D., & Willis, E. M. (2004). Complementary and alternative medicine: A sociological perspective. *Medical Journal of Australia*, *180*(4), 587–588.

Council on Linkages between Academia and Public Health Practice. (2010). *Core competencies for public health professionals*. Retrieved from http://www.phf .org/resourcestools/pages/core_public_health_competencies.aspx

Dickson, V. V., Clark, R. A., Rabelo-Silva, E. R., & Buck, H. G. (2013). Self-care and chronic disease. *Nursing Research and Practice*, *2013*, 1–2. doi: 10.1155/2013/827409

Gardiner, P., Phillips, R. S., Kemper, K. J., Legedza, A., Henlon, S., & Woolf, A. D. (2008). Dietary supplements: Inpatient policies in US children's hospitals. *Pediatrics*, *121*(4), e775–e781. doi: 10.1542/peds.2007-1898

Grandinetti, D. A. (2000). Doctors and the web: Help your patients surf the net safely. *Medical Economics*, *6*(5), 186–188.

Healthy People 2020. (n.d.). *Health communication and health information technology*. Retrieved from https://www.healthypeople.gov/2020/topics-objectives/ topic/health-communication-and-health-information-technology

Integrative Health Policy Consortium. (n.d.). *Frequently asked questions about Section 2706*. Retrieved from http://www.ihpc.org/wp-content/uploads/ section-2706-faq.pdf

Irvin, J. H., Domar, A. D., Clark, C., Zuttemzeister, P. C., & Friedman, R. (1996). The effects of relaxation response training on menopausal symptoms. *Journal of Psychosomatic Obstetrics & Gynecology*, *17*(4), 202–207.

Jacobson, J. S., Troxel, A. B., Evans, J., Klaus, I., Vahdat, L., Kinne, D., . . . Grann, V. R. (2001). Randomized trial of black cohosh for the treatment of hot flashes among women with a history of breast cancer. *Journal of Clinical Oncology*, *19*, 2739–2745.

Kantor, M. (2009). The role of rigorous scientific evaluation in the use and practice of complementary and alternative medicine. *Journal of the American College of Radiology*, 6(4), 254–262. doi: 10.1016/j.jacr.2008.09.012

Kroll, D. J. (2004). ASHP statement on the use of dietary supplements. *American Journal of Health-System Pharmacy*, 61(16), 1707–1711.

Kronenberg, F., Cushman, L. F., Wade, C. M., Kalmuss, D., & Chao, M. T. (2006). Race/Ethnicity and women's use of complementary and alternative medicine in the United States: Results of a national survey. *American Journal of Public Health*, 96(7), 1236–1242.

Kronenberg, F., & Fugh-Berman, A. F. (2002). Complementary and alternative medicine on menopausal symptoms: A review of randomized, controlled trials. *Annals of Internal Medicine*, 137, 805–813.

Lee, M. Y., Benn, R., Wimsatt, L., Cornman, J., Hedgecock, J., Gerik, S., . . . Haramati, A. (2007). Integrating complementary and alternative medicine instruction into health professions education: Organizational and instructional strategies. *Academic Medicine*, 82(10), 939–945.

Lee, S., Mountain, J., & Koenig, B. (2001). The meanings of "race" in the new genomics: Implications for health disparities research. *Yale Journal of Health Policy, Law, and Ethics*, 1, 33–75.

Mayo Clinic. (2014a). *Complementary and alternative medicine: Evaluate claims*. Retrieved from http://www.mayoclinic.org/alternative-medicine/ART-20046087

Mayo Clinic. (2014b). *Consumer health*. Retrieved from http://www.mayoclinic.org/healthy-lifestyle/consumer-health/basics/alternative-medicine/hlv-20049491

Micozzi, M. S. (2003). Integrative medicine in pharmacy and therapeutics. *Pharmacy and Therapeutics*, 28(10), 666–672.

Molassiotis, A., Fernadez-Ortega, P., Pud, D., Ozden, G., Scott, J. A., Panteli, V., . . . Patiraki, E. (2005). Use of complementary and alternative medicine in cancer patients: A European survey. *Annals of Oncology*, 16(4), 655–663.

National Center for Complementary and Integrative Health. (2012a). *Chiropractic: In depth*. Retrieved from http://www.nccih.nih.gov/health/chiropractic/introduction.htm

National Center for Complementary and Integrative Health. (2012b). *Naturopathy*. Retrieved from http://www.nccih.nih.gov/health/naturopathy

National Center for Complementary and Integrative Health. (2013a). *Are you considering complementary medicine?* Retrieved from https://nccih.nih.gov/health/decisions/consideringcam.htm

National Center for Complementary and Integrative Health. (2013b). *Complementary, alternative, or integrative health: What's in a name?* Retrieved from http://www.nccih.nih.gov/health/whatiscam

National Center for Complementary and Integrative Health. (2013c). *Homeopathy: An introduction.* Retrieved from http://www.nccih.nih.gov/health/homeopathy

National Center for Complementary and Integrative Health. (2013d). *Qi gong information.* Retrieved from http://www.nccih.nih.gov/taxonomy/term/249

National Center for Complementary and Integrative Health. (2013e). *Reiki: An introduction.* Retrieved from http://www.nccih.nih.gov/health/reiki/introduction.htm

National Center for Complementary and Integrative Health. (2013f). *Relaxation techniques for health: An introduction.* Retrieved from http://nccih.nih.gov/health/stress/relaxation.htm

National Center for Complementary and Integrative Health. (2014). *Natural products research: Information for researchers.* Retrieved from http://nccih.nih.gov/grants/naturalproducts

Post-White, J., Kinney, M. E., Savik, K., Gau, J. B., Wilcox, C., & Lerner. (2003). Therapeutic massage and healing touch improve symptoms in cancer. *Integrative Cancer Therapies, 2*(4), 332–344.

Purnell, L. D., & Paulanka, B. J. (2005). *Guide to culturally competent health care.* Philadelphia, PA: FA Davis.

Responsible Reform for the Middle Class. (n.d.). *The Patient Protection and Affordable Care Act. Section-by-section analysis.* Retrieved from http://www.dpc.senate.gov/healthreformbill/healthbill05.pdf

Trachtenberg, D. (2002). Alternative therapies and public health: Crisis or opportunity? *American Journal of Public Health, 92*(10), 1566.

Thernstrom, S. (1980). Religious affiliations of the populations in the United States. In *Harvard Encyclopedia of American Ethnic Groups*, 949–960. Cambridge, MA: Harvard University Press.

US Census Bureau (2012). *Population estimates.* Retrieved from http://www.census.gov/popest/

US Census Bureau. (2012). *US Census Bureau projections show a slower-growing, older, more diverse nation a half century from now.* Retrieved from https://www.census.gov/newsroom/releases/archives/population/cb12-243.html

Upchurch, D. M., & Chyu, L. (2005). Use of complementary and alternative medicine among American women. *Women's Health Issues, 15*(1), 5–13.

Ventola, C. L. (2010). Current issues regarding complementary and alternative medicine (CAM) in the United States. Part 2: Regulatory and safety concerns and proposed governmental policy changes with respect to dietary supplements. *Pharmacy and Therapeutics, 35*(9), 514–522.

Weitzman, S. (2008). Complementary and alternative (CAM) dietary therapies for cancer. *Pediatric Blood and Cancer, 50*(Suppl. 2), 494–497.

White House Commission on Complementary and Alternative Medicine Policy. (2002). Retrieved from http://www.whccamp.hhs.gov.

Whorton, J. C. (1999). The history of complementary and alternative medicine. In W. B. Jonas & J. S. Levin (Eds.), *The essentials of complementary and alternative medicine* (pp. 16–30). Philadelphia, PA: Lippincott Williams & Wilkins.

World Health Organization. (2014). *Traditional medicine: Definitions.* Retrieved from http://www.who.int/medicines/areas/traditional/definitions/en/

COMPLEMENTARY, ALTERNATIVE, AND INTEGRATIVE HEALTH APPROACHES AMONG WEST ASIAN AMERICAN COMMUNITIES

Gina Marie Piane and Brandon M. Eggleston

There are approximately three million immigrants from the West Asia region currently living in the United States. Many of these people have brought with them the medical traditions from their countries of origin, including complementary and alternative medicine (CAIH) practices, traditions and beliefs. The population of immigrants from India has increased dramatically since the 1990s and is now the second-largest immigrant group in the United States topped only by the Mexican population (Zong & Batalova, 2015a). In 2013, more than two million Indian-born immigrants—almost 5% of the foreign-born population—resided in the United States (Zong & Batalova, 2015a). In addition, in 2013, approximately 1.02 million immigrants from the Middle East and North Africa region, 2.5% of the nation's total, lived in the United States (Zong & Batalova, 2015b). A common theme in CAM medicine from this region is the coexistence of traditional and modern medicine.

The separation of CAM from modern allopathic medicine is not seen in many nations, as some countries are deeply connected with traditional culture, religion, and health behaviors and practices (Shaked, Renert, Mahuda, & Strous, 2004). The seamless integration of traditional medicine and allopathic medicine is clearly seen in the countries comprising the West Asia region.

LEARNING OBJECTIVES

At the completion of this chapter, students will be able to:

- Identify the complementary, alternative, and integrative health (CAM) practices most frequently used by West Asian American communities as described in the current literature.

- Synthesize the cultural roots and religious principles that led to the development of CAIH in West Asia.

- Gain cultural competence in understanding communities with high numbers of immigrants from West Asia who continue to practice ayurveda, Unani, and traditional Arabic and Islamic medicine.

- Evaluate the need for evidence related to the practice of complementary, alternative, and integrative health approaches in West Asia.

This chapter presents examples of CAIH categories that can be traced to this geographic region, including ayurvedic, Unani, and traditional Arabic and Islamic medicine (TAIM). This chapter also includes a description of the history of allopathic medicine and its introduction to the region. A discussion of CAIH in West Asia would not be complete without an exploration of the religious and cultural roots of Hinduism and Islam, which are also discussed in this chapter.

Theoretical Concepts

Overview

Medical systems evolved in West Asia from ancient disciplines that predate the germ theory of disease (Yesilada, 2011). Predominantly, these systems attribute disease to imbalance and promote health and wellness by maintaining and restoring balance through herbs, diet, and behavior. The medical systems sometimes called CAM techniques have a long history of practice in countries that make up West and Central Asia: India, Pakistan, Afghanistan, Bangladesh, Saudi Arabia, Iraq, Iran, Syria, Lebanon, Jordan, Israel/Palestine, Saudi Arabia, Qatar, Yemen, Oman, and the United Arab Emirates. CAM categories that can be traced to this geographic region include ayurveda, Unani, *siddha*, and TAIM.

Modalities

Ayurveda

Ayurveda has been amply discussed in Chapter 5 of this book. Therefore, this section just summarizes the major principles of ayurveda as a CAIH practice of West Indian Americans.

Records of ayurveda, the science of life, disease prevention, and longevity, were written more than 5,000 years ago. The ancient writing described medicinal herbs and healing techniques to treat various diseases, such as *vata*, or excessively vitiated gases; *pitta*, or fluids of the gall bladder and accumulated wastes; and *slesma*, phlegm or mucus in the mouth or throat. The Vedic religion included ancient ayurvedic healing techniques that were described in the four main books of spirituality. These books are known as the four Vedas: *Rik, Sama, Yajur,* and *Atharva* (Shakeel et al., 2011). The major concepts of ayurveda include: air (*akasa*); vital force (*vayu*); minerals, acids, and alkalies (*tejas*); water (*jala*); and organic substances and earthly matter (*prithvi*) (Shakeel et al., 2011).

Ayurveda posits that balance keeps the body healthy and that imbalance and impurities cause disease. Health and healing arise from "optimum balance between the body, mind and consciousness" (Shakeel et al., 2011, p. 30). The ayurvedic doctor studies the pulses of his or her patient for diagnosis and prescribes natural herbs and minerals that can be ingested or inhaled. The doctor may also prescribe yoga postures and *panchkarma* treatment, which consists of emesis, purgation, enema, nasal application of herbs, and bloodletting. *Panchkarma* is recommended three times a year to rejuvenate and revitalize the body (Shakeel et al., 2011).

Unani: The Greco-Arabic Healing Tradition

Greco-Arabic medicine arrived in India with the Muslims during the 18th century (Alavi, 2008). Using a similar explanatory model of health and wellness as ayurveda, Unani attributes disease to an imbalance of the four humors: phlegm (*balgham*), blood (*dam*), yellow bile (*safra*), and black bile (*sauda*).

This philosophical approach to health and wellness is based on the teachings of Hippocrates, Avicenna, and Galen. The practices are based on dichotomous pairs of humors, such as wet/dry and hot/cold, that promote healing and health. The Unani practitioner, after diagnosing a surplus or deficit of one of the four humors, seeks to reestablish harmony using herbs and other treatments, such as purging (*mushily*), sweating (*taareeq*), bath therapy (*hamman*), ripening (*munzij*), cupping (*mahajim*), and exercise (*riyazat*). Purging is the most common (Shakeel et al., 2011). Avicenna from Baghdad also included spinal manipulation in his manual, *The Book of Healing* (Pettman, 2007), as a practice of Unani. Traditional healers of Unani are known as *hakims*. Currently, they practice a variety of CAIH techniques, including chiropractic medicine, homeopathy, herbal medicine, and naturopathy.

Traditional Arabic and Islamic Medicine

Traditional Arabic and Islamic Medicine (TAIM) is comprised of CAM practices that consist of herbal medicine, other plant medicines, prophetic medicine, and meditation. TAIM is practiced in Western Asian countries such as Saudi Arabia, Iran, Iraq, Israel, Palestine, Yemen, and the United Arab Emirates. According to Azaizeh, Saad, Cooper, and Said (2010), TAIM is used widely by people of the Mediterranean to treat acute and chronic diseases; and for many who have faith in spiritual healers, TAIM is the first choice to combat depression, infertility, and epilepsy.

Herbal TAIM is based on a single plant species or a mixture of local plant species in small numbers, which sets it apart from traditional Chinese herbal therapies that use a large number of herb combinations (Azaizeh et al., 2010). TAIM practitioners administer remedies in the form of decoctions prepared by boiling parts of plants in water or infusing them in water or oil. Some remedies include inhalation of essential oils, juice, syrup, roasted plant material, fresh herbs in the form of salads or fruit, macerated plant parts, oil, sap, poultices, or pastes (Azaizeh et al., 2010).

Recent surveys conducted in the Middle East region found that many of the 200 to 250 plant species used in TAIM are in danger of eradication due to habitat loss, habitat degradation, and overharvesting (Azaizeh et al., 2010). Research has also revealed that younger TAIM practitioners have very limited knowledge of herbal medicine and may be resorting to supernatural methods of healing (Azaizeh et al., 2010). Al-Maissam, the Galilee Society's Medicinal Plants Center, which was established in 1999 in Shefa Amr, Israel, is seeking to preserve and rediscover the legacy of TAIM herbal medicine (Azaizeh et al., 2010).

Many Muslims who live in Western and Central Asia practice prophetic medicine as a form of TAIM. Prophetic medicine consists of a series of health recommendations given from the Prophet Muhammad and is a part of the *hadith* and is also found in the Qur'an (or Koran). These practices include the mandate of abstaining from the consumption of pork, alcohol, and other intoxicating substances. Prophetic medicine encourages a diet consisting of fruits, vegetables, dates, yogurt, and milk. Black seed and honey are recommended supplements for treating gastrointestinal and dermatological conditions and also for preventive medicine (Azaizeh, Fulder, Khalil, & Said, 2006).

The use of honey as medicine has been a part of Islamic culture for 1,400 years (Azaizeh et al., 2006). One of the original benefits of honey, according to Islamic tradition, is the treatment of stomach pain, including peptic ulcers. Additionally, honey also is used for pain or soreness in the throat and as a treatment for cold and coughs. Current research has identified honey as a natural remedy for decreasing inflammation and slowing the growth of bacteria, yeasts, and possibly viruses in the body (Azaizeh et al., 2006). Honey has also been used in traditional medicine in West Asia as a basic antiseptic ointment to sanitize and promote the healing of wounds (Azaizeh et al., 2006; Islam Web, 2014).

Black seed is another natural supplement used in prophetic medicine that has been used for centuries (Azaizeh et al., 2006; WebMD, 2015).

Historically known benefits and uses of black seed include relief from headache, nasal congestion, toothache, conjunctivitis (pink eye), and intestinal worms. Today in West Asia, black seed is often recommended for a variety of chronic conditions, such as cancer, emphysema, high blood pressure, gastrointestinal disorders, and high cholesterol. Black seed is currently used to treat acute illnesses, including dysentery, diarrhea, asthma, allergies, influenza, cough, and colds (WebMD, 2014). Some women also use black seed as a natural form of birth control, to start the menstruation cycle, and to increase milk production for nursing mothers (Sawahla, 2007; WebMD, 2015).

TAIM also includes the use of prayer as a technique to promote healing for those who suffer from both acute and chronic conditions. Some scholars have shown that prayer can be an effective treatment for a variety of conditions. However, the mechanism that explains the benefit of prayer has yet to be sufficiently explained for the scientific community to accept. Possible suggestions for how prayer promotes healing is through the placebo effect, where the positive thoughts of those who are praying for their own healing leads to improved function of many organs and systems in the human body. The improved function is largely a result of a combination of the sympathetic nervous response along with the adaptation and/or acquisition of positive health behaviors (Azaizeh et al., 2006).

The benefits of prayer for TAIM practitioners in Western Asia go beyond the metaphysical beliefs. Followers of Islam practice prayer in a specific position known as the *sujood*, where the person is on his or her knees and bows forward toward the ground on a mat or rug. The forward movement of this prayer position, which is practiced five times a day, is known to increase blood flow to both the brain and face. This is said to improve neurological function because of the increased amount of oxygen that is delivered to brain cells. Also, additional oxygen is delivered to the ears, nose, and throat, which decreases inflammation of the sinus cavities and pathways. Physicians and practitioners have reported decreased cases of sinusitis among Muslim patients who pray regularly because of the physical benefits of the *sujood* prayer position. Physicians also believe that the sinus pathways can drain more easily with the bowing forward movement of the *sujood* (Azaizeh et al., 2006).

TAIM has a long history of using cultural practices as a pathway to healing the mind, body, and spirit. These practices stem from Islamic traditions, and many even predate the Islamic faith (Azaizeh et al., 2006). Today many scholars are exploring the benefits of prophetic medicine and herbal supplements that have been used for centuries in Western Asia (Azaizeh, Fulder, Khalil, & Said, 2003). Herbal medicines are often credited with being the early and primary source of medicines and pharmaceuticals (Saad, Azaizeh, & Said, 2005). Many pharmaceuticals have been developed from traditional herbal medicine practices. TAIM in its current form is closely related to original European medicine and has contributed greatly to the development of allopathic medicine (Azaizeh et al., 2010). In addition to herbal remedies, TAIM has contributed to the discovery of the immune system, the introduction of microbiological science, and the separation of pharmacological science from medicine (Azaizeh et al., 2010).

Allopathic Medicine

As discussed by Arnold (1996), allopathic, or Western, medicine was introduced to India prior to the takeover of the country by the British Crown in 1858. It was first disseminated as the Indian Medical Service which provided medical assistance for officers and soldiers of the East India Company armies. Allopathic medicine had a limited reach in 19th-century India, due to the strong emphasis on the health of the army, coercion and imposition of medical practices rather than consultation, as well as resistance and lack of community participation by the people in India. In the years between the 1890s and the 1920s, successful campaigns against bubonic plague and other epidemics led to greater acceptance of allopathic medicine in India.

Despite its long history in the Indian subcontinent, however, allopathic medicine was not widely accepted by the general population. In fact, Arnold (1996) suggested that throughout the 1920s and 1930s, there were far more practitioners of the ayurvedic and Unani systems of Indian medicine than of allopathic medicine. According to Arnold, the failure of allopathic medicine to penetrate large areas of the countryside was due to the preference among rural Indians for a familiar system of medicine and way of understanding disease that is rooted in their own culture and also cheaper.

In India, ayurvedic medicine has long coexisted with allopathic medicine in the provision of mainstream healthcare (Janzen, 2002). Policy statements released by the government of India support medical pluralism—the policy of supporting many forms of treatment, including ayurveda, yoga, *siddha*, Unani, and homeopathy (AYUSH) (Jadhav, Mukherjee, & Thakur, 2013). Box 12.1 lists some of these policy statements and committees. India's school policy considers yoga to be an integral component of physical education (Arora & Sharma, 2013).

BOX 12.1   INDIAN GOVERNMENT COMMITTEES THAT SUPPORT INTEGRATIVE MEDICINE

Chopra Committee	1948
CG Pant Committee	1950
Dave Committee	1954
Mudalear Committee	1961
Udupa Committee	1968
National Health Policy	1983

Source: Jadhav, Mukherjee, & Thakur, 2013.

Cultural and Religious Influences on Medicine in West Asia

Hindu Principles

The most prevalent religion among India's 1.2 billion people is Hinduism, although 13% are Muslim and 2% are Christian (Arora & Sharma, 2014). Therefore, the Hindu religion, perhaps the world's oldest, has the greatest influence on Indian medicine and health behaviors, since healthcare decisions, social systems, customs, and practices are closely interwoven. *Karma* is a law of behavior and consequences in which the actions of one's past lives affect the circumstances in which one is born and lives in this life. Despite a complete understanding of the biological causes of illness, Indians often believe that illness is caused by karma (Alagiakrishnan & Chopra, 2014). Hinduism, unlike the major monotheistic religions, does not have a single holy text, a concept of a deity, a founder, a theological or moral system, a central religious authority, or the concept of a prophet. Hinduism is, however, based on five principles that guide behavior, as listed in Box 12.2.

Box 12.3 presents the 10 disciplines that serve as the basis for Hinduism. These disciplines guide human existence.

Islamic Principles

The Islamic faith is centered on the principle that the highest level of true human community can be achieved by submitting to the will of Allah through specific beliefs and practices. The beliefs of Islam come from the works of creation, prophets, holy writings, and divine revelation.

BOX 12.2   FIVE HINDU PRINCIPLES

1. God Exists: One Absolute OM. One Trinity: Brahma, Vishnu, Maheshwara (Shiva). Several divine forms.
2. All human beings are divine.
3. Unity of existence through love.
4. Religious harmony.
5. Knowledge of 3 Gs: Ganges (sacred river), Gita (sacred script), Gayatri (sacred mantra).

Source: Religious Tolerance.Org (2012).

BOX 12.3   TEN HINDU DISCIPLINES

1. *Satya* (truth). Consonance of thoughts, words, and deeds.
2. *Ahimsa* (nonviolence). Not to harm others whether in thought, word, or deed.
3. *Brahmacharya* (celibacy, nonadultery). Chastity in thought, word, and deed.
4. *Asteya* (no desire to possess or steal). Nonstealing, noncovetousness.
5. *Aparighara* (noncorrupt). Not to accept from others anything more than what is absolutely necessary for sustenance.
6. *Shaucha* (cleanliness). Purity and cleanliness.
7. *Santhosha* (contentment). Contentment, absence of greed, and cheerfulness.
8. *Swadhyaya* (reading of scriptures). Study of sacred literature and repetition of sacred mantras and prayers.
9. *Tapas* (austerity, perseverance, penance). Austerity in the form of service, control of speech and mind.
10. *Ishwarpranidhan* (regular prayers). Surrender of the fruits of one's actions, the surrender of one's very self.

Source: HinduNet Inc. (2003).

The Qur'an is considered by Muslims to be Allah's word, which was given to the Prophet Muhammad through a series of divine revelations between 610 and 632 CE (Yesilada, 2011). Islamic beliefs are considered to be a continuation of the teaching of previous prophets, including Adam, Abraham, Moses, Solomon, David, and Jesus. The Qur'an is seen not only as a holy text for religious and spiritual practices, but also as a text to be used in daily living and healing, which include the fields of medicine, nutrition, and health.

Islamic practices consist of the Five Pillars of Islam, as shown in Box 12.4, which are specific behavioral obligations that all Muslims must follow to demonstrate that they are true believers in God.

In traditional Islamic society, lifestyle, ideas, beliefs, and practices are strongly influenced by the family, community, and religion. Many times such influences lead to poor acceptance of the diagnosis and therapeutic measures of allopathic medicine (Niazi & Kalra, 2012). Niazi and Kalra (2012) contend, however, that traditional Islamic medicine, while not based on a biomedical model, is also not completely based on Islam. They have asserted that the treatments available in traditional Islamic medicine are based on the sociocultural milieu of the society. Their thesis is that the passivity associated with traditional Islamic medicine is actually contrary to the teaching of Islam, which includes a proactive role toward health. "One of the most basic concepts in Islam is a person's responsibility to his own body. According to the Islamic concepts, man does not own his own body; he merely uses it by the permission of Allah. By this concept, it is required of a Muslim to protect his body from disease and harm" (p. 35). The practice of using black seed and honey as well as other plant- and

---

BOX 12.4 THE FIVE PILLARS OF ISLAMIC PRACTICE

1. *Swam*, or fasting

2. *Iman*, or profession of faith

3. *Salah*, or prayer

4. *Zakah*, or purification

5. *Hajj*, or pilgrimage to Mecca

Source: Yesilada (2011).

animal-based medicines in Islam is unique to Western Asia countries because of the dry and often hot climate. Additional cultural influences come from previous empires and dynasties, including Persian, Ottoman, Greek, and Roman medicinal practices.

Prevalent Forms of Complementary, Alternative, and Integrative Health

The AYUSH, or traditional systems of medicine in India, include ayurveda, yoga, Unani, *siddha*, and homeopathy. AYUSH has a network in India including 787,000 registered practitioners and 501 recognized graduate and postgraduate colleges (Jadhav et al., 2013). Table 12.1 lists the disciplines related to AYUSH, including selected types of conditions for which they are used.

AYUSH medical systems are employed throughout the Indian subcontinent and West Asia. Forms of TAIM are more prevalent in West Asia. The use of CAM to maintain or restore health and wellness in West Asia varies by nation. The population of Palestine, for example, uses many CAM techniques; over 72% reported having used at least one CAM technique in one study (Sawahla, 2007). Palestinians, like people in many in other West Asian countries, commonly use prayer and herbal supplements as a part of their health and medical care. For instance, in Palestine the use of honey for many common ailments related to infectious diseases and other acute conditions is common. Scholars have had difficulty identifying a primary factor that determines the degree of CAIH use, but it is broadly associated with the traditions and cultural practices of Islam. In Palestine, middle-aged females with a low income are most likely to use CAM (Sawahla, 2007).

Table 12.1   Traditional Systems of Medicine in India

A	Ayurveda	Traditional Indian medicine	*Example:* Bitter melon to treat diabetes
Y	Yoga	Breath to movement	*Example:* Movement to relieve back pain
U	Unani	Traditional Arabic and Greek medicine	*Example: Khamiras* to treat heart disease
S	*Siddha*	Herbal medicine	*Example:* Mixture of leaves, flowers, fruit, and various roots to revitalize the body
H	Homeopathy	Dilutions to trigger the body's own immune response	*Example:* Dilute caffeine to treat insomnia

Source: Revathy, Rathinamala, & Murugesan (2012).

Consumer Issues

Worldwide, CAIH use among the general population is quite popular; estimates by nation range from 9% to 65% (Gupta, Gupta, Kapoor, Sharma, & Verma, 2014). Seventy percent of those who live in the developing world rely on CAM (Azaizeh et al., 2010). However, reportedly less than 40% of patients around the world discuss their use of CAM therapies with their primary care physicians (Gupta et al., 2014). Some CAIH users may not be aware of the limitations and, in some cases, risks associated with CAIH; they may assume that these products are inert or at least harmless (Gupta et al., 2014). Health professionals and health educators, in particular, need to be well versed in the use of CAIH by their clients/patients, but they need to be aware that those modalities may cause adverse reactions.

An example for consumer concern is the use of ayurvedic products. Gupta et al. (2014) found that ayurvedic drugs can be purchased over the counter in India and that both allopathic and ayurvedic practitioners prescribe allopathic drugs. They conclude that "cross-pathy" practices are common among allopathic and ayurveda practitioners. The researchers believed that patients throughout the nation would benefit from an optimal balanced and evidence-based use of the two systems. *Evidence-based use* refers to practitioners prescribing treatments, whether allopathic or ayurvedic, based on the results of scientific analysis and clinical trials. This method needs to be encouraged, especially in developing countries, such as India, with low doctor-patient ratios (Gupta et al., 2014). Another example of cross-pathy is that West Asian scholars and physicians have recently used CAM techniques to treat the side effects of allopathic treatments for cancer (Ayre et al., 2011), such as nausea, pain, digestive disorders, depression, anxiety, and stress-related conditions.

Despite the recommendations and wide use of ayurveda, Revathy et al. (2012) believe that in order to ensure the purity and clinical effects of ayurveda, *siddha*, and Unani (ASU) drugs, "authentication is a critical step for successful and reliable clinical applications and for further experimental studies" (p. 1). They examined the methods of "microscopy, spectroscopy, chromatography, chemometry, immunoassays, DNA fingerprinting, etc." as proper methods to authenticate drugs of plant, mineral, and animal origin. They are seeking to address problems with ASU drugs, which currently may vary in composition and properties. This is an issue that affects Indians as well as others throughout the world, since exports of ASU drugs are on the rise.

The relationship between CAIH usage and socioeconomic status (SES) in the United States is complex. Higher-SES patients may use mind-body therapies based on in-depth understanding of disease causation. They may also have the skills necessary to engage in patient-provider communication that empowers them (Brooks, Silverman, & Wallen, 2013). Lower-SES patients, however, may use CAM therapies as alternatives to allopathic medicine due to cost, familiarity, or difficulty in communication with allopathic providers.

Implications for Health Professionals

As CAIH use increases in popularity in the United States, health professionals need to understand how it can be integrated with allopathic medicine to achieve optimal health. This is true in all communities, as the use of CAIH is not specific to any one subculture. However, health professionals working in communities of more recent immigrants may need additional awareness of the theories and behaviors associated with CAIH use specific to the community. Communities with high numbers of immigrants from West Asia may continue to practice ayurveda, yoga, Unani, and TAIM. It is important for health professionals to recognize the value of spiritual and religious beliefs for the West Asian American communities.

Ayurveda and yoga are widely practiced in the United States. According to the National Center for Complementary and Integrative Health (NCCIH, 2015), "The percentage of adults who practice yoga has increased substantially from 5.1% in 2002 to 6.1% in 2007 and 9.5% in 2012." The 2007 National Health Interview Survey revealed that more than 200,000 US adults had used some form of ayurveda in the previous year (National Institutes of Health, 2013). In addition, the survey found yoga to be among the top 10 complementary health approaches used among US adults. Approximately 6% percent of US adults used yoga for health reasons (National Institutes of Health, 2014).

It is important to emphasize that CAM practices in India and West Asia are influenced by culture, religion, the structure of the society, economics, politics, and globalization. Both allopathic and CAM practices have evolved over their long history in West Asia. The side-by-side evolution has resulted in more integration and acceptance than in Western countries, such as the United States, where CAM practices receive more scrutiny and are viewed with more skepticism. Ning (2012) argued for a "more interdisciplinary dialogue to enhance a truly symmetrical system of medical pluralism in which a broader conceptual framework including diverse theories and methods can assess the validity of any therapy modality" (p. 151). She contended that both CAM practices and biomedical theories overlap and have evolved over time and claimed that the conventional dichotomy is false due to the "cross-fertilization" of CAM and allopathic medicine.

Caveat Emptor

According to the *Third Strategic Plan 2011–2015* from the National Center for Complementary and Alternative Medicine (NCCAM), now known as NCCIH, "the scope, self-care nature, and associated costs of CAM use in the United States reinforce the need to develop scientific evidence concerning the usefulness and safety—or lack thereof—of CAM interventions, and to ensure the public has access to accurate and timely evidence-based information" (2011, p. 2). As new modalities of CAIH emerge, new regulatory challenges arise. CAM practices such as Unani, *siddha*, and traditional Arabic/Islamic medicine are relatively new to the United States. Unani medicine is not a recognized health profession in the country (WebMD, 2015).

As more research is conducted on various medical modalities, more evidence-based information will be available for consumers to make informed decisions about. The three strategic plans produced by the NCCAM provide guidelines for the development of legislative mandates to regulate emerging alternative and complementary medical practices. The three goals and five objectives included in the 2011–2015 strategic plan can serve as guidelines for the development of research and regulatory actions for CAIH in the United States. These goals and objectives are presented in Box 12.5.

The World Health Organization (WHO, 2000) has cautioned consumers and health professionals about the need to increase their knowledge of emerging traditional CAM methods. WHO stated:

> Various practices of traditional medicine have been developed in different cultures in different regions without a parallel development of international standards and appropriate methods for evaluating traditional medicine. The challenge now is to ensure that traditional medicine is used properly and to determine how research and evaluation of traditional medicine should be carried out. Governments and researchers, among others, are increasingly requesting WHO to provide standards, technical guidance and information on these issues. (p. v)

Although Unani, *siddha*, and TAIM have been practiced for centuries in various parts of the world, this caution is still very applicable to their practice in the United States.

BOX 12.5   GOALS AND OBJECTIVES FROM THE NCCAM 2011–2015 STRATEGIC PLAN

Goals

1. Advance the science and practice of symptom management.

2. Develop effective, practical, personalized strategies for promoting health and well-being.

3. Enable better evidence-based decision making regarding CAM use and its integration into health care and health promotion.

Objectives

1. Advance research on mind and body interventions, practices, and disciplines.

2. Advance research on CAM natural products.

3. Increase understanding of "real-world" patterns and outcomes of CAM use and its integration into health care and health promotion.

4. Improve the capacity of the field to carry out rigorous research.

5. Develop and disseminate objective, evidence-based information on CAM Interventions.

Source: National Center for Complementary and Alternative Medicine (2011).

Conclusion

As scientists examine and evaluate CAIH treatments in West Asia, including ayurveda, Unani, *siddha*, yoga, homeopathy, and TAIM, they have discovered that some of these ancient practices have found their way into allopathic medicine. People throughout the world may benefit from additional effective treatment choices. Science and additional scrutiny may also reveal the dangers of certain practices that could be replaced with safer options. Medical pluralism should be the natural consequence of ever-increasing globalization.

Summary

- There are approximately three million immigrants from West Asia in the United States.

- CAM medicine and allopathic medicine are seamlessly intertwined in West Asia.

- West Asian medicine includes ayurveda, yoga, Unani, *siddha*, homeopathy, and traditional Arabic and Islamic medicine.

- West Asian medicine is influenced by Islamic and Hindu principles and cultures.

- As new modalities of complementary, alternative, and integrative health emerge, new regulatory challenges arise.

Case Study

Description

Jadhav et al. (2013) found that Indians with hemophilia are increasing their use of CAM. Those most likely to rely on CAM include the wealthier and more educated populations. Although the majority of people in their study used allopathic medicine, including the infusion of antihemophilic factor (the standard treatment recommended by the WHO), almost 40% of the patients used either ayurvedic or homeopathic remedies. Patients in the lowest income group and who were the least educated were more likely to rely on traditional spiritual healers.

Relying on ayurvedic or homeopathic treatment was overall more expensive than allopathic treatment. The authors concluded that the scarcity and cost of allopathic antihemophilic factor in India adversely influenced treatment protocols for people with hemophilia. Many educated, wealthy people with hemophilia were, therefore, resorting to episodic treatment and CAM.

Questions

1. What CAIH approaches were used by Indian people with hemophilia in the study presented in this case?

2. How does socioeconomic status influence the use of CAM among Indian persons with hemophilia in the study presented in this section?

3. Why should the medical and public health communities be concerned about the possible dangers of CAM use among people with hemophilia?

4. What recommendations would you provide to health professionals working with people with hemophilia in India?

KEY TERMS

Allopathic medicine. Western medicine based on the germ theory of disease. It is also called science-based medicine, evidence-based medicine, and modern medicine (MedicineNet, 2012).

Ayurveda (traditional Indian medicine). The science of life, disease prevention, and longevity, written more than 5,000 years ago (Shakeel et al., 2011).

AYUSH. The traditional systems of medicine in India, which include Ayurveda, yoga, Unani, *siddha*, and homeopathy (Arora & Sharma, 2013).

Traditional Arabic and Islamic medicine. TAIM practices that consist of herbal medicine, other plant medicines, prophetic medicine, and meditation (Azaizeh et al., 2008).

Unani medicine (Greco-Arabic healing tradition). Attributes disease to an imbalance of four humors: phlegm (*balgham*), blood (*dam*), yellow bile (*safra*), and black bile (*sauda*). Health and disease are the result of changes in elements such as air, earth, water, and fire (Pettman, 2007; WebMD, 2015).

References

Alagiakrishnan, K., & Chopra, A. (2014) *Health and healthcare of Asian Indian American elders*. Retrieved from http://web.stanford.edu/group/ethnoger/asianindian.html

Alavi, S. (2008). Medical culture in transition: Mughal gentleman physician and the native doctor in early colonial India. *Modern Asian Studies, 42*(5), 853–897. doi: 10.1017/S0026749X07002958

Arnold, D. (1996). The rise of Western medicine in India. *Lancet, 348*(9034), 1075–1078. Retrieved from http://ezproxy.nu.edu/login?url=http://search.proquest.com/docview/199014660?accountid=25320

Arora, V., & Sharma, A. (2013). *Is yoga religious? An Indian court mulls mandatory school exercises*. Retrieved from http://www.religionnews.com/2013/10/28/yoga-religious-indian-court-mulls-mandatory-school-exercises/

Azaizeh, H., Fulder, S., Khalil, K., & Said, O. (2003). Ethnobotanical knowledge of local Arab practitioners in the Middle Eastern region. *Fitoterapia, 74*, 98–108.

Azaizeh, H., Saad, B., Khalil, K., & Said, O. (2006). The state of the art of traditional Arab herbal medicine in the eastern region of the Mediterranean. *eCAM, 3*(2), 229–235. Retrieved from doi:10.1093/ecam/nel034

Azaizeh, H., Saad, B., Cooper, E., & Said, O. (2010) Traditional Arabic and Islamic medicine, a re-emerging health aid. *Evidence-Based Complementary and Alternative Medicine, 7*(4), 419–424. doi: 10.1093/ecam/nen039 DOI:10.1093%2Fecam%2Fnen039#pmc_ext

Ayre, E., Saleem, M., Shtayeh, A., Nejmi, M., Schiff, E., Hassan, E., & Silberman, M. (2011). Integrative oncology research in the Middle East: Weaving traditional and complementary medicine in supportive care. *Support Care Cancer, 20,* 557–564. doi:10.1007/s00520-011-1121-0

Brooks, A. T., Silverman, L., & Wallen, G. R. (2013). Shared decision making: A fundamental tenet in a conceptual framework of integrative healthcare delivery. *Integrative Medicine Insights, 8,* 29–36. doi:10.4137/IMI.S12783

Gupta, et al. (2014,). Allopathic vs. ayurvedic practices in tertiary care institutes of urban North India. *Indian Journal of Pharmacology, 39*(1). Academic OneFile.

Hao, X., & Chen, K. (2007). Integrating traditional medicine with biomedicine towards a patient centered healthcare system. *Chinese Journal of Integrative Medicine, 17*(2), 83–84.

HinduNet Inc. (2003). *Ethical and moral principles in Hinduism.* Retrieved from http://www.hindubooks.org/wehwk/chapter5/page3.htm

Islam Web. (2014). *The miracle of honey as alternative medicine.* Retrieved from http://main.islamweb.net/en/article/138095/

Jadhav, U., Mukherjee, K., & Thakur, H. (2013). Usage of complementary and alternative medicine among severe hemophilia patients in India. *Journal of Evidence-Based Complementary and Alternative Medicine, 18*(3), 191–197.

Janzen, J. (2002) *The social fabric of health: An introduction to medical anthropology.* Boston, MA: McGraw-Hill.

Lavery, S., Sullivan, K., Hill, C., Vowles, D., & Fyson, N. (1997). *Alternative healthcare: A comprehensive guide to therapies & remedies.* San Diego, CA: Thunder Bay Press.

MedicineNet. (2012). *Allopathic medicine.* Retrieved from http://www.medicinenet.com/script/main/art.asp?articlekey=33612

National Center for Complementary and Integrative Health. (2015). *What complementary and integrative approaches do Americans use?* Retrieved from https://nccih.nih.gov/research/statistics/NHIS/2012/key-findings

National Institutes of Health, National Center for Complementary and Alternative Medicine. (2013). *Ayurvedic medicine: An introduction.* Retrieved from http://nccam.nih.gov/health/ayurveda/introduction.htm

National Center for Complementary and Alternative Medicine. (2011). *Third strategic plan 2011–2015: Exploring the science of complementary and alternative medicine.* Retrieved from https://nccih.nih.gov/sites/nccam.nih.gov/files/about/plans/2011/NCCAM_SP_508.pdf

National Institutes of Health, National Center for Complementary and Alternative Medicine. (2013). *Yoga.* Retrieved from http://nccam.nih.gov/health yoga

Niazi, A. K., & Kalra, S. (2012). Patient centred care in diabetology: An Islamic perspective from South Asia. *Journal of Diabetes and Metabolic Disorders, 29,* 30. Academic OneFile. Web. 3 Apr. 2014.

Ning, A. (2012). How "alternative" is CAM? Rethinking conventional dichotomies between biomedicine and complementary/alternative medicine. *Health (London)*. doi: 10.1177/1363459312447252.

Pettman, E. (2007). A history of manipulative therapy. *Journal of Manual and Manipulative Therapies, 15*(3), 165–174.

ReligiousTolerance.org. (2012). *Hinduism: The world's third largest religion.* Retrieved from http://www.religioustolerance.org/hinduism.htm

Revathy, S. S., Rathinamala, R., & Murugesan, M. (2012). Authentication methods for drugs used in ayurveda, siddha and Unani systems of medicine: An overview. *International Journal of Pharmaceutical Sciences and Research, 3*(8), 2352–2361. Retrieved from http://ezproxy.nu.edu/login?url=http://search.proquest.com/docview/1034724026?accountid=25320

Saad, B., Azaizeh, H., & Said, O. (2005). Tradition and perspectives of Arab herbal medicine: A review. *eCam, 2*(4), 475–479.

Sawalha, A. (2007). Complementary and alternative medicine use in Palestine. *Journal of Alternative and Complementary Medicine, 13*(2), 263–269.

Shaked, G., Renert, N., Mahuda, I., & Strous, R. D. (2004). Psychiatric care in the Middle East: A mental health supermarket in the town of Lod. *Psychiatric Rehabiliation Journal, 27*(3), 207–211.

Shakeel, M., Dilanawaz, P., Ziyaurrrahman, Safura, K., & Chanderprakash, B. (2011). Alternative system of medicine in India: A review. *International Research Journal of Pharmacy, 2*(4), 2937.

WebMD. (2015). *Unani medicine.* Retrieved from http://www.webmd.com/vitamins-supplements/ingredientmono-1212-unani%20medicine.aspx?activeingredientid=1212&activeingredientname=unani%20medicine

World Health Organization. (2000). *General guidelines for methodologies on research and evaluation of traditional medicine.* Report WHO/EDM/TRM/2000.1. http://apps.who.int/iris/bitstream/10665/66783/1/WHO_EDM_TRM_2000.1.pdf

Yesilada, E. (2011). The contribution of traditional medicine in the healthcare system of the Middle East. *Chinese Journal of Integrative Medicine, 17*(2), 95–98.

Zong, J., & Batalova, J. (2015a, May 6). Indian immigrants in the United States. *Migration Policy Institute Online Journal.*

Zong, J., & Batalova, J. (2015b, June 3). Middle Eastern and North African immigrants in the United States. *Migration Policy Institute Online Journal.*

COMPLEMENTARY, ALTERNATIVE, AND INTEGRATIVE HEALTH

Beyond the Paradigm of CAM

Helda Pinzón-Pérez, Miguel A. Pérez, and Raffy R. Luquis

Maintaining good health and avoiding disease appear to be goals pursued by many throughout the history of humankind. Practices designed to prevent the onset of disease, including amulets, talismans, and spells, have been widely documented among cultures. Many of those practices continue to this day (Spector, 2009). Similarly, for much of human history, nature, gods, deities, and other spiritual beings were often believed to be responsible for a person's health and well-being. In some societies, it was often believed that chanting and sacrifices could be used to convince deities to grant the favor of good health (Last, 1993; Turner, 2003).

This chapter integrates the various concepts presented throughout the book with an analysis of the historical evolution of health, the evolving concept of wellness, and the influence of culture in the adoption of complementary, alternative, and integrative health. This chapter further discusses the use of the term *complementary, alternative, and integrative health* (CAIH) to reflect the growing emphasis on health and wellness as they relate to complementary and alternative medicine (CAM). The chapter also includes a discussion of a new paradigm for CAM in the 21st century.

LEARNING OBJECTIVES

At the completion of this chapter, students will be able to:

- Describe the relationship between culture and health.

- Understand the interaction between health and wellness as they relate to complementary and alternative medicine.

- Identify the principles and limitations of the use of complementary, alternative, and integrative health (CAIH).

- Identify the major consumer health issues related to complementary, alternative, and integrative health.

- Explain the role of CAM in the Affordable Care Act.

- Discuss the foundation for a new way of thinking about CAM in the 21st century.

Theoretical Concepts

Overview

Evolution of the Concept of Health and Wellness

The 1947 definition of health by the World Health Organization (WHO) has served for many years as the framework for the understanding of emerging forms of healthcare. This definition looks at health as "the complete physical, mental, and social well-being and not merely the absence of infirmity" (WHO, 2003). According to Sartorious (2006), historical definitions of health vary from defining health as the absence of infirmity, to contemporary conceptualizations in which health is seen as a state of being able to cope with the challenges of life. Modern definitions look at health as a state of inner balance and equilibrium with the social and physical environment.

The WHO's definition is still used and has relevance today, even though it has not been officially amended since 1948. It reflects the integration of the various domains of well-being.

CAIH therapies are based not only on the concept of health but also on the paradigm of wellness. The National Wellness Institute (NWI) defined this term as a self-initiated and rational process that evolves from the desire of individuals to achieve full potential. A state of well-being involves an active process in which human beings are aware of their health needs and make choices to achieve a successful existence (NWI, 2014).

CAIH looks for means to restore the balance of the various dimensions of wellness. The NWI (2014) described wellness as a balance between the physical, social, intellectual, spiritual, emotional, and occupational dimensions of human nature. Most societies around the world have developed their own definitions of health and disease. It is this evolving definition and the contributions from many cultures that make health and disease complicated states for individuals to comprehend. For purposes of this chapter, the authors employ the WHO's definition of health and the NWI's definition of wellness, while incorporating cultural and historical contributions to the development of these concepts. This section focuses on the contributions of several cultures to the current understanding of health and disease.

Modalities

The Egyptians

The ancient Egyptians believed that personal hygiene was related to good health; therefore, it is not surprising that most Egyptian homes had baths and toilets despite the lack of running water. Ancient Egyptians are known to have used amulets to promote good health. These amulets represented Egyptian deities and served very specific health-related purposes. Egyptians also used nets to protect themselves from mosquitoes, and it is believed that they used makeup around the eyes to protect themselves from disease (Nordqvist, 2012a).

The ancient Egyptians introduced the channel theory, which suggests that health was the result of unblocked channels in the human body that allowed for good health, and they believed that any blockage in those channels would result in disease. The Ebers Papyrus, dating to around 1550 BC, contained information specifying that the human heart is the center of the body supply and that there are blood vessels, akin to what we now know as arteries and veins, attached to each portion of the human body. The papyrus also contains incantations designed to drive away evil spirits that cause disease and infirmity (Nordqvist, 2012a).

The Edwin Smith Papyrus is a medical text based on scientific principles as practiced in ancient Egypt and contains information on medical treatments. Furthermore, this papyrus provides detailed information about treatments, including the closing of wounds with sutures, and suggests the use of honey to prevent and cure infections. Another Egyptian medical textbook, the Kahun Gynecological Papyrus, focuses on women's health issues, including contraception, pregnancy, and other fertility issues (New York Academy of Medicine, 2005).

The Greeks

The ancient Greeks incorporated lifestyle as means for attainment of well-being. They believed that health was a personal matter and that their gods played a big role in maintaining good health. It is therefore not surprising that, in Greek society, the pillars of health were exercise, nutrition, and sleep (Kumar, 2007). In fact, the ancient Greeks developed the Olympics as a means to celebrate health achievements and to explore the wonders of the human body.

The ancient Greeks believed that Asclepius, or Asklepious, was the god of healing. According to their beliefs, Asclepius had two daughters, Panacea, known as the goddess of healing, and Hygea, known as the goddess of health. Together, Asclepius, Panacea, and Hygea provided the ancient Greeks with the protection they needed to maintain their health status.

Not everyone in ancient Greece, however, adhered to or relied on the gods to provide for good health. Some scientists, including Hippocrates, rejected outright the spiritual explanations for health and disease and instead advanced the humoral theory as an explanation for disease and infirmity. They suggested that any imbalance of the four humors—blood, phlegm, black bile, and yellow bile—would result in disease (Dargie, 2007; Edelstein & Edelstein, 1967; Westmoreland, 2007).

The Romans

The ancient Romans saw health as the result of cleanliness and hygiene. For this society, prevention of illness was more important than curing disease. The adoption of prevention methods to minimize risk was of paramount importance for Roman society (Kumar, 2007). The ancient Romans believed that poor health (illness) could be traced to natural causes, including bad water and sewage. Given these beliefs, it is not surprising that the Romans invested significant resources in draining swamps to get rid of mosquitoes and in building public baths to ensure that everyone had access to bathing facilities and practiced good hygiene. Evidence suggests that public toilets were linked to Rome's sewage system in an effort to curtail the spread of disease (Kumar, 2007).

Mental health was one of the major contributions of ancient Roman society to the evolving definition of health and disease. The phrase "a sound mind in a sound body" can be traced to the ancient Romans. Similarly, the Romans provided the foundation for what we now know as clinics and hospitals and utilized a variety of herbal medicines, including fennel to address nervous conditions, egg yolks to treat dysentery, willow as an antiseptic, unwashed wool for sores, and opium and scopolamine, which they derived from henbane, as painkillers (Nordqvist, 2012b).

The Chinese

The Chinese culture sees health as the balance between body, mind, and spirit. This balance, as described by Chin (2005), could be internal and external, between hot and cold, and between emptiness and excess (Centers for Disease Control and Prevention [CDC], 2008). Chinese populations adhere to the belief in the yin and yang, which are complementary forces that attract each other to maintain a state of equilibrium in the body. The yin is defined as the female, negative, and passive principle found in nature. The yang is conceptualized as the male, positive, and active natural force (Spector, 2009).

Traditional Chinese medicine (TCM) originated more than 3,000 years ago and is one of the of the most ancient healing practices known to humans (Nestler, 2002). It is based on the holistic principle of harmony with the universe, the philosophy of yin-yang, and the Five Elements (Xua &Yangb,

2009). In addition to yin and yang, TCM includes the concepts of the "five zang organs and six fu organs, qi (vital energy), blood, and meridians.... It differentiates syndromes according to the eight principles (yin, yang, exterior, interior, cold, heat, deficiency (xu) and excess (shi)" (p. 133). The goal of a health practitioner is to restore balance between the yin and the yang and bring harmony back to the body. Practices such as acupuncture, Chinese massage, and Chinese herbology are very important components of TCM and are used to restore balance. Acupuncture is used, for example, to stimulate the body, release energy blockages, and restore balance in the body; herbs are used to restore balance based on each herb's energy classifications (Nestler, 2002; Xua & Yangb, 2009).

Islamic Cultures

Islamic cultures have contributed to the historical evolution of the concept of health. During the Islamic Umayyad period (661-750), it was widely believed that Allah would treat illnesses. These views started changing by AD 900, when Islamic societies started increasing their focus on purity and cleanliness.

The Persian physician Muhammad ibn Zakariyā Rāzī (Al-Razi), also known as the father of pediatrics, was the first scholar to distinguish measles from smallpox. He is also believed to be the first physician who wrote about allergies and immunology and who discovered asthma as a pathological entity. Other notable Islamic scientists who have contributed to the advancement of health and medicine include Ibn al-Haytham, the first scientist to describe the eye as an optical instrument, and Ahmad ibn Abi al-Ash'ath, an Iraqi doctor, who is believed to have conducted experiments on gastric physiology centuries before Western doctors undertook similar work. Islamic societies used poppy to relieve pain, hemp for earaches and to assist during childbirth, and mercury chloride to disinfect wounds (Conrad, 1993; Nordqvist, 2012c).

The prohibitions against the consumption of pork and alcohol and other mind-altering substances, along with the encouragement of regular consumption of fruits and vegetables, are part of traditional Islamic medical practices. Islamic views shaped the understanding of health, wellness, and disease by emphasizing the interaction of lifestyle and health outcomes.

The Jewish Tradition

The Jewish tradition has provided additional contributions to the under-standing of health. Jewish beliefs see health as a wholeness that integrates the body, mind, and spirit. Jewish religious laws dictate specific rules to maintain health, such as adherence to a kosher diet, which involves specific methods of preparation for beef and other foods as well as the avoidance of certain foods, such as pork and gelatin, and food combinations, such as beef and dairy products (Ehman, 2012).

Given the evolving nature of the definition and practice of health, and as illustrated by the practices just described above, different cultures have developed healing methods different from those of allopathic medicine. In fact, the terms *complementary and alternative medicine* may be misleading, given the fact that, in many cultures, there are the primary form of treatment. In this chapter, those terms are used as a reference point to describe healing practices not widely accepted by allopathic practitioners.

Culture, Health, and CAIH

Culture plays a major role in health and illness. In the United States, variations in health needs, the leading causes of death, and health disparities have been associated with cultural and ethnic background. Discussing patterns of health and illness for the major ethno-cultural groups in the United States helps illustrate the influence of culture on health.

The term *culture* can be defined in multiple ways. For example, Spector (2009) defined culture as the "sum of beliefs, practices, habits, likes, dislikes, norms, customs, rituals, and so forth that we have learned from our families during the years of socialization" (p. 9). Culture "involves shared customs, values, social rules of behavior, rituals, and traditions, and perceptions of human nature and natural events" (US Department of Health and Human Services, 2003, p. 8).

Individuals' cultures influence their beliefs, practices, expected behaviors, communication, and perceptions of health and well-being. For example, some Hispanics/Latinos believe that illness is a punishment from God for previous or current sinful behaviors or wrongdoing (Diaz-Cuellar & Evans, 2014); consequently, they protect their health with prayers, by wearing religious artifacts, and by keeping relics at home (Spector, 2009). Still other Hispanics/Latinos believe in herbal remedies and folk healing practices based on their indigenous cultural heritage (Ortiz, Shields, Clauson, & Clay, 2007).

In June 2014, the United States was the third most populous nation in the world, after China and India, with a population of 318,287,221 people (US Census Bureau, 2014b). Data from 2012 revealed that the largest racial groups were White (77.9%), African Americans (13.1%), Asian Americans (5.1%), Native Americans or Alaskan Natives (1.2%), Native Hawaiian and Pacific Islanders (0.2%), and two or more races (2.4%). By ethnicity, the breakdown was non-Hispanics/Latinos of any race (83.1%) and Hispanics/Latinos of any race (16.9%) (US Census Bureau, 2014a). In this section, we provide a brief overview of the health issues affecting the major racial and ethnic groups in the United States. More information is presented elsewhere in this volume.

American Indians and Alaskan Natives believe that health occurs because of a harmony with nature, and illness and is the result of instability between natural and supernatural forces (Diaz-Cuellar & Evans, 2014). Asian populations attribute illness to an imbalance between the yin and the yang, and they engage in practices such as acupuncture to restore this balance (CDC, 2008). These examples show how cultural beliefs influence the views of health and illness among different populations. Healthcare providers must understand the relationship between culture and health to effectively work with and serve diverse populations.

American Indian and Alaskan Native populations in the United States are defined as people having aboriginal roots from North, Central, and South America and who maintain tribal affiliations and belong to one of the 656 federally recognized tribes or other tribes without federal recognition. Most American Indians and Alaskan Natives believe that illness has its roots in spiritual problems and that everyone and everything in nature is interrelated. For these groups, the role of traditional healers is vital, as they restore harmony with god, also known as the Great Mystery (American Cancer Society, 2008). In 2009, the five major causes of death for this group were heart disease, cancer, unintentional injuries, diabetes, and chronic liver disease and cirrhosis (CDC, 2013a). According to the CDC, "geographic isolation, economic factors, and suspicion toward traditional spiritual beliefs are some of the reasons why health among [American Indians and Alaskan Natives] is poorer than other groups, [along with] cultural barriers, geographic isolation, inadequate sewage disposal, and economic factors" (CDC, 2013a). As examples of health disparities for this group, in 2009, members of this group had one of the highest prevalence rates of binge drinking; in 2007, they had the highest rates of motor vehicle–related deaths; and in 2009, they had the highest prevalence of smoking compared to other ethno-cultural groups.

Asian American populations in the United States are defined as people with origins in the Far East, Southeast Asia, or the Indian subcontinent, including, for example, Cambodia, China, India, Japan, Korea, Malaysia, Pakistan, the Philippine Islands, Thailand, and Vietnam (CDC, 2013b). In 2010, the three largest subgroups were Chinese, Filipinos, and Asian Indians. Traditional cultural beliefs in this group include the concepts of the yin and yang (natural opposites that complement each other), *qi* or *chi* (energy force), and hot and cold theory of disease (yin is cold and yang is hot) (Salimbene, 2000). For this cultural group, the head is viewed as the most important part of the body, and it should not be touched without the person's or the parents' permission; blood is viewed as a vital component that should not be drawn; and medical procedures, such as a venipuncture, are perceived as weakening the person's natural balance (Salimbene, 2000). The five major causes of death in 2010 for this group were cancer, heart disease, stroke, unintentional injuries, and diabetes. Examples of health disparities for this group include being the least likely group to have a Pap smear test (only 68% of women) and being at risk for chronic obstructive pulmonary disease, hepatitis B, HIV/AIDS, smoking, and tuberculosis (CDC, 2013b).

Black or African American populations in the United States are defined as people with origins in any of the Black racial groups of Africa (CDC, 2014a). Traditional cultural beliefs of this group include the use of roots and medicinal plants to treat disease, the utilization of copper and silver to prevent illness, and the use of prayer and spiritual healing (Spector, 2009). The five major causes of death in 2010 for this group were heart disease, cancer, stroke, diabetes, and unintentional injuries. Examples of health disparities for this group are the presence of the highest rates of heart disease, stroke, and hypertension compared to other ethno-racial groups, high rates of diabetes and obesity, as well as high rates of infant mortality and homicide (CDC, 2014a).

Hispanic Latino populations are defined as persons "of Cuban, Mexican, Puerto Rican, South or Central American, or other Spanish culture or origin, regardless of race" (CDC, 2013c). Members of this group believe in the strong relationship between religious values and health. The "hot and cold" theory of disease is of paramount importance for their understanding of health. Disease is the result of the imbalance of body humors, such as hot and cold. Natural healers such as *sobanderos* (massage healers) and *curanderos* (traditional healers) are in charge of restoring the balance between these body humors (Spector, 2009). The five major causes of death in 2009 for this group were cancer, heart disease, unintentional injuries, stroke, and diabetes. Examples of health disparities for this group include large gaps in income and education, lower influenza vaccination rates, and higher uninsured rates as compared to other ethno-cultural groups (CDC, 2013c).

Native Hawaiian and Other Pacific Islanders are defined as people with origins in Hawaii, Guam, Samoa, and other Pacific islands (CDC, 2013d). Cultural health-related beliefs in this group include the concept of *lokahi*, which refers to balance of the physical, mental, and spiritual realms of the human being. Members of this group also believe that illness results from a lack of harmony with the environment, which includes ancestors, *ohana* (family members), and god(s). Health, for members of this group, is also the result of *aloha* (love, compassion) and *malama* (taking care of others) (Stanford School of Medicine, 2014). The five major causes of death in 2010 for this group were cancer, heart disease, stroke, unintentional injuries, and diabetes. Examples of health disparities for this group include higher cancer death rates, lower five-year survival rates for all cancers, high infant mortality rates, and greater prevalence of diabetes as compared to other groups (CDC, 2013d).

White or Caucasian populations were defined for the 2010 census as persons "having origins in any of the original peoples of Europe, the Middle East, or North Africa" (Humes, Jones, & Ramirez, 2011, p. 3). The White/ Caucasian category also includes Irish, German, Italian, Lebanese, Arab, Moroccan, and Caucasian peoples (Humes et al., 2011). Members of this group believe in the value of herbal medicine, diet, and meditation to restore and maintain health. Specific subgroups, such as Italians, believe in culturally bound syndromes such as the evil eye (*malocchio*) and curses (*castiga*) (Spector, 2009). The leading causes of death in 2010 for this group were heart disease, cancer, and chronic lower respiratory disease. Examples of health disparities for this group include 12.7% of people under 65 years without health insurance as of 2010, and 33.5% of women compared to 34.7% of men over the age of 20 who are obese (CDC, 2014b).

CAIH Overview

The National Center for Complementary and Alternative Medicine (NCCAM), known since December 2014 as the National Center for Complementary and Integrative Health (NCCIH), is the guiding agency regarding CAIH in the United States. This agency has worked in collaboration with the CDC on CAM research.

The 2012 National Health Interview Survey (NHIS) is a research initiative conducted by the National Center for Health Statistics (NCHS) from the CDC. The 2002, 2007, and 2012 surveys have provided specific data regarding CAM use among Americans (NCCIH, 2015c).

The 2012 NHIS showed that 33.2% of US adults used complementary health approaches. According to the same survey, 11.6% of US children ages 4 to 17 used complementary health approaches; the 2007 NHIS indicated that 12.0% of US children used them (NCCIH, 2015d). From the 2007 NHIS, it was estimated that 38.3% of US adults and 11.8% of US children used CAM (Barnes, Bloom, & Nahim, 2008). Although rates are different ethnic groups in the United States have different rates, these figures pale in comparison to the 70% to 80% of the world's population who use traditional medicine as their primary form of medicine as reported by WHO (2014).

Given the increasing interest in CAM, it is not surprising that during the last three decades, holistic health and CAM principles have attracted the attention of health educators, anthropologists, sociologists, and medical professionals as they seek not only to better understand CAM, but to find ways to incorporate CAM into the healthcare system. In response to these increasing rates, the American Medical Association and the American Holistic Nurses Association have encouraged members to become better informed about CAM practices. The Consortium of Academic Health Centers for Integrative Medicine has promoted the incorporation of CAM courses in medical schools as a result of the National Institutes of Health education project, which since 1999 has promoted medical training in CAM (NCCAM, 2014a).

Principles and Use of CAIH

In the Western paradigm of health, allopathic medicine is the only established and reliable form of treatment. CAIH often is regarded as an occasional treatment method, when in fact millions of people around the world rely on it as their primary form of care. Furthermore, many of the treatments classified as CAM have been in existence far longer than Western medicine. They are important to many individuals who rely on them either because of culture, because they are effective, or because access to other forms of treatment is limited or not financially feasible. Finally, it is important to note that for many individuals around the world, it is Western, or allopathic, medicine, with its reliance on the germ theory, that is considered to be complementary or alternative.

CAM represents an alternative paradigm to the understanding of health and wellness. Allopathic medicine establishes one treatment modality over others and often continues to perpetuate the separation between mind and body. Box 13.1 presents some commonly used definitions related to CAM concepts.

For ease of discussion, the authors utilize allopathic medicine as the "gold standard" and use it as the foundation to compare other forms of treatment. However, the term *integrative medicine* is gaining acceptance in the medical and healthcare community because it integrates alternative and conventional medicine with an emphasis on healthy lifestyles.

BOX 13.1   COMMONLY USED DEFINITIONS RELATED TO CAM

Alternative medicine. "Using a non-mainstream approach in place of conventional medicine" (NCCAM, 2013e). An example is to use homeopathy instead of chemotherapy.

    Complementary medicine. Practices that use "a nonmainstream approach together with conventional medicine." Examples include natural products, such as dietary supplements, herbs, and probiotics, as well as mind and body practices, such as meditation, chiropractic, acupuncture, and massage (NCCAM, 2013c). An example of complementary medicine is the use of meditation after surgery to relieve discomfort.

    Integrative medicine. Related to "the combination of mainstream medical therapies and CAM therapies for which there is some high-quality scientific evidence of safety and effectiveness" (Lemley, 2014). An example is combining naturopathic treatments with radiotherapy for some cancer cases.

Source: Lemley, 2014; NCAAM 2013b, c.

The NCCAM (2013e) grouped CAM practices into four major groups:

1. *Natural products* (e.g., herbal medicines, botanicals, vitamins, minerals, and probiotics)

2. *Mind and body medicine* (e.g., meditation, yoga, acupuncture, deep-breathing exercises, qi gong, and tai chi, among others)

3. *Manipulative and body-based practices* (e.g., spinal manipulation, osteopathic manipulation, and massage therapy)

4. *Other CAM practices* (e.g., movement therapies, such as the Feldenkrais method, Alexander technique, Trager psychophysical integration; traditional healing practices, such as *curanderism* and shamanism; manipulation of energy fields, such as magnet therapy, reiki, and healing touch; and whole medical systems, such as ayurveda, homeopathy, TCM, and naturopathy)

This classification serves as the basis to assess the value of these therapies for multiple pathological conditions.

Limits of CAM and the Placebo Effect

CAIH looks for the means to restore the balance of the various dimensions of wellness. Although several studies have shown scientific evidence for the benefit of some CAIH therapies and treatment, scientific data supporting the efficacy of many CAM treatment modalities is lacking (NCCAM, 2008).

A critical view of CAIH is a healthy position for healthcare providers, health educators, and anyone interested in using CAM, as it allows them to recognize the benefits and risks associated with these practices. Healthcare providers and health educators must become knowledgeable regarding the limits of CAIH in treating or healing chronic health conditions and other health problems. For example, results from the National Interview Survey showed that most people used CAM modalities for the treatment of back pain; yet the scientific evidence on whether these therapies help back pain is limited (NCCAM, 2011a).

Researchers have found promising evidence on the benefits of acupuncture, massage, spinal manipulation, progressive relaxation, and yoga for chronic low back pain; however, research study results provide limited or no evidence for the use of some CAIH therapies, such as herbal remedies, for this condition. In addition, just because a treatment is beneficial for one condition, it is not necessarily beneficial for other similar conditions. For instance, previous research studies provided evidence on the benefits of acupuncture for arthritis and headaches, but not for neck pain (NCCAM, 2011a).

When identifying the risks and benefits of CAIH therapies, it is important to acknowledge that research study methodology and limitations may hinder conclusions on the effectiveness of CAIH modalities. Williams et al. (2009) found that yoga decreased functional disability, pain, and depression in people with chronic low back pain; nonetheless, the limitations of their study (i.e., self-report instrument and differential demands between treatment/control groups) may have hindered conclusions on the effectiveness of this modality.

Research studies on the effect of complementary health practices and cancer have shown similar results. Although the use of CAM would not cure cancer, some CAIH approaches have shown potential benefits on the management of cancer symptoms or treatment of side effects (NCCAM, 2013b). Acupuncture, massage therapy, mindfulness-based stress reduction, some herbs, and yoga may help people manage cancer symptoms or the side effects of treatment. There is some evidence that acupuncture, ginger, and massage therapy may help relieve the symptoms of nausea in cancer patients; but the limited amount of rigorous research restricts conclusions regarding the benefits of these CAM practices. Likewise, the benefits of mindfulness-based stress reduction on patients' anxiety, stress, fatigue, and general mood have been limited to patients with early-stage cancer (NCCAM, 2013b).

According to the WHO (2014), in a survey of 142 countries, CAM use can be risky due to the lack of structured regulation for its use, the variability in the quality of the products, and the availability of CAM remedies without prescriptions by knowledgeable and accredited CAM professionals. The WHO (2014) has emphasized the value of weighing the benefits and risks associated with CAM. The benefits of acupuncture for pain relief have been demonstrated by various studies; as a result, "90% of pain clinics in the United Kingdom and 70% in Germany include acupuncture as a form of treatment." Other benefits documented for CAM include medicinal combinations of the Chinese herb *Artemisia annua*, also known as sweet wormwood or sweet annie, which is now one of the most cost-effective treatments for malaria. Yet CAIH risks have been documented by the National Research Institute on Complementary and Alternative Medicine in Norway, which conducted a study that revealed cases of pneumothorax caused by inappropriate acupuncture techniques and cases of paralysis resulting from manual therapies.

Individuals using CAIH need to be cognizant of and take into account the placebo effect, defined as a "measurable, observable, or felt improvement in health or behavior not attributable to a medication or invasive treatment that has been administered" (Carroll, 2013, p. 1). This effect can have an impact on whether a medical treatment is considered to produce positive results. In relation to CAIH, the placebo effect refers to the positive response to a substance that has not had a documented therapeutic value.

Critics of CAM effectiveness have looked at the placebo effect as a major reason for the perceived benefits of these practices. Due to the unproven nature of many CAM modalities, the placebo effect may account for some of its outcomes. Although the placebo effect has been found relevant in the effectiveness of some CAM practices (Wechsler et al., 2011), it has also been found to influence the effectiveness of some mainstream allopathic treatments for depression, sleep disorders, and irritable bowel syndrome (WebMD, 2015).

A recent study on the placebo effect on patients with asthma showed that while patients reported a significant and equal improvement on symptoms with albuterol (drug), placebo inhaler, and sham acupuncture, data showed that lung function improved only after treatment with albuterol (Wechsler et al., 2011). Results from this study suggest that it is important for health professionals to use clinical assessments in addition to patient self-reported outcomes when a CAIH modality is used. Similarly, research has found that factors such as empathy and social learning, emotion and motivation, spirituality and healing rituals, and conditions and expectancy are important in understanding the placebo effect in patients. Thus, more rigorous research is needed to understand the intricacies of the placebo effect, CAIH use, and clinical outcomes (NCCAM, 2011b).

Josephine Briggs, director of the NCCAM, published a provocative analysis of CAM and the placebo effect and the importance of conducting research on this topic. She based her reflection on the benefits of tai chi in fibromyalgia. She referred to an editorial in the *New England Journal of Medicine* in which tai chi was described as a complex intervention involving "multiple components: exercise, breathing, meditation, relaxation, and a practitioner." She added:

> How do you control for all of these variables when designing a study? Some CAM proponents will say that it is the combination that makes the intervention work; many conventional researchers will say you must isolate the components to identify the active "ingredient." Critics will say it is all just the placebo effect—you expect the intervention to work, and so it does. . . . In the meantime, we are also interested in understanding and exploring the many components of the placebo effect: what role does expectation play? How important is the patient-provider interaction in health? What is the mind-body connection and how can it be harnessed to promote health and well-being? (Briggs, 2010)

In addition to the need to be vigilant about the scientific validity of CAIH modalities, users, including healthcare providers, need to support the WHO's (2014) call for governments around the world to produce regulations that allow CAM consumers to get accurate information. Consumers need to be informed on CAM benefits and risks and make informed decisions based on a risk-benefit assessment.

Consumer Issues

Informed consumers are those who make decisions based on a body of knowledge that is congruent with scientific discovery and evidence-based findings. Informed consumers of CAIH are those who are knowledgeable regarding the benefits and risks of their CAIH selections and consult with their healthcare providers about those interests and concerns. Box 13.2 contains recommendations for the safe use of CAM products and services.

According to the NCCAM (2013e):

> As with any treatment, it is important to consider safety before using complementary health products and practices. Safety depends on the specific therapy, and each complementary product or practice should be considered on its own. Mind and body practices such as meditation and yoga, for example, are generally considered to be safe in healthy people, when practiced appropriately.

BOX 13.2   BE AN INFORMED CONSUMER: NCCAM/NCCIH RECOMMENDATIONS

- *Take charge of your health by being an informed consumer.* Find out and consider what scientific studies have been done on the safety and effectiveness of the complementary product or practice that interests you. Discuss the information with your healthcare provider before making a decision.

- If you are considering a therapy provided by a complementary medicine practitioner, such as acupuncture, choose the practitioner as carefully as you would choose a conventional healthcare provider.

- If you are considering a dietary supplement, such as an herbal product, find out about any potential side effects or interactions with medications you may be taking.

- Complementary products or practices that have not been proven safe and effective should never be used as a replacement for conventional medical treatment or as a reason to postpone seeing a healthcare provider about any health problem.

- *Tell all your healthcare providers about any complementary approaches you use.* Give them a full picture of what you do to manage your health. This will help ensure coordinated and safe care.

- *Talk with your healthcare providers.* Tell them about the product or practice you are considering and ask any questions you may have about safety, effectiveness, or interactions with medications (prescription or nonprescription) or dietary supplements.

- *Visit the NCCAM website* (nccam.nih.gov) *now known as the National Center for Complementary and Integrative Health* (https://nccih.nih.gov/). The "Health Information" page has information on specific complementary therapies and links to other online sources of information. The website also has contact information for the NCCAM/NCCIH Clearinghouse, where information specialists are available to assist you in searching the scientific literature and to suggest useful NCCAM/NCCIH publications. You can also find information from NCCAM/NCCIH on Facebook, Twitter, and YouTube.

- *Visit your local library or a medical library.* Ask the reference librarian to help you find scientific journals and trustworthy books with information on the therapy that interests you.

Source: National Center for Complementary and Alternative Medicine (2013a).

The NCCIH encourages consumers to talk with their providers about their use of CAM, so they can receive coordinated and safe care. Box 13.3 presents some recommendations on how to talk with your provider about CAM.

One area of major concern in relation to consumers is the use of dietary supplements. According to the NCCAM (2013d), "Natural products such

BOX 13.3 PATIENT TIPS FOR DISCUSSING CAM WITH PROVIDERS

- When completing patient history forms, be sure to include all therapies and treatments you use. Make a list in advance.
- Tell your healthcare providers about all therapies or treatments—including over-the-counter and prescription medicines, as well as dietary and herbal supplements.
- Don't wait for your providers to ask. Be proactive.
- If you are considering a new complementary health practice, ask your healthcare providers about its safety, effectiveness, and possible interactions with medications (both prescription and nonprescription).

Source: National Center for Complementary and Alternative Medicine (2012b).

BOX 13.4 WHAT CONSUMERS NEED TO KNOW ABOUT DIETARY SUPPLEMENTS

1. *Take charge of your health by being an informed consumer.* The standards for marketing supplements are very different from the standards for drugs. For example, marketers of a supplement do not have to prove to the Food and Drug Administration that it is safe or that it works before it arrives on grocery store shelves. Find out what the scientific evidence says about the safety of a dietary supplement and whether it works.

2. *"Natural" does not necessarily mean "safe."* For example, the herbs comfrey and kava can cause serious harm to the liver. Also, when you see the term *standardized* (or *verified* or *certified*) on the bottle, it does not necessarily guarantee product quality or consistency.

3. *Interactions are possible.* Some dietary supplements may interact with medications (prescription or over-the-counter) or other dietary supplements, and some may have side effects on their own. Research has shown that St. John's wort interacts with many medications in ways that can interfere with their intended effects, including antidepressants, birth control pills, antiretrovirals used to treat HIV infection, and others.

4. *Be aware of the potential for contamination.* Some supplements have been found to contain hidden prescription drugs or other compounds, particularly in dietary supplements marketed for weight loss, sexual health including erectile dysfunction, and athletic performance or body building.

5. *Talk to your healthcare providers.* Tell them about any complementary health products or practices you use, including dietary supplements. This will help give them a full picture of what you are doing to manage your health and will help ensure coordinated and safe care.

Source: Adapted from National Center for Complementary and Alternative Medicine (2012c).

as herbal medicines or botanicals are often sold as dietary supplements and are readily available to consumers; however, there is a lot we don't know about the safety of many of these products, in part because a manufacturer does not have to prove the safety and effectiveness of a dietary supplement before it is available to the public." Two major concerns in the use of dietary supplements are the possibility of drug interactions and the possibility of product contamination. Box 13.4 lists concepts consumers need to know about dietary supplements.

Implications for Health Professionals

According to the 2012 NHIS, the 10 most common complementary health approaches used by adults in the United States were: natural products (17.7%); deep breathing (10.9%); yoga, tai chi, or qi gong (10.1%); chiropractic or osteopathic manipulation (8.4%); meditation (8.0%); massage (6.9%); special diets (3.0%); homeopathy (2.2%), progressive relaxation (2.1%); and guided imagery (1.7%). Fish oil was the most commonly used natural product used by adults (7.8%) and children (1.1%) as reported in the 2012 survey, compared to echinacea, which was the most commonly used natural product in the 2007 survey (NCCIH, 2015a).

The 2012 NHIS revealed that 28.9% of males and 37.4% of females use complementary and integrative approaches. In the 2007 NHIS, 31.4% of males and 39.4% of female respondents used CAM (Clarke, Black, Stussman, Barnes, & Nahin, 2015). By age, the highest use was in the 50–59 years old group (44.1%), followed by the 60–69 years old group (41%). Twelve percent of children in the United States used some form of CAM. The most common CAM therapies used by adults in the United States were: natural products (17.7%), deep breathing (12.7%), meditation (9.4%), chiropractic/osteopathic (8.6%), massage (8.3%), and yoga (6.1%). The most common CAM therapies used by children were: natural products (3.9%), chiropractic and osteopathic (2.8%), deep breathing (2.2%), and yoga (2.1%) (Barnes, Bloom, & Nahin et al., 2008). These results pose multiple challenges to healthcare providers, as they will frequently be confronted with the reality of CAM use among their patients.

The leading role of nursing professionals in holistic health is worth mentioning in this section. Nurses are healthcare providers who have historically incorporated many of the principles of holistic healing in their practice. Nursing theorists such as Madeleine Leininger, Jean Watson, Margaret Newman, Martha Rogers, and Dorothea Orem, among others, have advocated for the emphasis given in nursing to holistic healthcare approaches. The American Holistic Nurses Association (AHNA) is a professional organization that has led the pathway for holistic caring. Since 1998, AHNA has defined holistic nursing as "all nursing practice that has healing the whole person as its goal" (2015). This professional organization promotes the education of nurses, other healthcare professionals, and the public at large on complementary, alternative, and holistic healing with the ultimate goal to improve healthcare delivery by embracing multicultural and diversity perspectives in health.

The need for effective communication between consumers and healthcare providers is relevant in CAM. The WHO (2014) described the risks associated with gingko biloba, an herbal medicine used to increase blood circulation. Some cases of excess bleeding during surgical operations arose when patients did not inform their providers about their use of gingko biloba.

Among healthcare providers, health educators play a major role in educating populations about responsible use of CAM services. Health educators promote healthy lifestyles and wellness through education about behaviors and prevention of diseases (National Commission for Health Education Credentialing, 2008). As more people are exploring CAM modalities, health educators and other healthcare professionals must be knowledgeable about these healing modalities in order to educate consumers appropriately.

Health educators have embraced holistic views of health, healing, and integrated medicine; hence, many of them know the concepts associated with CAM. Nonetheless, Pinzón-Pérez (2014) stated that there is limited literature on the application of CAM in the field of health education. She suggested health educators must become knowledgeable about the scientific and cultural basis of different CAM practices, develop professional skills, and conduct additional research in this area to fully understand and apply concepts of CAM in health education and health promotion (Pinzón-Pérez, 2005, 2014).

There is a growing need to educate health educators and other healthcare providers on CAM (Association of American Medical Colleges, 2012). Barzanzky and Etzel (2003) indicated that 45 medical schools offered courses on CAM in the 1996–1997 academic year and 98 medical schools offered such courses in the 2002–2003 academic year. Among family nurse practitioners, a study conducted by Burman (2003) revealed that 98.5% of respondents reported having CAM-related instruction integrated into existing courses. In pharmacy schools, it has been reported that 73% of the participating surveyed schools were offering instruction in CAM (National Research Council, 2005). Although progress has been made toward educating the healthcare workforce in the United States on CAIH, there is still a need to increase course offerings on this subject matter. In addition, there is also a need to educate consumers on the guidelines to be followed when selecting CAIH services.

Caveat Emptor

The pursuit of optimal health and the avoidance of disease seem embedded into the very nature of human existence. Humans tend to relentlessly pursue a survival status and adopt health practices that are congruent with their understanding of health and disease.

In today's society, many factors contribute to good health. Factors that the WHO (2012) has called social determinants of health and has defined as "the conditions in which people are born, grow, live, work and age" contribute to the health of individuals in all societies. Evidence suggests, however, that rich and poor alike continue to strive to attain optimal health status.

CAIH products have been used around the world for years. Scientific testing has validated their use and has proven many of them to be effective, while it has also demonstrated the controversial nature of many others. Efficacy, safety, potency, testing, and regulation are among the many issues faced by the scientific community. Consumers in today's information society are faced with many choices and many questions. While we cannot provide definite answers to many of the questions faced by today's consumers, we do encourage an open mind and a critical evaluation of products currently labeled as CAM.

CAIH products and services continue to be controversial and are derided by many who do not understand the science behind them. In reality, some practices are questionable and are not backed by scientific evidence. However, completely ignoring their place in the healthcare needs of individuals is as myopic as blind faith in them.

Affordable Care Act and CAM

The enactment of the Patient Protection and Affordable Care Act (ACA) in 2010 (US Department of Health and Human Services, n.d.) has increased the emphasis on health promotion and disease prevention by making preventive care more accessible and affordable for many Americans. The ACA includes CAM providers in the list of health professionals that are part of the healthcare workforce.

In addition, the law establishes the development and implementation of interdisciplinary, interprofessional care plans that integrate clinical and community preventive and health promotion services for patients, including the support for primary care providers to coordinate the appropriate use of CAIH approaches to those who request such services.

Furthermore, Section 2706 of the ACA indicates that insurance providers cannot discriminate against any state-licensed health provider. While the law emphasizes licensed CAM providers, it is important to note that credentialing and licensing of complementary and alternative health practitioners vary from discipline to discipline and from state to state (NCCAM, 2013b). Thus, healthcare professionals, health educators, and consumers alike must understand state and local laws concerning CAIH practitioners and be careful when recommending or selecting these providers (NCCAM, 2013b).

WHO's Strategy for Traditional and Complementary Medicine

The *WHO Traditional Medicine Strategy 2014–2023* was developed to respond to the 2009 World Health Assembly WHA62.13 resolution on traditional medicine (TM). This strategy proposed policy and regulatory changes for traditional medicine and complementary medicine (T&CM) around the world.

The strategy proposed actions in the following areas:

> *Policy*—integrate TM within national health care systems, where feasible, by developing and implementing national TM policies and programmes; *safety, efficacy and quality*—promote the safety, efficacy and quality of TM by expanding the knowledge base, and providing guidance on regulatory and quality assurance standards; *access*—increase the availability and affordability of TM, with an emphasis on access for poor populations; (and) *rational use*—promote therapeutically sound use of appropriate TM by practitioners and consumers. (WHO, 2012, p. 11)

The guidelines provided by this strategy involve recommendations such as: (1) building the knowledge base of conventional and traditional practitioners on T&CM; (2) developing national policies that acknowledge the potential of T&CM; (3) strengthening the control and regulations of T&CM products, practices, and practitioners to ensure quality and consumer safety; (4) promoting universal health coverage by incorporating T&CM into clients' medical management; and (5) helping users make informed decisions by knowing the benefits and risks associated with T&CM. These recommendations are vital for the United States to develop a national agenda congruent with the goals and plans of other nations around the world.

New Ways of Thinking about Complementary and Alternative Medicine in the 21st Century

In 2005, Pinzón-Pérez discussed the need for more comprehensive terminology on CAM issues. She advocated for the use of terms such as *complementary and alternative healing* or *integrative healing*. According to Pinzón-Pérez, the use of the term *healing* instead of *medicine* expands the realm of these terms and makes them encompass various models of healthcare. Pinzón-Pérez considered integrative healing as the use of mainstream and complementary/alternative health promotion and disease prevention mechanisms to achieve or restore wellness.

Recently, the term *integrative medicine* has gained acceptance. According to Lemley (2014), integrative medicine is a philosophical concept that provides an integration of conventional medicine and alternative therapies. With the 2014 change in the name of the NCCAM to the National Center for Complementary and Integrative Health, the term *integrative medicine* was revised to reflect the growing need to include all health fields. The term *complementary and integrative health* was proposed, since it embraces the multidisciplinary nature of complementary and alternative healing practices.

Although no consensus has been achieved, the term *complementary, alternative, and integrative health (CAIH)* may respond to the need for unifying terminology. This term is proposed to reflect a new paradigm for health professionals to understand CAIH in the 21st century. The acronym *CAIH* enhances professional understanding of alternative and integrative models of care and emphasizes health and wellness rather than the medical model. Regardless of the terminology used, health professionals need to become proficient on nonallopathic healing methods used by many around the world and continue to explore the evolving definition of health and healing.

Conclusion

With the name change of the NCCAM to NCCIH, a new paradigm has emerged for CAIH. This new paradigm emphasizes health and wellness. This book has used the term *complementary, alternative, and integrative health (CAIH)* to reflect such paradigm change. Because the term *CAM* has been used in the literature, this book has used it when reporting on published data. CAM use has been described among various cultures throughout history. Several CAM therapies have been described as effective mechanisms used by the Egyptians, Greeks, and Romans, among other societies. Today's scientific paradigm has questioned the effectiveness of CAM therapies. The variability in the effectiveness of CAM therapies described in research studies emphasizes the importance of dialogue between healthcare providers and consumers. Health professionals should emphasize the importance of clients consulting with their healthcare providers before using CAIH approaches. CAIH therapies, like any other form of care, have side effects, contraindications, and potentiation effects that may positively or negatively affect health outcomes.

Summary

- The historical definition of health has varied from its understanding as the absence of infirmity to contemporary conceptualizations in which health is seen as a state of being able to cope with the challenges of life.

- Wellness is defined as a self-initiated and rational process that evolves from the desire of individuals to achieve full potential. The WHO's 1948 definition of health as the complete physical, mental, and social well-being and not merely the absence of infirmity continues to serve as the framework for the practice of medicine, health promotion, and health education around the world. Consumers of health services and healthcare providers need to be cognizant that this is not the only accepted definition of health and that new conceptualizations continue to appear. The cultural understanding of health and disease is very relevant in the health field and is of paramount importance in the discussion of CAIH practices.

- Section 2706 of the Patient Protection and Affordable Care Act indicates that insurance plans cannot discriminate against any state-licensed health provider. This includes licensed CAIH providers who are part of the healthcare workforce.

- Professional organizations, such as the American Medical Association, the American Holistic Nurses Association, and the Consortium of Academic Health Centers for Integrative Medicine, have advocated for discussion on ways to incorporate CAM into the healthcare system. These organizations have emphasized the importance of including CAM courses in the training of health personnel.

- The NCCAM changed its name to NCCIH. It is the leading federal agency on CAM in the United States. It is one of the 27 institutes and centers of the National Institutes of Health within the US Department of Health and Human Services.

- There is a variety of terms being used to refer to CAM. The term *complementary and integrative health* has recently been used by the

NCCIH. This book proposes the term *complementary, alternative, and integrative health* as one that may respond to the need for unifying terminology. The acronym *CAIH* enhances professional understanding of alternative and integrative models of care and emphasizes health and wellness.

- There is an urgent need for informed consumers, particularly as it relates to CAIH practices. Informed consumers are those who make decisions based on a body of knowledge that is congruent with scientific discovery and evidence-based findings. Informed consumers of CAIH are those who are knowledgeable regarding the benefits and risks of their CAIH selections and who discuss with their healthcare providers their interests and concerns about CAIH approaches.

Case Study

Description

A group of healthcare professionals and community representatives are writing a grant proposal to get funding for a grassroots initiative involving the creation of a training center on complementary, alternative, and integrative health. This training center will provide continuing education for health professionals and community members living in a rural area of California. The proposal should actively involve the community.

Questions

1. Where can this group of health professionals and community members get data on CAM use in the United States?

2. What CAM statistics could be relevant in this grant proposal?

3. What theoretical considerations can be used to convey the need for the proposed center to address complementary, alternative, and integrative health approaches?

4. What cultural considerations should this group of healthcare professionals and community members consider when writing the grant proposal?

5. What could be the role of health professionals in the grant proposal?

6. What could be the role of the community in the grant proposal?

7. What information/sections from the Affordable Care Act could be used to support this grant proposal?

KEY TERMS

Alternative medicine. Nonmainstream approaches used in place of conventional medicine (NCAAM, 2013b, c).

Complementary medicine. Nonmainstream approaches used together with conventional medicine (NCAAM, 2013b, c).

Complementary, alternative, and integrative health (CAIH). Term used to denote complementary, alternative, and integrative approaches to prevent and manage disease as well as to maintain or restore health and wellness. This term is congruent with the 2014 name change of the National Center for Complementary and Alternative Medicine [NCCAM] to National Center for Complementary and Integrative Health [NCCIH] (NCCIH, 2015a).

Culture. Shared customs, values, social rules of behavior, rituals, traditions, and perceptions of human nature and natural events (US Department of Health and Human Services, 2003).

Health. Complete physical, mental, and social well-being, not merely the absence of infirmity (WHO, 2003).

Integrative health. Incorporation of complementary approaches into mainstream healthcare (NCCIH, 2015a).

Integrative medicine. Combination of mainstream medical therapies and CAM therapies (NCAAM, 2013c, e).

References

American Cancer Society. (2008). *Native American healing*. Retrieved from http://www.cancer.org/treatment/treatmentsandsideeffects/complementary andalternativemedicine/mindbodyandspirit/native-american-healing?sitearea= ETO

American Holistic Nurses Association. (2015). *Who we are*. Retrieved from http://www.ahna.org/About-Us

Association of American Medical Colleges. (2012). *More medical schools offer instruction in complementary and alternative therapies*. Retrieved from https://www.aamc.org/newsroom/reporter/feb2012/273812/therapies.html

Barnes, P. M., Bloom, B., & Nahin, R. L. (2008). Complementary and alternative medicine use among adults and children: United States, 2007. *National Health Statistics Report, 12*. Retrieved from https://nccih.nih.gov/news/camstats/2007#pdf

Briggs, J. (2010). *Director's page: Maybe it's all placebo?* Retrieved from http://nccam.nih.gov/about/offices/od/2010-08.htm

Carroll, R. (2013). *Placebo effect*. Retrieved from http://skepdic.com/placebo.html

Centers for Disease Control and Prevention. (2008). *Overview of Chinese culture. Promoting cultural sensitivity: Chinese guide.* Retrieved from http://www.cdc.gov/tb/publications/guidestoolkits/ethnographicguides/China/chapters/chapter2.pdf

Centers for Disease Control and Prevention. (2013a). *American Indian & Alaska Native populations.* Retrieved from http://www.cdc.gov/minorityhealth/populations/REMP/aian.html

Centers for Disease Control and Prevention. (2013b). *Asian American populations.* Retrieved from http://www.cdc.gov/minorityhealth/populations/REMP/asian.html

Centers for Disease Control and Prevention. (2013c). *Hispanic or Latino populations.* Retrieved from http://www.cdc.gov/minorityhealth/populations/REMP/hispanic.html

Centers for Disease Control and Prevention. (2013d). *Native Hawaiian & other Pacific Islander populations.* Retrieved from http://www.cdc.gov/minorityhealth/populations/REMP/nhopi.html

Centers for Disease Control and Prevention. (2014a). *Black or African American populations.* Retrieved from http://www.cdc.gov/minorityhealth/populations/REMP/black.html

Centers for Disease Control and Prevention. (2014b). *Health of White non-Hispanic population.* Retrieved from http://www.cdc.gov/nchs/fastats/white-health.htm

Clarke, T. C., Black, L. I., Stussman, B. J., Barnes, P. M., & Nahin, R. L. (2015, February 10). Trends in the use of complementary health approaches among adults: United States 2002–2012. *National Health Statistics Reports, 79.*

Conrad, L. I. (1993). Arab-Islamic medicine. In W. F. Bynum & R. Porter (Eds.), *Companion encyclopedia of the history of medicine*, pp. 676–727. London, UK: Routledge.

Dargie, R. (2007). *Ancient Greece health and disease (Changing times: ancient Greece).* Mankato, MI: Capstone.

Department of Health and Human Services. (n.d.). *HealthCare.gov. Read the Affordable Care Act.* Retrieved from https://www.healthcare.gov/where-can-i-read-the-affordable-care-act/

Diaz-Cuellar, A. L., & Evans, S. F. (2014). Diversity and health education. In M. Pérez & R. Luquis (Eds.), *Cultural competence in health education and health promotion* (2nd ed., pp. 87–118). San Francisco, CA: Jossey-Bass.

Edelstein, E., & Edelstein, L. (1967). *Asclepius: A collection and interpretation of the testimonies.* Baltimore, MD: Johns Hopkins University Press.

Ehman, J. (2012). *Religious diversity: Practical points for health care providers.* Retrieved from http://www.uphs.upenn.edu/pastoral/resed/diversity_points.html

Humes, K., Jones, N., & Ramirez, R. (2011). *US Census Bureau overview of race and Hispanic origin: 2010 Census Briefs.* Retrieved from http://www.census.gov/prod/cen2010/briefs/c2010br-02.pdf

Kumar, S. (2007). *History of public health.* Retrieved from http://www.priory.com/history_of_medicine/public_health.htm

Last, M. (1993). *Non-Western concepts of disease*. In W. F. Bynum & R. Porter (Eds.), *Companion encyclopaedia of the history of medicine*, pp. 634–660. London, UK: Routledge.

Lemley, B. (2014). *What is integrative medicine?* Retrieved from http://www.drweil .com/drw/u/ART02054/Andrew-Weil-Integrative-Medicine.html

National Center for Complementary and Alternative Medicine. (2008). *The use of complementary and alternative medicine in the United States.* Retrieved from http://nccam.nih.gov/news/camstats/2007/camsurvey_fs1.htm

National Center for Complementary and Alternative Medicine. (2011a). *Chronic pain and CAM: At a glance*. Retrieved from http://nccih.nih.gov/sites/nccam .nih.gov/files/D456_05-14-2012.pdf

National Center for Complementary and Alternative Medicine. (2011b). *Potential roles of the placebo effect in health care*. Retrieved from http://nccam.nih.gov/ research/results/spotlight/051711.htm

National Center for Complementary and Alternative Medicine. (2012a). *Informed Consumer*. Retrieved from http://nccam.nih.gov/timetotalk/forpatients.htm

National Center for Complementary and Alternative Medicine. (2012b). *Patients tips for discussing CAM with providers..* Retrieved from https://nccih.nih.gov/ news/2008/060608.htm

National Center for Complementary and Alternative Medicine. (2012c). *5 Tips: What Consumers Need to Know about Dietary Supplements*. Retrieved from http://nccam.nih.gov/health/tips/supplements

National Center for Complementary and Alternative Medicine. (2013a). *Are you considering a complementary health approach?* Retrieved from http://nccam .nih.gov/health/decisions/consideringcam.htm

National Center for Complementary and Alternative Medicine. (2013b). *Cancer and complementary health approaches*. Retrieved from http://nccam.nih.gov/ health/cancer/camcancer.htm

National Center for Complementary and Alternative Medicine. (2013c). *Credentialing: Understanding the education, training, regulation, and licensing of complementary health practitioners*. Retrieved from http://nccam.nih .gov/health/decisions/credentialing.htm

National Center for Complementary and Alternative Medicine. (2013d). Safe use of complementary health products and practices. Retrieved from http://nccam .nih.gov/health/safety

National Center for Complementary and Alternative Medicine. (2013e). *Complementary, Alternative, or Integrative Health: What's In a Name?* Retrieved from https://nccih.nih.gov/health/integrative-health

National Center for Complementary and Alternative Medicine. (2014a). *About research training and career development*. Retrieved from http://nccam.nih.gov/ training/about

National Center for Complementary and Alternative Medicine. (2014b). *NCCAM facts-at-a-glance and mission*. Retrieved from http://nccam.nih.gov/about/ ataglance

National Center for Complementary and Integrative Health. (2015a). *Complementary, alternative, or integrative health: What's in a name?* Retrieved from https://nccih.nih.gov/health/integrative-health

National Center for Complementary and Integrative Health. (2015b). *National Center for Complementary and Integrative Health: NIH turning discovery into health. NCCIH facts-at-a-glance and mission.* Retrieved from https://nccih.nih.gov/about/ataglance

National Center for Complementary and Integrative Health. (2015c). *Statistics from the National Health Interview Survey.* Retrieved from https://nccih.nih.gov/research/statistics/NHIS

National Center for Complementary and Integrative Health. (2015d). *What complementary and integrative approaches do Americans use?* Retrieved from https://nccih.nih.gov/research/statistics/NHIS/2012/key-findings

National Commission for Health Education Credentialing. (2008). *Health education profession.* Retrieved from http://www.nchec.org/credentialing/profession/

National Research Council. (2005). *Complementary and alternative medicine in the United States.* Washington, DC: National Academies Press, 2005.

National Wellness Institute. (2014). *The six dimensions of wellness.* Retrieved from http://www.nationalwellness.org/?page=Six_Dimensions

Nestler, G. (2002). Traditional Chinese medicine. *Medical Clinics of North America, 86*(1), 63–73.

New York Academy of Medicine. (2005). *Academy papyrus to be exhibited at the Metropolitan Museum of Art.* Retrieved from http://www.nyam.org/news/press-releases/2005/2493.html

Nordqvist, C. (2012a). *What is ancient Egyptian medicine?* Retrieved from http://www.medicalnewstoday.com/info/medicine/ancient-egyptian-medicine.php

Nordqvist, C. (2012b). *What is ancient Roman medicine?* Retrieved from http://www.medicalnewstoday.com/info/medicine/ancient-roman-medicine.php

Nordqvist, C. (2012c). *What is medieval Islamic medicine?* Retrieved from http://www.medicalnewstoday.com/info/medicine/medieval-islamic-medicine.php

Ortiz, B., Shields, K., Clauson, K., & Clay, P. (2007). Complementary and alternative medicine use among Hispanics in the United States. *Annals of Pharmacotherapy, 41*, 994–1004.

Pinzón-Pérez, H. (2005). Complementary and alternative medicine, holistic health, and integrative healing: Applications in health education. *American Journal of Health Education, 36*(3), 174–178.

Pinzón-Pérez, H. (2014). *Complementary and alternative medicine in culturally competent health education.* In M. Pérez & R. Luquis (Eds.), *Cultural competence in health education and health promotion* (2nd ed., pp. 87–118). San Francisco, CA: Jossey-Bass.

Salimbene, S. (2000). *What language does your patient hurt in?: A practical guide to culturally competent patient care.* Retrieved from http://www.diversityresources.com/health/asian.html

Sartorius, N. (2006). The meanings of health and its promotion. *Croatian Medical Journal, 47*(4), 662–664.

Spector, R. (2009). *Cultural diversity in health and illness* (7th ed.). Upper Saddle River, NJ: Pearson Education.

Stanford School of Medicine. (2014). Culturally appropriate care for Native: Fund of Knowledge. Retrieved from https://geriatrics.stanford.edu/ethnomed/hawaiian_pacific_islander/fund.html

Turner, B. S. (2003). *Changing concepts of health and illness*. In R. Albrecht, R. Fitzpatrick, & S. C. Scrimshaw (Eds.), *The handbook of social studies in health and medicine*. London, UK: Sage.

US Census Bureau. (2014a). *Quick facts United States*. Retrieved from http://quickfacts.census.gov/qfd/states/00000.html

US Census Bureau. (2014b). *US and world population clock*. Retrieved from http://www.census.gov/popclock/

US Department of Health and Human Services. (2003). *Developing cultural competence in disaster mental health programs: Guiding principles and recommendations*. DHHS Pub. No. SMA 3828. Rockville, MD: Center for Mental Health Services, Substance Abuse and Mental Health Services Administration. Retrieved from https://store.samhsa.gov/shin/content/SMA03-3828/SMA03-3828.pdf

US Department of Health and Human Services. (n.d.). *The Affordable Care Act, Section by Section*. Retrieved from http://www.hhs.gov/healthcare/rights/law/index.html

WebMD. (2015). *What is the placebo effect?* Retrieved from http://www.webmd.com/pain-management/what-is-the-placebo-effect

Wechsler, M. E., Kelley, J. M., Boyd, I. O., Dutile, S., Marigowda. G., Kirsch. I., . . . Kaptchuk, T. J. (2011). Active albuterol or placebo, sham acupuncture, or no intervention in asthma. *New England Journal of Medicine, 365*(2), 119–26. doi: 10.1056/NEJMoa1103319

Westmoreland, P.L. (2007). *Ancient Greek beliefs*. San Ysidro, CA: Lee and Vance.

Williams, K., Abildso, C., Steinberg, L., Doyle, E., Epstein, B., Smith, D., . . . Cooper, L. (2009). Evaluation of the effectiveness and efficacy of Iyengar yoga therapy on chronic low back pain. *Spine, 34*(19), 2066–2076.

World Health Organization. (2003). *WHO definition of health*. In Preamble to the Constitution of the World Health Organization. Retrieved from http://www.who.int/about/definition/en/print.html

World Health Organization. (2004). *New WHO guidelines to promote proper use of alternative medicines*. News release. Retrieved from http://www.who.int/mediacentre/news/releases/2004/pr44/en/

World Health Organization. (2012). *What are social determinants of health?* Retrieved from http://www.who.int/social_determinants/sdh_definition/en/

World Health Organization. (2013). *WHO traditional medicine strategy 2014–2023*. Retrieved from http://apps.who.int/iris/bitstream/10665/92455/1/9789241506090_eng.pdf?ua=1&ua=1

Xua, J., & Yangb, Y. (2009). Traditional Chinese medicine in the Chinese health care system. *Health Policy, 90*, 133–139.

INDEX

A

Abies balsamea. See Balsam fir

ACA. *See* Affordable Care Act

Acer saccharinum. See Silver maple

Achilleamillefolium. See Common yarrow; Western yarrow

Acorus calamus L. See Calamus

Acupressure: benefits of, 100; cautions and contraindications of, 101; defined, 112; history of, 98–99; Jin Shin Do, 100; Ohashiatsu, 100; regulation of, 110; research on, 99; shiatsu, 99; tui na, 99–100; types of, 99–100; Watsu, 100

Acupuncture, 4; Asian Americans using, 271; benefits of, 97; defined, 285; history of, 94–97; meridian model in, 95; NCCAOM and, 105; regulation of, 109–110; risks of, 98; side effects of, 98; 12 meridians in, 95

Affordable Care Act (ACA): American Indians impacted by, 195; CAM/CAIH under, 10–11, 341–342; defined, 23; section 2706 of, 299

Africa: Hispanics/Latinos health beliefs influenced by, 210–211; spiritual practices of, 158–160

African Americans: CAIH approaches among, 235–253; case study, 253; caveat emptor for health care use by, 249–251; consumer issues with for health care use by, 243–245; defined, 253; health professionals, implications of, 245–249; herbal supplements used by, 240–243; modalities in use with, 238–243; population in US of, 235; prayer among, 240; theoretical concepts with, 236–238

Aiga, 270

Air (Akasa), 306

Ajo. See Garlic

Akasa. *See* Air

Alaska natives: CAIH approaches among, 177–197; causes of "disease" vary greatly among, 181; caveat emptor for health care use by, 194–195; consumer issues with for health care use by, 192; health and wellness perceptions with, 179–181; health professionals, implications of, 192–194; medicinal plants used by, 185–187; modalities in use with, 182–191; theoretical concepts with, 178–182

Allopathic medicine: bridging gap between CAIH and, 1, 18–19; defined, 23, 320

Alnum serrulata. See Hazel alderdler

Aloe vera. *See Savila*

Aloha (Love, compassion), 269–270

Alternative medicine: CAM related definition of, 333; defined, 283–284, 299, 346

American Indian Religious Freedom Act of 1978, 195

American Indians: CAIH approaches among, 177–197; case study, 196–197; causes of "disease" vary greatly among, 181; caveat emptor for health care use by, 194–195; chanting of, 188; consumer issues with for health care use by, 192; crystals of, 189; dance ceremonies of, 190–191; diversity of, 177; healing ceremonies of, 190; health and wellness perceptions with, 179–181; health professionals, implications of, 192–194; heterogeneity of, 178–179; medicinal plants used by, 185–187; medicine wheel, 180; modalities in use with, 182–191; pipe ceremonies of, 188–189; plant-based healing practices of, 183–184; smudging of, 191; spiritual healing practices of, 184–191; sweat lodge ceremonies of, 188; theoretical concepts with, 178–182; tobacco used for ceremonial purposes, 184, 188; vision quest of, 189–190

American red raspberry (*Rubus ideaeus L.*), 185

American Tai chi and Qigong Association, 45

Anis estrella (Star anise), 218

ANS. *See* Autonomic nervous system

Anthemis cotula. See Stinking chamomile

Apple cider vinegar, African Americans using, 242

Aromatherapy, 127

Arroyo willow (*Salix lasiolepis*), 186

Art therapy, 130

Artemisia californica. See Coastal sagebrush

Artemisia tridentate. See Big sagebrush

Asarum candadense L. See Canadian wild ginger